HANDBOOK OF GASTROENTEROLOGIC PROCEDURES

FIFTH EDITION

Todd H. Baron, MD
Professor of Medicine
Division of Gastroenterology and Hepatology
University of North Carolina School of Medicine
Chapel Hill, North Carolina

Ryan J. Law, DO
Assistant Professor of Medicine
Division of Gastroenterology
University of Michigan School of Medicine
Ann Arbor, Michigan

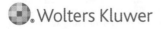 Wolters Kluwer

Philadelphia • Baltimore • New York • London
Buenos Aires • Hong Kong • Sydney • Tokyo

Acquisitions Editor: Nicole Dernoski
Development Editor: Sean McGuire
Editorial Coordinator: Julie Kostelnik
Marketing Manager: Phyllis Hitner
Production Project Manager: Kim Cox
Design Coordinator: Elaine Kasmer
Manufacturing Coordinator: Beth Welsh
Prepress Vendor: TNQ Technologies

Fifth edition

9 8 7 6 5 4 3 2 1

Printed in China

Library of Congress Cataloging-in-Publication Data

ISBN-13: 978-1-975111-65-6

Cataloging in Publication data available on request from publisher.

For my wife, Beatrice, who has been there for me from college to present, to my mentor Richard Kozarek, and to those colleagues who have helped me along the way.

—Todd H. Baron, MD

For my wife Laura and daughter Jocelyn, to my parents Bruce and Marjorie, to friends and colleagues who have supported me throughout my career, and, last but not least, to my mentor and friend Todd Baron who has taught me so much about the world of therapeutic endoscopy.

—Ryan Law, DO

Acknowledgments

We would like to first, and foremost, thank our families for their unending support throughout the creation of this book. We would like to acknowledge all of the hard work by our editorial team at Wolters Kluwer and the publishing team at TNQ Technologies. Without the constant push to continue forward momentum, this project would not have been successful. Finally, we would like to thank our friends and colleagues from around the world who have served as contributors to this work. The fifth edition of the *Handbook of Gastroenterologic Procedures* will serve as technical reference for endoscopic interventions, and without the tireless efforts of our contributors, this would not have been possible.

Preface

We are most pleased to offer the fifth edition of the *Handbook of Gastroenterologic Procedures*. Initially created as a reliable and concise resource for almost all of the gastroenterological (GI) procedures commonly used in clinical practice and academic training programs, the fifth edition offers a significant update to include cutting-edge procedures and techniques in evolution. The handbook aims for a broad readership, including physicians, nurses, technicians, and students, to provide a wide range of procedural details not easy to find elsewhere and in a standardized format. Thus, we have maintained the basic format for the chapters, with section headings relating to indications, contraindications, patient preparation, procedure techniques, and adverse events.

This updated edition retains all similarities of the prior edition, but the procedural landscape in GI has changed dramatically since the fourth edition was published. To account for this evolution, we have made important enhancements and modifications. The rapid growth in technology coupled with the trend in endoscopy as a diagnostic and therapeutic discipline has produced an unprecedented increase in the range of procedures now available. We have taken care to include procedures that are commonly used or are growing rapidly in their application frequency. The fifth edition has over 50 chapters on endoscopic techniques; however, we are still able to retain the smaller book size compatible with our goal to provide a concise, direct, and easy-to-access handbook for practicing endoscopists. We have recruited recognized experts within the field of endoscopy to contribute to this book with a goal of providing accurate, up-to-date, high-fidelity information on the given topic.

The handbook is not intended nor is it sufficient to provide complete endoscopic information or a description of all possible endoscopic procedures. Instead, it serves as a supplement to more comprehensive endoscopy textbooks by providing the essential information and helpful tips regarding the most prevalent endoscopic procedures in practice today. All chapters have been extensively revised, rewritten, in some cases removed, or added since the previous edition. We have added several new chapters to reflect significant growth in the field of endoscopy, including cutting-edge techniques in therapeutic endoscopic ultrasound, endoscopic submucosal dissection, third space endoscopy (i.e., peroral endoscopic myotomy [POEM]), and bariatric endoscopy.

Perhaps one of the most unique aspects to this handbook is the continued inclusion of chapters devoted to nonendoscopic procedures, such as the insertion of the Minnesota tube for refractory variceal bleeding; esophageal, small bowel, and ano-rectal motility testing; percutaneous liver biopsy; paracentesis; feeding tube placement; and hydrogen breath testing for disac-charidase deficiency or bacterial overgrowth. This compendium of information is not easily found in any one resource.

Finally, we include chapters that contain generic information relating to the organization and function of the endoscopy unit, preprocedure planning and bowel preps, and analgesia and seda-tion (including the use of propofol).

We hope that this fifth edition will continue to serve many purposes for all of us involved in the diagnosis, treatment, and care of patients with gastrointestinal disorders.

Todd H. Baron, MD
Ryan J. Law, DO

Contributors

Hiroyuki Aihara, MD, PhD
Assistant Professor of Medicine
Gastroenterology, Hepatology,
    and Endoscopy
Brigham and Womens Hospital
Boston, Massachusetts

Harry R. Aslanian, MD
Professor
Section of Digestive Diseases
Yale School of Medicine
New Haven, Connecticut

Jason R. Baker, PhD
Associate Director, GI
    Physiology Laboratory
Division of Gastroenterology
University of Michigan
Ann Arbor, Michigan

Subhas Banerjee, MD
Professor
Division of Gastroenterology
    and Hepatology
Stanford University
Palo Alto, California

Monique T. Barakat, MD
Instructor
Division of Gastroenterology
    and Hepatology
Stanford University
Palo Alto, California

Todd H. Baron, MD
Professor of Medicine
Division of Gastroenterology
    and Hepatology
University of North Carolina
    School of Medicine
Chapel Hill, North Carolina

Michael C. Bennett, MD
Assistant Professor
Division of Gastroenterology
Washington University
St. Louis, Missouri

Sean Bhalla, MD
Gastroenterology Fellow
Division of Gastroenterology
University of Michigan
Ann Arbor, Michigan

John C. Byrn, MD
Associate Professor of Surgery
Colon and Rectal Surgery
University of Michigan
Ann Arbor, Michigan

Dustin A. Carlson, MD
Assistant Professor of Medicine
Division of Gastroenterology
    and Hepatology
Northwestern University
Chicago, Illinois

David R. Cave, MD
Professor
Department of Gastroenterology
University of Massachusetts
    Medical School
Worcester, Massachusetts

Joan W. Chen, MD, MS
Assistant Professor of Medicine
Division of Gastroenterology
University of Michigan
Ann Arbor, Michigan

Enad Dawod, MD
Resident
Weill Cornell Medical College
New York, New York

Qais Dawod, MD
Department of Gastroenterology
     and Hepatology
Weill Cornell Medical College
New York, New York

Ana DeRoo, MD
Surgery Resident
Department of Surgery
University of Michigan
Ann Arbor, Michigan

David L. Diehl, MD, FACP, FASGE
Division of Gastroenterology
Geisinger
Danville, Pennsylvania

Rami El Abiad, MD
Associate Professor
James A. Clifton Digestive
     Health Center
University of Iowa
Iowa City, Iowa

Larissa Fujii-Lau, MD
Faculty Physician
Department of
     Gastroenterology
The Queen's Medical Center
Honolulu, Hawaii

Norio Fukami, MD
Consultant
Division of Gastroenterology
     and Hepatology
Mayo Clinic
Scottsdale, Arizona

Sarah Gerken, MD
Instructor
Department of Anesthesiology
University of Toledo
Toledo, Ohio

Karthik Gnanapandithan, MD, MS
Hospitalist
Yale New Haven Health
Northeast Medical Group
New Haven, Connecticut

Mishita Goel, MBBS
Resident Physician
Department of Medicine
Wayne State University
Detroit, Michigan

Ian S. Grimm, MD
Professor
Division of Gastroenterology
     and Hepatology
University of North Carolina
Chapel Hill, North Carolina

Kimberly N. Harer, MD
Clinical Lecturer
Division of Gastroenterology
University of Michigan
Ann Arbor, Michigan

William L. Hasler, MD
Professor
Division of Gastroenterology
University of Michigan
Ann Arbor, Michigan

Tadd K. Hiatt, MD
Assistant Professor of Medicine
Division of Gastroenterology
University of Michigan
Ann Arbor, Michigan

Amy Hosmer, MD
Assistant Professor
Division of Gastroenterology,
 Hepatology and Nutrition
The Ohio State University
Columbus, Ohio

Donovan Inniss, BS
Medical Student
University of Michigan Medical
 School
Ann Arbor, Michigan

Shayan Irani, MD
Faculty Physician
Digestive Disease Institute
Virginia Mason Medical Center
Seattle, Washington

Theodore W. James, MD
Fellow
Division of Gastroenterology
 and Hepatology
University of North Carolina
Chapel Hill, North Carolina

Salmaan A. Jawaid, MD
Advanced Endoscopy Fellow
Division of Gastroenterology,
 Hepatology, and Nutrition
University of Florida
Gainesville, Florida

Allon Kahn, MD
Associate Consultant
Division of Gastroenterology
 and Hepatology
Mayo Clinic
Scottsdale, Arizona

Sergey V. Kantsevoy, MD, PhD
Faculty Physician
Director, The Center for
 Therapeutic Endoscopy
Mercy Hospital
Baltimore, Maryland

Rajesh Keswani, MD, MS
Associate Professor of Medicine
Digestive Health Center
Northwestern Medicine
Chicago, Illinois

Mouen A. Khashab, MD
Associate Professor
Division of Gastroenterology
 and Hepatology
Johns Hopkins University
Baltimore, Maryland

**Richard A. Kozarek, MD, FACG,
 FASGE, AGAF, FACP**
Faculty Physician
Executive Director, Digestive
 Disease Institute
Virginia Mason Medical Center
Seattle, Washington

Richard S. Kwon, MD, MS
Associate Professor
Division of Gastroenterology
University of Michigan
Ann Arbor, Michigan

Ryan Law, DO
Assistant Professor
Division of Gastroenterology
University of Michigan
Ann Arbor, Michigan

Allen A. Lee, MD
Clinical Lecturer
Division of Gastroenterology
University of Michigan
Ann Arbor, Michigan

Cadman L. Leggett, MD
Consultant
Division of Gastroenterology
    and Hepatology
Mayo Clinic
Rochester, Minnesota

Laura E. Lehrian, DO
Assistant Professor
Department of Anesthesia
University of Michigan
Ann Arbor, Michigan

Amar Mandalia, MD
Gastroenterology Fellow
Division of Gastroenterology
University of Michigan
Ann Arbor, Michigan

Maen Masadeh, MD
Advanced Endoscopy Fellow
Division of Gastroenterology
University of California-San
    Francisco
San Francisco, California

Stephen McClave, MD
Professor
Division of Gastroenterology,
    Hepatology, and Nutrition
University of Louisville
Louisville, Kentucky

Sarah K. McGill, MD
Assistant Professor
Division of Gastroenterology
    and Hepatology
University of North Carolina
Chapel Hill, North Carolina

Shaffer R.S. Mok, MD, MBS
Digestive Health Institute
University Hospitals
Westlake, Ohio

**Thiruvengadam Muniraj, MD,
    MRCP, PhD**
Assistant Professor
Section of Digestive Diseases
Yale School of Medicine
New Haven, Connecticut

V. Raman Muthusamy, MD
Professor
Division of Digestive Diseases
David Geffen School of Medicine
University of California-Los
    Angeles
Los Angeles, California

**Jose M. Nieto, DO, AGAF, FACP,
    FACG, FASGE**
Staff Physician
Borland Groover
Jacksonville, Florida

Makoto Nishimura, MD
Staff Physician
Division of Gastroenterology,
    Hepatology and Nutrition
    Services
Memorial Sloan Kettering
    Cancer Center
New York, New York

**Keith L. Obstein, MD, MPH,
    FASGE, FACG, AGAF**
Associate Professor
Department of
    Gastroenterology,
    Hepatology, and Nutrition
Vanderbilt University Medical
    Center
Nashville, Tennessee

Endashaw Omer, MD
Assistant Professor
Division of Gastroenterology,
    Hepatology, and Nutrition
University of Louisville
Louisville, Kentucky

Woo Hyun Paik, MD, PhD
Professor
Department of
   Gastroenterology
Seoul National University
   Hospital
Seoul, Korea

John E. Pandolfino, MD, MSCI
Professor of Medicine
Digestive Health Center
Northwestern Medicine
Chicago, Illinois

Do Hyun Park, MD, PhD
Professor
Department of
   Gastroenterology
Asan Medical Center
Seoul, Korea

Arpan H. Patel, MD
Staff Gastroenterologist
Mid Atlantic Permanente
   Medical Group
Rockville, Maryland

Dhyanesh A. Patel, MD
Assistant Professor
Department of
   Gastroenterology,
   Hepatology, and Nutrition
Vanderbilt University Medical
   Center
Nashville, Tennessee

Vilas R. Patwardhan, MD
Assistant Professor of Medicine
Division of Gastroenterology/
   Liver Center
Beth Israel Deaconess Medical
   Center
Boston, Massachusetts

Manuel Perez-Miranda, MD, PhD
Associate Professor
Valladolid University Medical
   School
Head of Department
Department of Gastroenterology
   and Hepatology
Hospital Universitario Rio
   Hortega
Valladolid, Spain

Bret T. Petersen, MD
Consultant
Division of Gastroenterology
   and Hepatology
Mayo Clinic
Rochester, Minnesota

Cyrus Piraka, MD
Faculty Physician
Department of
   Gastroenterology
Henry Ford Hospital
Detroit, Michigan

Anoop Prabhu, MD
Assistant Professor of Medicine
University of Michigan
Ann Arbor, Michigan

Andrew J. Read, MD
Clinical Lecturer
Division of Gastroenterology
University of Michigan
Ann Arbor, Michigan

Chanakyaram A. Reddy, MD
Fellow
Division of Gastroenterology
University of Michigan
Ann Arbor, Michigan

Michael D. Rice, MD
Assistant Professor
Division of Gastroenterology
University of Michigan
Ann Arbor, Michigan

Melinda C. Rogers, MD
Staff Physician
Ohio Gastroenterology Group
Columbus, Ohio

Nadav Sahar, MD
Assistant Professor
Division of Gastroenterology
and Hepatology
University of Iowa
Iowa City, Iowa

Allison R. Schulman, MD, MPH
Assistant Professor of Medicine
Division of Gastroenterology
University of Michigan
Ann Arbor, Michigan

Shreya Sengupta, MD
Department of
Gastroenterology,
Hepatology and Nutrition
The Cleveland Clinic
Cleveland, Ohio

Reem Z. Sharaiha, MD, MSc
Associate Professor
Department of Gastroenterology
and Hepatology
Weill Cornell Medical College
New York, New York

Uzma D. Siddiqui, MD
Associate Professor of Medicine
Center for Endoscopic Research
and Therapeutics
University of Chicago
Chicago, Illinois

Sumit Singla, MD
Faculty Physician
Department of
Gastroenterology
Henry Ford Hospital
Detroit, Michigan

Aaron J. Small, MD
Staff Gastroenterologist
Hawaii Health Partners
Aiea, Hawaii

Arjun R. Sondhi, MD
Advanced Endoscopy Fellow
Division of Gastroenterology
University of Michigan
Ann Arbor, Michigan

Daniel S. Strand, MD
Assistant Professor
Division of Gastroenterology
and Hepatology
University of Virginia
Charlottesville, Virginia

Shelby Sullivan, MD
Associate Professor
Division of Gastroenterology
University of Colorado
Aurora, Colorado

Elliot B. Tapper, MD
Assistant Professor of Medicine
Division of Gastroenterology
University of Michigan
Ann Arbor, Michigan

Anna Tavakkoli, MD, MSc
Assistant Professor
Division of Gastrointestinal and
Liver Diseases
University of Texas-
Southwestern
Dallas, Texas

Monica A. Tincopa, MD, MSc
Clinical Lecturer
Division of Gastroenterology
University of Michigan
Ann Arbor, Michigan

Joseph R. Triggs, MD, PhD
Advanced Endoscopy Fellow
Division of Gastroenterology
University of Pennsylvania
Philadelphia, Pennsylvania

Edward Villa, MD
Division of Gastroenterology
    and Hepatology
University of Illinois Health
Chicago, Illinois

Andrew Y. Wang, MD
Professor
Division of Gastroenterology
    and Hepatology
University of Virginia
Charlottesville, Virginia

Jessica X. Yu, MD, MS
Assistant Professor
Division of Gastroenterology
    and Hepatology
Oregon Health Sciences
    University
Portland, Oregon

Contents

Preface vii
Acknowledgments v

I. PREPARATION OF THE PATIENT 1

1. Pre-procedure Assessment of Patients Undergoing Gastrointestinal Procedures 3
   Bret T. Petersen, MD

2. Analgesia and Sedation 15
   Laura E. Lehrian, DO and Sarah Gerken, MD

3. Bowel Preps 21
   Tadd K. Hiatt, MD

4. Management of Anticoagulation and Antithrombotics 27
   Arjun R. Sondhi, MD

II. UPPER ENDOSCOPY PROCEDURES 39

5. Esophagogastroduodenoscopy 41
   Arpan H. Patel, MD

6. Dilation of the Esophagus: Wire-guided Bougie (Savary, American) and Balloon Dilators 51
   Chanakyaram A. Reddy, MD and Joan W. Chen, MD, MS

7. Feeding Tubes (Nasogastric, Nasoduodenal, and Nasojejunal) 59
   Dhyanesh A. Patel, MD and Keith L. Obstein, MD, MPH, FASGE, FACG, AGAF

8. Percutaneous Endoscopic Gastrostomy (PEG), Percutaneous Endoscopic Gastrostomy and Jejunostomy (PEGJ), and Direct Percutaneous Endoscopic Jejunostomy (DPEJ) 73
   Endashaw Omer, MD and Stephen McClave, MD

9. Ablation Therapy for Barrett Esophagus 87
   Allon Kahn, MD and Cadman L. Leggett, MD

10. Endoscopic Mucosal Resection of Esophageal Lesions 99
    Sumit Singla, MD and Cyrus Piraka, MD

11. Endoscopic Management of Foreign Bodies of the Upper Gastrointestinal Tract 109
    Dustin A. Carlson, MD

12. Pneumatic Dilation for Achalasia 119
    Anna Tavakkoli, MD, MSc

13. Placement of Esophageal Self-Expandable Metal Stents 127
    Anna Tavakkoli, MD, MSc and Ryan Law, DO

III. SMALL BOWEL ENDOSCOPY PROCEDURES **133**

14. Push Enteroscopy   135
Michael D. Rice, MD and Andrew J. Read, MD

15. Deep Enteroscopy   145
Andrew J. Read, MD, Ryan Law, DO and Michael D. Rice, MD

16. Placement of Enteral Self-Expandable Metal Stents   159
Aaron J. Small, MD and Shayan Irani, MD

17. Endoscopic Mucosal Resection of Duodenal Lesions   169
Richard S. Kwon, MD, MS

18. Capsule Endoscopy   179
Salmaan A. Jawaid, MD and David R. Cave, MD

IV. COLONOSCOPY PROCEDURES **189**

19. Basic Colonoscopy   191
Mishita Goel, MBBS and Rajesh Keswani, MD, MS

20. Anoscopy and Rigid Sigmoidoscopy   203
Ana DeRoo, MD and John C. Byrn, MD

21. The Role of Endoscopy in the Management of Hemorrhoids   213
Shaffer R.S. Mok, MD, MBS and David L. Diehl, MD, FACP, FASGE

22. Polypectomy, Endoscopic Mucosal Resection, and Tattooing in the Colon   227
Sarah K. McGill, MD, Theodore W. James, MD and Ian S. Grimm, MD

23. Colonic Decompression   241
Karthik Gnanapandithan, MD, MS, Thiruvengadam Muniraj, MD, MRCP, PhD and Harry R. Aslanian, MD

24. Placement of Colonic Self-Expandable Metal Stents   247
Amy Hosmer, MD

V. ENDOSCOPIC RETROGRADE CHOLANGIOPANCREATOGRAPHY **253**

25. Basics of ERCP   255
Larissa Fujii-Lau, MD

26. Endoscopic Sphincterotomy   269
Todd H. Baron, MD

27. Management of Biliary Lithiasis   279
Sean Bhalla, MD and Ryan Law, DO

28. Management of Biliary and Pancreatic Ductal Obstruction: Endoprosthesis and Nasobiliary/Nasopancreatic Drain Placement   287
Nadav Sahar, MD and Richard A. Kozarek, MD, FACG, FASGE, AGAF, FACP

VI. ENDOSCOPIC ULTRASOUND **299**

29. Basics of Endoscopic Ultrasound   301
Monique T. Barakat, MD and Subhas Banerjee, MD

30. Endoscopic Ultrasound-Guided Fine Needle Aspiration and Biopsy   311
Melinda C. Rogers, MD and V. Raman Muthusamy, MD

31. Endoscopic Ultrasound-Guided Liver Biopsy   325
Enad Dawod, MD and Jose M. Nieto, DO, AGAF, FACP, FACG, FASGE

32. EUS-Guided Drainage of Pancreatic Collections and Necrosectomy   335
Ryan Law, DO and Todd H. Baron, MD

33. EUS-Guided Biliary Drainage   341
Woo Hyun Paik, MD, PhD and Do Hyun Park, MD, PhD

34. EUS-Guided Pancreatic Duct Drainage   353
Manuel Perez-Miranda, MD, PhD

VII. ENDOSCOPIC THERAPY FOR HEMOSTASIS 363

35. Injection Therapy for Hemostasis   365
Jessica X. Yu, MD, MS

36. Bipolar Probe, Heater Probe, and Argon Plasma Coagulation   371
Anoop Prabhu, MD

37. Clips and Loops   379
Hiroyuki Aihara, MD, PhD

38. Injection Therapy of Esophageal and Gastric Varices   385
Edward Villa, MD and Uzma D. Siddiqui, MD

39. Endoscopic Variceal Ligation   395
Vilas R. Patwardhan, MD and Elliot B. Tapper, MD

40. Balloon Tamponade   403
Donovan Inniss, BS and Monica A. Tincopa, MD, MSc

VIII. BARIATRIC ENDOSCOPY 411

41. Intragastric Balloon Placement for Weight Loss   413
Michael C. Bennett, MD and Shelby Sullivan, MD

42. Endoscopic Suturing   427
Qais Dawod, MD and Reem Z. Sharaiha, MD, MSc

43. Transoral Outlet Reduction (TORe)   437
Allison R. Schulman, MD, MPH

44. Endoscopic Management of Postsurgical Adverse Events   445
Amar Mandalia, MD and Allison R. Schulman, MD, MPH

IX. ENDOSCOPIC SUBMUCOSAL DISSECTION AND PERORAL ENDOSCOPIC MYOTOMY 459

45. Esophageal Endoscopic Submucosal Dissection   461
Daniel S. Strand, MD and Andrew Y. Wang, MD

46. Gastric Endoscopic Submucosal Dissection   471
Makoto Nishimura, MD and Norio Fukami, MD

47. Colon Endoscopic Submucosal Dissection   481
Sergey V. Kantsevoy, MD, PhD

48. Esophageal Peroral Endoscopic Myotomy   491
Amy Hosmer, MD and Ryan Law, DO

49. Gastric Per-Oral Endoscopic Myotomy   499
Maen Masadeh, MD, Rami El Abiad, MD and Mouen A. Khashab, MD

X. PERCUTANEOUS GASTROINTESTINAL-RELATED PROCEDURES..................................... 509

50. Abdominal Paracentesis 511
   Shreya Sengupta, MD
51. Percutaneous Liver Biopsy 519
   Shreya Sengupta, MD

XI. TESTS OF GASTROINTESTINAL FUNCTION............ 525

52. Esophageal Manometry 527
   Joseph R. Triggs, MD, PhD and John E. Pandolfino, MD, MSCI
53. Ambulatory 24-Hour Esophageal pH Monitoring 537
   Jason R. Baker, PhD
54. Small Bowel Motility Testing: Manometry and Scintigraphy 547
   Kimberly N. Harer, MD and William L. Hasler, MD
55. Anorectal Manometry and Biofeedback 561
   Jason R. Baker, PhD
56. Hydrogen Breath Tests for Diagnosis of Carbohydrate Malabsorption and Small Intestinal Bacterial Overgrowth 571
   Allen A. Lee, MD and Jason R. Baker, PhD

Index 581

PART ONE

Preparation of the Patient

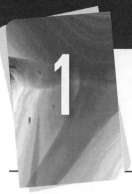

Pre-procedure Assessment of Patients Undergoing Gastrointestinal Procedures

Bret T. Petersen, MD

Prior to performing an endoscopic procedure, careful consideration of the indications, risks, contraindications, preparation, timing, and environment for the procedure should be undertaken, and consent must be obtained from the fully informed and collaborative patient or an appropriate responsible representative. In most cases, this is a straightforward process, but in some instances, procedural planning must be altered by the issues or needs identified in the preprocedure evaluation. National guidelines define quality measures for preprocedural aspects of care, including elements relevant to all procedure types (Table 1.1)[1] and others unique to each of the major procedure types (esophagogastroduodenoscopy [EGD],[2] colonoscopy,[3] endoscopic retrograde cholangiopancreatoscopy [ERCP],[4] and endoscopic ultrasonography [EUS][5]). Among them, the most important "priority indicators" identified for preprocedure care in all procedures include (1) documented performance for a "standard" or broadly accepted indication in at least 80% of cases, (2) appropriate use of prophylactic antibiotics in at least 98% of cases, and (3) appropriate management and documentation of antithrombotic therapy before and after the procedure in at least 98% of cases.

INDICATIONS

Most procedures are performed for relatively standard, well-defined indications that identify the symptom, sign, or pathology for which investigation is planned (e.g., nausea, abdominal pain, bile leak, known or suspected polyp, bleeding, etc.) and for which intervention or subsequent alteration of management is anticipated. Indications should not be defined solely by a planned intervention (e.g., polypectomy, sphincterotomy, stent placement). Procedures should not be undertaken out of curiosity or for documentation or evaluation of a prior result unless the findings or outcome will be likely to influence subsequent care or improve the patient's well-being.[6]

TABLE 1.1 Preprocedure Quality Indicators for Gastrointestinal Endoscopy Procedures	
Quality Indicator	**Performance Target (%)**
ALL PROCEDURES	
1. *Frequency with which* endoscopy is performed for an indication that is included in a published standard list of appropriate indications, and the indication is documented **(priority indicator). (Performance target > 80%).**	>80
2. ... informed consent is obtained and fully documented.	>98
3. ... preprocedure history and directed physical examination are performed and documented.	>98
4. ... risk for adverse events is assessed and documented before sedation is started.	>98
5. ... prophylactic antibiotics are administered for appropriate indication **(priority indicator)**.	>98
6. ... a sedation plan is documented.	>98
7. ... management of antithrombotic therapy is formulated and documented before the procedure **(priority indicator)**.	N/A
8. ... a team pause is conducted and documented.	>98
9. ... endoscopy is performed by an individual who is fully trained and credentialed to perform that particular procedure.	>98
Esophagogastroduodenoscopy (EGD)	
... a proton pump inhibitor is used for suspected peptic ulcer bleeding **(priority indicator)**.	
COLONOSCOPY	
... colonoscopies follow recommended postpolypectomy and postcancer resection surveillance intervals and 10-y intervals between screening colonoscopies in average-risk patients who have negative examination results and adequate bowel cleansing **(priority indicator)**.	>90%

Key *priority indicators* are identified for all procedures and appended for specific procedures. All are process indicators defined by frequency with which an indicator is met among all procedures of the type. Performance targets are proposed for minimal frequency of meeting the specific indicator in practice.

(Data from ASGE/ACG Task Force on Quality in Endoscopy, Rizk MK, Sawhney MS, Cohen J, et al. Quality indicators common to all GI endoscopic procedures. *Gastrointest Endosc.* 2015;81:3-16; ASGE/ACG Task Force on Quality in Endoscopy, Park WG, Shaheen NJ, Cohen J, et al. Quality indicators for EGD. *Gastrointest Endosc.* 2015;81:17-30; and ASGE/ACG Task Force on Quality in Endoscopy, Rex DK, Schoenfeld PS, Cohen J, et al. Quality Measures or Colonoscopy. *Gastrointest Endosc.* 2015;81:31-53.)

PREPROCEDURE ASSESSMENT

While GI endoscopy is generally considered minimally invasive, risks are engendered by the administration of sedation and analgesia, passage of the endoscope through the upper airway, tissue sampling, therapeutic maneuvers involving cutting, thermal ablation, stretching, or potential tearing of tissues, and sometimes prolonged immobility.[7] Assessment of a patient's candidacy for endoscopy includes consideration of tolerance for these standard maneuvers for common and severe complications involving potential vasodilation, dehydration, agitation, suppression of ventilation, bleeding, or infection. Hence, attention should be paid to preexisting comorbidities that might be exacerbated by these stresses.

The preprocedure assessment should, at minimum, document current medications, allergies, history of prior anesthesia or sedation tolerance and adverse events, history of other specific risk factors for endoscopy or sedation, and contemporary cardiorespiratory and airway examinations. Examination for adequacy of the airway should document the presence of facial, oropharyngeal, or dental deformities which might impede resuscitative measures in the event of need for supportive ventilation or airway rescue. The Mallampati Score provides a standardized visual assessment of the oral airway, as a means of estimating potential difficulty in establishing endotracheal intubation (Fig. 1.1). No specific laboratory testing,[8] imaging, or cardiovascular studies are required for patients who are generally well and lack important risks discussed below.

Cardiovascular and respiratory: Cardiopulmonary risks for endoscopy are predominantly related to patient characteristics and vary little by individual procedure type beyond overall complexity and duration.[9] Numerous indices have been described to estimate cardiopulmonary risks during sedation or anesthesia, primarily for surgery. The American Society for Anesthesiology (ASA) Score (range 1-5) is the most universally applied index and is now a standard expectation before administration of sedation or anesthesia (Table 1.2).[10] Numerous specific cardiac or pulmonary limitations should be identified and noted before electing to proceed with endoscopy (Table 1.3).[9] Their presence should prompt attention to the stability or severity of symptoms at the time of endoscopy and consideration whether intervention is required to limit the procedure risk by optimizing the patient's status and/or altering the planned timing, monitoring, sedation, or location for the procedure. Preprocedure chest x-rays are not routinely recommended but should be considered in those with new signs or symptoms of pulmonary compromise or decompensated heart failure.

Coagulation status: Assessment of coagulation parameters (international normalized ratio [INR], prothrombin time [PT], activated partial thromboplastin time [aPTT]) or platelet counts is not recommended unless the patient has a history of severe chronic liver disease, malnutrition, prolonged obstructive jaundice, suspected thrombocytopenia from disease or

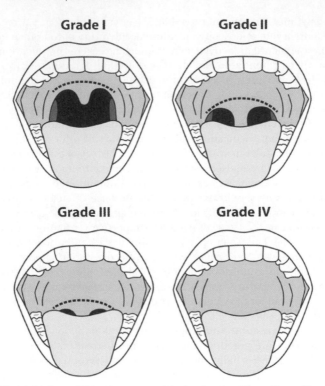

FIG. 1.1 Mallampati Score Assessment of the Oropharyngeal Upper Airway. Class I: soft palate, fauces, uvula, pillars. Class II: soft palate, fauces, portion of uvula. Class III: soft palate, base of uvula. Class IV: hard palate only. (Reprinted from Vargo JJ, DeLegge MH, Feld AD, Gerstenberger PD, Kwo PY, et al. Multisociety sedation curriculum for gastrointestinal endoscopy. *Gastrointest Endosc.* 2012;76(1):e1-e25 with permission from Elsevier.)

TABLE 1.2	ASA (American Society for Anesthesiology) Physical Status Classification System—for Assessment of Risk During Anesthesia, Adapted
Class 1	Normal healthy patient
Class 2	Mild systemic disease
Class 3	Severe systemic disease
Class 4	Severe system disease that is a constant threat to life
Class 5	Moribund and not expected to live without procedure

(ASA Physical Status Classification System, approved by the American Society of Anesthesiology House of Delegates, October 23, 2019, is reprinted with permission of the American Society of Anesthesiologists, 1061 American Lane, Schaumburg, Illinois 60173-4973.)

TABLE 1.3	Health History That Should Be Identified During Preprocedure Assessment of Cardiovascular and Pulmonary Status

Patients Age

Impaired exercise tolerance due to angina or dyspnea—preventing climbing a flight of stairs or brisk walking

Current, recent, or prior myocardial infarction (MI) or stroke

Current, recent, or prior congestive heart failure (CHF)

Nonsinus cardiac rhythm disorder

Uncontrolled hypertension or pulse

Severe chronic obstructive pulmonary disease

Active pneumonia

Sleep apnea

Obesity

Home oxygen use

Renal failure

Diabetes

(Reprinted from Homagnuolo J, Cotton PB, Eisen G, et al. Identifying and reporting risk factors for adverse events in endoscopy. Part I: cardiopulmonary events. *Gastrointest Endosc.* 2011;73(3):579-585. Copyright © 2011 Elsevier. With permission.)

chemotherapy, history of a bleeding disorder, prior bleeding after procedures or dental care, or ongoing therapy with anticoagulants.

PERIPROCEDURAL PLANNING

Once an endoscopic examination is determined to be appropriate, planning should address preprocedure preparations, including dietary constraints, evacuation of bowel contents, management of daily medications, administration of prophylactic antibiotics, and optimal timing and location of the procedure. When significant complicating comorbidities have been identified during the patient assessment (outlined above), consultation with anesthesia professionals should be undertaken to consider whether additional assessment or deferral for an interval of stabilization is advisable. This might prompt noninvasive cardiovascular studies, improved diuresis, cardiac rate control, or pulmonary therapy. Discussion might also prompt relocation from outpatient settings to hospital settings with greater intensity of monitoring.

Standardized fasting intervals prior to administration of sedation have been published by the American Society of Anesthesiology.[11,12] To ensure a high likelihood of an empty stomach at the time of endoscopy, patients should avoid intake of rich solid foods for at least 8 hours, versus 6 hours for a light meal (without meat, fatty, or fried foods), full liquids, or infant formula,

4 hours for breast milk, and 2 hours for clear liquids. Some disease states such as gastroparesis or suspected upper gut obstruction should prompt guidance for even longer intervals.

Prophylactic antibiotics are indicated prior to endoscopic procedures for a limited number of specific indications (Table 1.4),[13] most of which relate to the underlying pathology being addressed, invasiveness of the procedure, or specific patient comorbidities. Antibiotics are most strongly indicated

TABLE 1.4	Guidance for Prophylactic Antibiotics Before Gastrointestinal Endoscopy
Antibiotics advised	**Antibiotic Recommendation**

Prophylaxis against infective endocarditis in patients with cardiac conditions with highest risk of adverse outcome undergoing endoscopic procedures at high risk of inducing bacteremia (esophageal dilation, ERCP):
■ Prosthetic cardiac valve
■ History of infectious endocarditis
■ Cardiac transplant with valvulopathy
■ Congenital heart disease *with*:
  ● Unrepaired cyanotic lesion, including with palliative shunts and conduits
  ● Complete repair with prosthetic material or device, for 6 mo after surgery
  ● Repaired CHD with residual defects at site of prosthetic patch or device
	Advised—include coverage for enterococci—e.g., penicillin, ampicillin, piperacillin, or vancomycin

ERCP for biliary obstruction with anticipated incomplete drainage (especially primary sclerosing cholangitis and hilar strictures)	Advised before and 3-5 d after procedure—include coverage for enteric pathogens and enterococci
ERCP in liver transplant patients	Advised before and after procedure—include coverage for enteric pathogens and enterococci
ERCP in patients with necrotizing pancreatitis	Advised before and after
PEG or PEJ placement for nutritional support	Advised preprocedure—use coverage for cutaneous organisms (Cefazolin 1 gm IV, 30 min prior)
Cirrhosis with acute gastrointestinal bleeding, *independent of plans for endoscopy*	Advised on admission— (ceftriaxone IV or equivalent coverage)
Antibiotics *suggested*:	
Colonoscopy in patients on peritoneal dialysis	Suggested by ip or iv route prior
EUS-FNA of mediastinal or pancreatic cysts	Suggested prior and 3-5 d after

TABLE 1.4 Guidance for Prophylactic Antibiotics Before Gastrointestinal Endoscopy—(Continued)

Antibiotics advised	Antibiotic Recommendation
ERCP in patients with biliary or pancreatic duct leaks	Suggested prior and 3-5 d after
Any procedure in patient with profound immunosuppression or neutropenia (<500 cells/µL)	Individualize coverage decisions
Antibiotics not recommended:	
ERCP without obstruction or with anticipation of complete relief of obstruction	NA
Diagnostic EUS, or EUS + FNA of solid lesions	NA
Any procedure in patients with orthopedic prostheses	NA
Any procedure in patients with vascular grafts or nonvalvular prostheses, including electronic devices	NA

CHD, coronary heart disease; ERCP, endoscopic retrograde cholangiopancreatoscopy; EUS-FNA, endoscopic ultrasound–guided fine needle aspiration; PEG/PEJ, percutaneous endoscopic gastrostomy/jejunostomy.

(Adapted from ASGE Standards of Practice Committee, Khashab MA, Chithadi KV, Acosta RD, et al. Antibiotic prophylaxis for GI endoscopy. *Gastrointest Endosc.* 2015;81(1):81-89. Copyright © 2015 American Society for Gastrointestinal Endoscopy. With permission.)

for percutaneous endoscopic gastrostomy (PEG) or jejunostomy (PEJ) placement[14] and before injecting or accessing closed or extraluminal spaces that cannot be fully drained, including during ERCP for biliary or pancreatic leaks, pancreatic cysts, necrotizing pancreatitis, or complex biliary obstruction that is at high risk for incomplete resolution (e.g., hilar disease and sclerosing cholangitis). Prophylactic antibiotics are also prudent for patients with profound immunosuppression or severe chemotherapy-induced neutropenia (<1000), as they experience higher rates of procedural bacteremia. Antibiotics are indicated for prevention of bacterial endocarditis only when procedures which induce higher rates of bacteremia (esophageal stricture dilation, variceal therapy, and intervention for biliary obstruction) are performed in patients with high-risk cardiovascular lesions or grafts.[15]

Diabetes confers increased risks for delayed gastric emptying and suboptimal bowel preparation. Clear guidance is required for diabetic patients to ensure optimal bowel preparation and safely manage their insulin or other antihyperglycemic agents during the periprocedural interval. For elective procedures, baseline hemoglobin a1c levels within the prior 3 months should be < 8%. Higher levels should prompt referral to the primary physician for improved glycemic control before rescheduling of the procedure.

While fasting prior to endoscopy, patients should withhold their noninsulin diabetes medications and check fasting blood glucose levels every 1 to 2 hours to monitor for hypo- or hyperglycemia. For patients on insulin, consider decreasing basal doses by 25% to 50% while fasting and document the last dose and time of insulin administered. For patients on basal plus bolus doses, ensure receipt of usual basal doses only in the 24 hours before the procedure. Thereafter manage blood glucose as indicated by serial glucose measurements, targeting for fasting and before meal blood glucose levels of <140 mg/dL and random blood glucose levels of <180 mg/dL. Levels ≤70 mg/dL should be treated for hypoglycemia. Levels ≥140 mg/dL in stable patients with good vascular perfusion and procedure duration <2 hours should be treated with subcutaneous correction scale insulin not treat more frequently than every 2 hours. Intravenous insulin infusions can be considered for longer procedures, in unstable patients, or those with uncontrolled levels after first correction dosing.[16]

Age-related alterations in standard practices are often employed for patients in the pediatric[17] and geriatric[18] age groups to enhance the safety and efficacy of both preparation and procedural care. Standard fasting intervals based on food or liquid type are similar across the age spectrum. For children, preparation must attend to the emotional well-being of both the parents and the child. Scheduled morning procedures reduce prolonged fasting intervals, which can be more challenging for both young children and the elderly. Numerous considerations, including patient positioning, airway management, and titrated weight-based medication dosing require age-specific training and equipment availability for the care of children.

Preoperative assessment and preparation of the geriatric patient differ little from other adults, with the exception of screening for and documentation of depression or reduced cognitive abilities that may affect the patient's capacity to understand the procedure indications and guidance. Those patients with profound new or unexpected psychiatric or cognitive impairment should be referred for evaluation prior to elective endoscopy.[19]

Commonly employed split-dose, polyethylene glycol–based, balanced-electrolyte bowel preparations are advisable for elderly individuals, to avoid the potentially harmful fluid and electrolyte shifts notably seen with phosphate- or magnesium-based preparations.

Pregnant patients require assessment of necessity and suitability for endoscopy of both the mother (the patient) and child, including safety of medications, anesthesia, and commonly, fluoroscopy or radiography.[20] Informed consent should include both procedural and sedation risks for both the mother and the

TABLE 1.5	General Principles Guiding Endoscopy in Pregnancy

- Always obtain a preoperative consultation with an obstetrician, regardless of fetal gestational age.
- Proceed only when a strong indication is present, particularly in high-risk pregnancies.
- Defer endoscopy to second trimester whenever possible.
- Use lowest effective dose of sedative medications and category B drugs whenever possible.
- Minimize procedure time.
- Position patient in left pelvic tilt or left lateral position to avoid vena cava or aortic compression.
- Individualize monitoring of fetal heart rate based upon gestational age of the fetus.
- Before 24 wk of gestation, confirm the presence of the fetal heart rate by Doppler before sedation is begun and after the endoscopic procedure.
- After 24 wk of fetal gestation, if possible have a qualified individual monitor the fetal heart rate and uterine contractions before, during, and after the procedure and have obstetric support readily available in case of fetal distress or a pregnancy-related complication.
- After 24 wk of fetal gestation, at a minimum, simultaneously monitor electronic fetal heart rate and uterine contractions before, during, and after the procedure, ideally at an institution with neonatal and pediatric services.
- Endoscopy is contraindicated in placental abruption, imminent delivery, ruptured membranes, or uncontrolled eclampsia.

(Modified from ASGE Standards of Practice Committee, Shergill AK, Ben-Menachem T, Chandrasekhara V, et al. Guidelines for endoscopy in pregnant and lactating women. *Gastrointest Endosc.* 2012;76(1):18-24. Copyright © 2012 American Society for Gastrointestinal Endoscopy. With permission.)

fetus, as the fetus is highly sensitive to changes in maternal oxygenation and blood pressure, which can cause fetal hypoxia and demise. While therapeutic endoscopy offers a safer alternative to many surgical interventions during pregnancy, the risks of fetal hypoxia, premature birth, and exposure to teratogenic medications and ionizing radiation require attention to general principles of endoscopy in pregnancy that are outlined in Table 1.5.

INFORMED CONSENT

Obtaining informed consent to employ a procedure, test, or therapy involves a combination of an appropriate level of disclosure and voluntary decision-making by the competent patient or their representative. Standards for disclosure vary by state but generally expect either the disclosure of information expected by the reasonable lay person or provided by the average physician in a similar situation.[21] The *process* of gaining informed consent should generally entail a conversation between the performing physician or their participating colleague or trainee and the patient or their representative. Generally expected elements of the conversation include the discussion of indication for the procedure and its major components, the major and common risks and potential complications and their management, the alternatives to the procedure, and the potential consequences of not performing the procedure. For gastrointestinal endoscopy, consent must address both the procedure and the proposed sedation or anesthesia. Patients should be afforded the opportunity to ask questions and should be given allowance to decline without prejudice against subsequent or alternate care. Once obtained, signed documentation of the consent to proceed should be obtained for all procedures or interventions with greater-than-minimal risk but not generally for insertion of intravenous catheters, nasogastric tubes, or enemas. Institutions and practices vary greatly in the detail pertaining to risks and complications included in the printed consent document, depending on their legal guidance and state of practice.

Settings in which procedures can proceed in the absence of consent include (1) emergent situations without a lucid patient or time for contacting a patient representative, (2) a patient's voluntary waiver of information prior to consent, which should itself be documented, (3) when a legal mandate is made to proceed, and rarely, (4) when so-called "therapeutic privilege" is claimed, deeming provision of full information about a treatment or procedure to be a risk to the patient's well-being. Lastly, consent can be declined by the patient and refusals to proceed should also be documented, given likely professional opinions that a given procedure is appropriate for the benefit of the patient.

References

1. ASGE/ACG Task Force on Quality in Endoscopy, Rizk MK, Sawhney MS, Cohen J, et al. Quality indicators common to all GI endoscopic procedures. *Gastrointest Endosc.* 2015;81:3-16.
2. ASGE/ACG Task Force on Quality in Endoscopy, Park WG, Shaheen NJ, Cohen J, et al. Quality indicators for EGD. *Gastrointest Endosc.* 2015;81:17-30.
3. ASGE/ACG Task Force on Quality in Endoscopy, Rex DK, Schoenfeld PS, Cohen J, et al. Quality measures or colonoscopy. *Gastrointest Endosc.* 2015;81:31-53.
4. ASGE/ACG Task Force on Quality in Endoscopy, Adler DG, Lieb JG, Cohen J, et al. Quality indicators for ERCP. *Gastrointest Endosc.* 2015;81:54-66.
5. ASGE/ACG Task Force on Quality in Endoscopy, Wani S, Wallace MB, Cohen J, et al. Quality indicators for EUS. *Gastrointest Endosc.* 2015;81:67-80.
6. ASGE Standards of Practice Committee, Early D, Ben-Menachem T, Decker A, et al. Appropriate use of GI endoscopy. *Gastrointest Endosc.* 2012;75:1127-1131.
7. Romagnuolo J, Cotton PB, Eisen G, et al. Identifying and reporting risk factors for adverse events in endoscopy. Part II: noncardiopulmonary events. *Gastrointest Endosc.* 2011;73:586-597.
8. ASGE Standards of Practice Committee, Pasha SF, Acosta R, Chandrasekhara V, et al. Routine laboratory testing before endoscopic procedures. *Gastrointest Endosc.* 2014;80:28-33.

9. Romagnuolo J, Cotton PB, Eisen G, et al. Identifying and reporting risk factors for adverse events in endoscopy. Part I: cardiopulmonary events. *Gastrointest Endosc*. 2011;73:579-585.

10. American Society for Anesthesiology. *ASA Physical Status Classification Update, Approved by the American Society of Anesthesiology House of Delegates.* October 23, 2019. Available at https://www.asahq.org/standards-and-guidelines/asa-physical-status-classification-system. Accessed December 3, 2019.

11. American Society for Anesthesiology. Practice guidelines for preoperative fasting and the use of pharmacologic agents to reduce the risk of pulmonary aspiration: application to healthy patients undergoing elective procedures. *Anesthesiology*. 2017;126:376-393.

12. ASGE Standards of Practice Committee, Early DS, Lightdale JR, Vargo JJ, et al. Guidelines for sedation and anesthesia in GI endoscopy. *Gastrointest Endosc*. 2018;87:327-337.

13. ASGE Standards of Practice Committee, Khashab MA, Chithadi KV, Acosta RD, et al. Antibiotic prophylaxis for GI endoscopy. *Gastrointest Endosc*. 2015;81:81-89.

14. Lipp A, Lusardi G. Systemic antimicrobial prophylaxis for percutaneous endoscopic gastrostomy. *Cochrane Database Syst Rev*. 2013;(11):CD005571. Available at https://www.ncbi.nlm.nih.gov/pmc/articles/PMC6823215/pdf/CD005571.pdf. Accessed December 3, 2019.

15. Wilson W, Taubert KA, Gewitz M, et al. Prevention of infective endocarditis: guidelines from the American Heart Association: a guideline from the American Heart Association Rheumatic Fever, Endocarditis, and Kawasaki Disease Committee, Council on Cardiovascular Disease in the Young, and the Council on Clinical Cardiology, Council on Cardiovascular Surgery and Anesthesia, and the Quality of Care and Outcomes Research Interdisciplinary Working Group. *Circulation*. 2007;116:1736-1754.

16. Apsey HA, Knight AM, Pearson KK, et al. Periprocedural Glycemic Control (Adult). ASK Mayo Expert Institutional Website. https://askmayoexpert.mayoclinic.org/topic/clinical-answers/gnt-20152511/cpm-20152508. Accessed May 4, 2019.

17. ASGE Standards of Practice Committee, Lightdale JR, Acosta R, Shergill AK, et al. Modifications in endoscopic practice for pediatric patients. *Gastrointest Endosc*. 2014;79:699-710.

18. ASGE Standards of Practice Committee, Early DS, Acosta R, Chandrasekhara V, et al. Modifications in endoscopic practice for the elderly. *Gastrointest Endosc*. 2013;78:1-7.

19. Chow WB, Rosenthal RA, Merkow RP, et al. Optimal preoperative assessment of the geriatric surgical patient: a best practices guideline from the American College of Surgeons national surgical quality improvement program and the American Geriatrics Society. *J Am Coll Surg*. 2012;215:453-466.

20. ASGE Standards of Practice Committee, Shergill AK, Ben-Menachem T, Chandrasekhara V, et al. Guidelines for endoscopy in pregnant and lactating women. *Gastrointest Endosc*. 2012;76:18-24.

21. ASGE Standards of Practice Committee, Zuckerman M, Shen B, Harrison E, et al. Informed consent for GI endoscopy. *Gastrointest Endosc*. 2007;66:213-218.

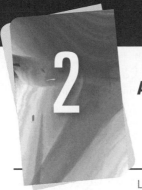

2

Analgesia and Sedation

Laura E. Lehrian, DO
Sarah Gerken, MD

The need for anesthesia, analgesia, or sedation provided for gastroenterological procedures has evolved in parallel with the types of procedures being performed, as well as with the increasing complexity of patients requiring those procedures. The goal of sedation or anesthesia in endoscopic procedures is to achieve an appropriate level of patient comfort during the procedure, while maintaining hemodynamic stability and patient safety. Practice guidelines for nonanesthesiologists providing sedation have been published by the American Society of Anesthesiologists (ASA) Committee for Sedation and Analgesia by Non-Anesthesiologists, and the guidelines have been approved by the American Society for Gastrointestinal Endoscopy (ASGE).[1]

To strike a balance between sedation and safety, the physician responsible for patient care must understand the patient factors that can influence the course of the procedure, as well as the sedation they are providing. Prior to performing a procedure, a thorough evaluation of preexisting medical comorbidities, current medications and drug allergies, previous sedation/anesthesia history, current vital signs, as well as a history and physical should be undertaken. Many factors can influence a patient's response to sedation medications and these include, but are not limited to, disease states of organ systems (renal, hepatic, neurologic, cardiac, and respiratory impairment), obstructive sleep apnea, obesity, substance abuse, and chronic use of certain medications (opioids, benzodiazepines, etc.). The ASA has provided a patient physical status classification that reflects a patient's comorbid conditions and general fitness for undergoing anesthesia and procedures; a recent study demonstrated that an increasing ASA classification was associated with higher prevalence of serious adverse events for upper endoscopy.[2]

ASA CLASSIFICATION

I   The patient is normal and healthy.

II   The patient has mild systemic disease that does not limit activities (e.g., controlled hypertension or controlled diabetes without systemic sequelae).

III The patient has moderate or severe systemic disease that does not limit activities (e.g., stable angina or diabetes with systemic sequelae).

IV   The patient has severe systemic disease that is a constant threat to life (e.g., severe congestive heart failure, end-stage renal failure).

V   The patient is moribund and is at a substantial risk of death within 24 hours (with or without a procedure).

E   Emergency status: in addition to indicating the underlying ASA status (I-V), any patient undergoing an emergency procedure is indicated by suffix "E."

Patients with a history of problems with anesthesia or sedation, stridor, snoring or obstructive sleep apnea, rheumatoid arthritis, or certain chromosomal abnormalities may present problems with airway management, if that were to become necessary. In addition to those conditions, patients with certain physical characteristics can be associated with difficult airway management. Some of these characteristics may include a short, thick neck; limited head and neck mobility; dysmorphic facial features; small mouth opening; a high, arched palate; micrognathia; and retrognathia.[3]

The Mallampati Classification

Class I	Hard palate, soft palate, uvula
Class II	Hard palate, soft palate, portion of uvula
Class III	Hard palate, soft palate, base of uvula
Class IV	Hard palate only

The sedation level required for each procedure and each patient will vary every time. Levels of sedation are described from minimal sedation (anxiolysis) to general anesthesia. With increasing sedation, there will be increasing requirements to be able to intervene and rescue a patient if a level of sedation becomes deeper than intended. In minimal sedation, a patient is able to respond to commands and respiratory and cardiovascular status is unaffected. Moderate sedation (formerly "conscious" sedation) will allow a patient to respond purposefully to light stimuli as well as to verbal commands, with unaffected respiratory and cardiovascular functions. Deep sedation results in a patient who cannot be easily aroused but can respond purposefully with repeated or painful stimulation; here, the ability to maintain a patent airway and spontaneous ventilation may be inadequate and may require ventilatory support. General anesthesia results in loss of consciousness during which time patients are not arousable even to painful stimuli; here, assistance in maintaining the airway is typically necessary, and it is important to note that cardiovascular function may be impaired.

	Minimal Sedation/ Anxiolysis	Moderate Sedation	Deep Sedation	General Anesthesia
Responsiveness	Patient responds to verbal commands	Patient has a purposeful response to verbal or tactile stimuli	Patient has a purposeful response to painful stimuli	Patient is unarousable to painful stimuli
Airway	Maintains patient airway	Maintains patient airway	Intervention may be required	Intervention often required
Ventilation	Spontaneous	Adequate spontaneous ventilation	Spontaneous ventilation may be inadequate	Spontaneous ventilation frequently inadequate
Cardiovascular function	Unaffected	Usually Unaffected	Usually Unaffected	Possibly affected

Ensuring the patient has had an appropriate period of fasting prior to sedation will help to reduce the likelihood of pulmonary aspiration; current recommendations include 2 hours of fasting for clear liquids and 6 hours for light meals in otherwise-healthy patients. Patients with conditions that impair gastric emptying (e.g., gastroparesis, prior vagotomy) or heavy, greasy meals may require longer fasting times (8 hours). Additionally, patients experiencing significant upper GI bleeding at the time of the procedure represent a higher aspiration risk.

Fasting Guidelines

Clear liquids (nonparticulate)	2 hr
Human breast milk	4 hr
Nonhuman milk or formula	6 hr
Light meal	6 hr
Heavy meal	8 hr

Prior to starting a procedure, adequate preparation must be undertaken to ensure a safe environment in which to perform the endoscopy. This includes proper monitoring equipment (e.g., pulse oximetry, noninvasive blood pressure) during the procedure, appropriately trained personnel to administer medications to and monitor the patient, a reliable source of oxygen, reliable suction, as well as appropriate recovery care. Emergency supplies such as defibrillators, advanced airway management equipment, resuscitation medications, as well as pharmacologic antagonists for opioids and benzodiazepines (naloxone and flumazenil, respectively) which should be immediately available at all times.

During minimal or moderate sedation, there should be a designated individual present during the procedure who is responsible for monitoring the patient throughout; this individual should be trained to recognize apnea and airway obstruction. Provided the individual is not a member of the procedural team and that the patient's vital signs and level of sedation/analgesia are adequate, this individual may assist with minor, interruptible tasks. It is recommended that any physician administering or monitoring deep sedation is dedicated to that task; therefore any nonanesthesiologist physician performing the sedation must be different from the individual performing the procedure. The nonanesthesiologist physician administering deep sedation will also be required to have certification in advanced cardiac life support (ACLS).

Prolonged or complex procedures may require deeper levels of sedation such as monitored anesthesia care (MAC) or general anesthesia; consultation with an anesthesiologist is recommended for cases such as these and for patients with substantial medical comorbidities.[1] Regardless of the type of sedation chosen, routine monitoring of cardiopulmonary status, including heart rate, blood pressure, and oxygen saturation, is recommended. As the primary causes of morbidity associated with sedation include medication-induced respiratory depression and airway obstruction, monitoring of end-tidal carbon dioxide should be considered in cases where deep sedation is anticipated or intended.[3]

For minimal and moderate sedation, the use of benzodiazepines and opioids, either alone or in combination, remains the standard of care. Midazolam, with its favorable profile of fast onset of action, short duration of action, and amnestic properties, is the most commonly used benzodiazepine. The dose of benzodiazepine needed for sedation will vary based on several factors including the patient's weight, age, and comorbidities. A typical starting dose for midazolam is 1 mg IV, with additional, incremental dosing, over at least a 2-minute period of time, to reach desired level of sedation. It is important to remember that, although a single dose of midazolam has a duration of less than 2 hours in healthy adults, half-life elimination will be prolonged by factors such as renal impairment, cirrhosis, congestive heart failure, obesity, as well as being elderly.

The addition of an opiate such as fentanyl or meperidine will provide analgesia, as well as sedation, by acting synergistically with the benzodiazepine. Due to active metabolites that can accumulate in patients with renal impairment, meperidine is infrequently used in routine sedation. Small doses of fentanyl, starting at 25 to 50 μg IV, can be given slowly over 1 to 2 minutes with an analgesic response time of approximately 3 to 5 minutes expected. Maximal respiratory depressant effects may not be seen for several minutes, therefore repeated dosing should be titrated with caution.

Conscious Sedation	Midazolam	Fentanyl	Propofol	Benadryl
Initial dose	0.5-1 mg IV	25-50 μg IV slowly over 1-2 min	0.5 mg/kg IV slowly over 3-5 min	10-25 mg IV
Maintenance dose	0.5-1 mg IV, may repeat ~25% initial dose every 2-3 min until desired effect, up to total 0.01-0.1 mg/kg	May give small, repeat boluses, every 15-30 min, up to 0.5-2 μg/kg IV	25-100 μg/kg/min IV	Typical dose totals range from 25 to 50 mg IV

In addition to benzodiazepines and opioids, propofol is a commonly used adjunct for sedation. Propofol-mediated sedation is limited nationally, with regulations of its administration occurring at state, regional, and local levels. In the United States, propofol sedation is typically performed by individuals trained in the administration of general anesthesia, who are not simultaneously involved in the procedure. During the administration of propofol, patients should be monitored, without interruption, to assess the level of consciousness and to identify early signs of hypotension, bradycardia, apnea, oxygen desaturation, and/or airway obstruction. Administration of combinations of drugs including sedatives and analgesics may increase the likelihood of adverse outcomes.[4] In healthy adults, sedation can be achieved with a small bolus of propofol of 0.5 mg/kg IV over 3 to 5 minutes, followed by an IV infusion of 25 to 75 μg/kg/min. If needed, small boluses of 10 to 20 mg may be administered to deepen sedation for particularly stimulating portions of the procedure.

The addition of diphenhydramine as an adjunct, to achieve sedation, is not uncommon. Typical doses for the off-label use of this medication tend to range from 25 to 50 mg IV.

For clinical scenarios in which oversedation, unplanned respiratory depression, or unwanted side effects are encountered, use of appropriate antagonists are indicated. Naloxone should be readily available to counteract opioid effects; initial doses of 0.4

to 2 mg IV can be given, with repeat dosing every 2 to 3 minutes. If a patient has a history of chronic opioid use, smaller initial doses of 0.1 to 0.2 mg IV can be considered, in order to avoid precipitating acute withdrawal symptoms. Similarly, flumazenil is utilized for reversal of benzodiazepines. A dose of 0.2 mg IV should be administered initially, with repeat dosing every minute, up to 1 mg, until patient reaches the desired level of consciousness. Resedation may occur in patients, so repeated dosing of naloxone and/or flumazenil may be necessary.

References

1. ASGE Standards of Practice Committee, Early DS, Lightdale JR, Vargo JJ II, et al. Guidelines for sedation and anesthesia in GI endoscopy. *Gastrointest Endosc.* 2018;87:327-337.
2. Enestvedt BK, Eisen GM, Holub J, et al. Is the American Society of Anesthesiologists classification useful in risk stratification for endoscopic procedures? *Gastrointest Endosc.* 2013;77:464-471.
3. American Society of Anesthesiologists. Practice guidelines for moderate procedural sedation and analgesia 2018: a report by the American Society of Anesthesiologists Task Force on Moderate Procedural Sedation and Analgesia, the American Association of Oral and Maxillofacial Surgeons, American College of Radiology, American Dental Association, American Society of Dentist Anesthesiologists, and Society of Interventional Radiology. *Anesthesiology.* 2018;128:437-479.
4. *Statement on Safe Use of Propofol.* American Society of Anesthesiologists; 2014.

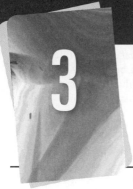

3

Bowel Preps

Tadd K. Hiatt, MD

GENERAL CONSIDERATIONS

Adequate bowel preparation is necessary for all endoscopic procedures. Ease of patient administration and adequate patient compliance with the prep instructions are important to achieve successful bowel cleansing. This chapter will provide an overview of the various bowel preparatory regimens utilized in current gastrointestinal (GI) practice.

UPPER ENDOSCOPY

Fasting prior to upper endoscopy is required for nearly all elective cases. Relative contraindications for upper endoscopy include known esophageal, gastric, or duodenal perforation; severe strictures and tortuosity of the esophagus; and large diverticula involving the cervical esophagus.

Preparation for upper endoscopy consists of nothing by mouth 6 hours before the procedure. Occasionally when a large blood clot or bezoar is located in the stomach, a promotility agent such as erythromycin 250 mg IV may be given in advance of the procedure in an attempt to clear the gastric contents.[1] Large-bore orogastric or nasogastric lavage may also be beneficial in those situations.[2]

PHYSIOLOGIC STUDIES

The preparation for the performance of physiologic studies also depends upon the indication for the procedure. Individuals undergoing 24-hour pH studies may need to discontinue all acid-suppressive medicines or may need to be tested while on their standard dose. Subjects should refrain from taking motility-altering agents such as narcotics prior to undergoing esophageal, gastric, or small bowel motility studies. Most physiologic studies require that the patient take nothing by mouth 6 hours before the procedure.

There are no absolute contraindications to the performance of motility studies. Relative contraindications include patient anxiety and an inability to cooperate with the procedure.

CAPSULE ENDOSCOPY

The preparation for capsule endoscopy is similar to upper endoscopy. Individuals are typically instructed to take nothing by mouth 6 hours before the procedure. However, protocols vary from institution to institution, with many recommending that colonoscopy bowel preparation be utilized to clear the small bowel contents and improve visualization.

Absolute contraindications to capsule endoscopy include a high-grade stricture or obstruction. Severe motility disorders, such as scleroderma, are relative contraindications. In selected patients where luminal pathology is suspected, a patency capsule is often utilized to ensure safe passage to the colon.[3]

DEEP ENTEROSCOPY

Although video capsule endoscopy is theoretically able to visualize the entire small intestine, push enteroscopy or deep enteroscopy (single-balloon enteroscopy or double-balloon enteroscopy) is required to obtain biopsy specimens or perform therapeutic interventions in the area between the ampulla of Vater and the ileocecal valve.

As far as preparation for these procedures is concerned, a fasting-only approach is typically adequate for a push enteroscopy or lesions targeted in the proximal to mid-jejunum. Deep enteroscopy, however, requires a full bowel prep.[4]

FLEXIBLE SIGMOIDOSCOPY

The preparation of the bowel for sigmoidoscopy is determined by the indication. If the sigmoidoscopy is being used to evaluate chronic diarrhea, then the procedure is occasionally performed on an unprepped colon. If the procedure is being performed for colorectal cancer screening or as a diagnostic tool, then a colonic preparation is necessary.

In many circumstances, flexible sigmoidoscopy is utilized for polyp removal or for treatment of radiation proctitis. Prior to such interventions (or others that involve thermal therapy), a full bowel prep is recommended to minimize the risk of bowel explosion.

When a bowel prep is required, purgatory agents may consist of enemas or oral laxatives, and the patient takes nothing by mouth for 6 hours prior to the procedure. Several studies have compared the efficacy of enema preparations to oral regimens.

The results of these studies have been variable with regard to patient acceptance and quality of preparation. Of note, sodium phosphate enemas should be used with caution in individuals with renal impairment, partial colonic obstruction, or ileus because of the risk of fatal hyperphosphatemia.[5]

COLONOSCOPY

Adequate bowel preparation for colonoscopy results in higher adenoma detection and cecal intubation rates, shorter procedure time, decreased risk of electrocautery, and longer required intervals between examinations. Bowel cleansing is a prerequisite for all colonoscopic evaluations, except when it is unsafe due to obstruction, peritonitis, toxic or fulminant colitis, acute diverticulitis, ileus, or known bowel perforation.[6,7]

1. General considerations:
   a. It has been shown that effective patient education improves the quality of the bowel preparation. This could include counseling, written instructions in their native language, visual aids, and/or smartphone applications.
   b. Dietary modifications are important with any bowel preparation regimen. Most commonly, patients should maintain a clear liquid diet the day before the procedure. This consists of water, strained fruit juices, clear broths, coffee, tea, and noncarbonated clear drinks such as Gatorade or Sprite. Red liquids should be avoided as they can be mistaken for blood or may obscure mucosal details. In addition, it is often recommended that patients maintain a low-residue diet (avoiding seeds in particular) for several days leading up to the colonoscopy. This is especially important in those with underlying constipation.
   c. A split-dose preparation has been shown to result in a higher-quality colonoscopic examination. This involves taking half of the standard dose of the bowel preparation on the day prior to the procedure, and the second half on the day of the procedure, 3 to 8 hours before the start of the procedure.
2. Isosmotic agents:
   a. Polyethylene glycol (PEG-ELS). Marketed as GoLytely, this prep is designed as osmotically balanced to minimize fluid and electrolyte shifts. The large volume and poor taste has been shown to limit completion of the prep in 5% to 15% of patients; however, it is generally well tolerated. The tolerance may be improved by the addition of flavorings, as well as chilling the solution. PEG-ELS is considered safe for patient with preexisting electrolyte imbalances, as well as those with renal failure, heart failure, and advanced liver disease.

   b. Sulfate-free PEG-ELS. Marketed as Nulytely, this is comparable to Golytely in terms of effective bowel cleaning and safety. This was designed without sodium sulfate in order to improve the taste and overall patient tolerance.

   c. Low-volume PEG preparations. Marketed as Moviprep, this has been shown to be effective and is the only low-volume PEG-ELS commercially available preparation. This should be used with caution in patients with glucose-6-phosphate dehydrogenase deficiency, as it may provoke hemolysis in these patients.

3. Hypo-osmotic agents:

   a. PEG-3350 (Miralax): Combined with a sports drink, this is not FDA approved but is widely used due to its low-volume (2-L) and good patient tolerance. Studies looking at prep quality have been mixed. More importantly, rare reports of hyponatremia have raised concerns and have limited widespread use.

4. Hyperosmotic agents:

   a. Oral sodium sulfate. Marketed commonly as Suprep, this prep involves a split-dose of a small volume of prep solution (12 ounces) in addition to water. There are limited safety data, but this has been shown in several studies to be well tolerated and effective. Another commercially available product is Suclear, which is a combination of oral sodium sulfate and 2-L of PEG-ELS. While effective, this had a slightly higher rate of vomiting and discomfort compared to PEG-ELS + bisacodyl.

   b. Magnesium citrate. Not recommended for routine colonoscopy preparation due to limited efficacy data and potential renal toxicity.

   c. Sodium phosphate. Marketed as Osmoprep or Visicol, this is a low-volume pill-based prep that is also not recommended for routine use due to potential for renal toxicity and electrolyte abnormalities.

References

1. Barkun AN, Bardou M, Martel M, Gralnek IM, Sung JJ. Prokinetics in acute upper GI bleeding: a meta-analysis. *Gastrointest Endosc.* 2010;72(6):1138-1145.
2. Laine L, Jensen D. Management of patients with ulcer bleeding. *Am J Gastroenterol.* 2012;107:345-360.
3. Bandorski D, Kurniawan N, Baltes P, et al. Contraindications for video capsule endoscopy. *World J Gastroenterol.* 2016;22(45):9898-9908.
4. Gerson L. Capsule endoscopy and deep enteroscopy. *GIE Sept.* 2013;78(3):439-443.
5. Kolts BE. A comparison of the effectiveness and patient tolerance of oral sodium phosphate, castor oil, and standard electrolyte lavage for colonoscopy or sigmoidoscopy preparation. *Am J Gastroenterol.* 1993;88:1218-1223.

6. Johnson DA, Barkun AN, Cohen LB, et al. Optimizing adequacy of bowel cleansing for colonoscopy: recommendations from the US Multi-Society Task Force on Colorectal Cancer. *Am J Gastroenterol.* 2014;109:1528-1545.
7. Saltzman JR, Cash BD, Pasha SF, et al. Bowel preparation before colonoscopy. *Gastrointest Endosc.* 2015;81(4):781-794.

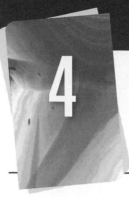

4

Management of Anticoagulation and Antithrombotics

Arjun R. Sondhi, MD

An increasing number of patients require antithrombotics (antiplatelets and/or anticoagulants), which are also increasing in number and complexity, requiring endoscopists to understand the indications, metabolism, bleeding risk, and thrombosis risk surrounding the use and interruption of these medications in low- and high-bleeding-risk procedures. This provides a summary of multiple guidelines, recognizing many of these are based on observational studies or the expert opinion.[1-4] With the growing interest in improving the knowledge base and accessibility to antithrombotic management resources, consider use of a free, validated online tool (www.endoaid.net) to assist in real-time management of antithrombotics.[5,6] This decision support is based on the 2016 American Society of Gastrointestinal Endoscopy (ASGE).

PROCEDURAL RISK

While antithrombotics increase the risk of gastrointestinal (GI) bleeding, there is a large body of evidence supporting their use in a variety of conditions. There are competing interests—maintaining vascular patency with use of these medications but avoiding procedure-related GI bleeding by interrupting the medication. These competing interests have been stratified as low risk and high risk.[1,4] An ultra-high-risk category has also been described.[3] The main risk factor for periprocedural bleeding is the type of procedure.[2] The bleeding risk of endoscopy without biopsy or intervention is very low, even in the setting of antithrombotics, but the risk significantly increases with interventions, especially with more invasive endoscopic approaches (e.g., large lesion endoscopic mucosal resection [EMR], per-oral endoscopic myotomy [POEM], and endoscopic submucosal dissection [ESD]). Table 4.1 stratifies procedural bleeding risk.

TABLE 4.1	Bleeding Risk Stratification of Procedures[3,4]	
Low Risk	**High Risk**	**Ultra High Risk**
Upper or lower endoscopy with or without cold forceps biopsy	Polypectomy	Endoscopic submucosal dissection (ESD)
Endoscopic ultrasound (EUS) without fine needle aspiration (FNA)	ERCP with sphincterotomy	Endoscopic mucosal resection (EMR) of polyps >2 cm
Endoscopic retrograde cholangiopancreatography (ERCP) with or without pancreatobiliary stenting or papillary dilation but without sphincterotomy	Pneumatic or bougie dilation	Per-oral endoscopic myotomy (POEM)
Push or diagnostic balloon-assisted enteroscopy (BAE)	Therapeutic BAE	
Video capsule endoscopy	Variceal sclerotherapy or band ligation	
Esophageal, enteral, or colonic stenting	Percutaneous endoscopic gastrostomy or jejunostomy	
Argon plasma coagulation	EUS with FNA	
Barrett's ablation	Endoscopic hemostasis	
	Tumor ablation	
	Cyst gastrostomy	
	Ampullectomy	
	EMR	

From Chan FKL, Goh KL, Reddy N, et al. Management of patients on antithrombotic agents undergoing emergency and elective endoscopy: joint Asian Pacific Association of Gastroenterology (APAGE) and Asian Pacific Society for Digestive Endoscopy (APSDE) practice guidelines. *Gut.* 2018;67(3):405-417. doi:10.1136/gutjnl-2017-315131. Epub January 13, 2018. Review. PMID: 29331946 and Acosta RD, Abraham NS, Chandrasekhara V, et al. The management of antithrombotic agents for patients undergoing GI endoscopy. *Gastrointest Endosc.* 2016;83(1):3-16. doi:10.1016/j.gie.2015.09.035. Epub November 24, 2015. PMID: 26621548.

THROMBOSIS RISK

Conditions carrying risk of thrombosis or requiring antithrombotics include atrial fibrillation (AF), cardiac valvular replacements, deep vein thrombosis and venous thromboembolism, cerebral artery thrombosis, percutaneous coronary intervention (PCI) or other vascular stenting, acute coronary syndromes, cerebrovascular accident (CVA), transient ischemic attack (TIA), and a genetic or acquired (e.g., malignancy) hypercoaguable state.[2] Complicating this, the objective measurement of severity of bleeding is difficult.[2] For example, a 2002 ASGE guideline designated a procedure as low risk of bleeding if the rate was ≤1.5%,[7] but this definition is not standardized and has not appeared in later iterations of the ASGE's antithrombotic guidelines.

Of particular mention is AF, as this is one of the most common reasons for anticoagulation, and the prevalence of this condition increases with age. The CHA_2DS_2-VASc (C2V) score quantifies the risk of AF-related CVA. The C2V score is calculated as a sum of points associated with the below patient attributes:

- *C*ongestive heart failure = 1 point
- *H*ypertension = 1 point
- *A*ge 75 years or greater = 2 points
- *D*iabetes = 1 point
- *S*troke or TIA = 2 points
- *V*ascular disease = 1 point
- *A*ge 65 to 74 years = 1 point
- *S*ex *c*ategory (female gender) = 1 point

The annual risk of AF-related CVA generally increases with an increasing C2V score.[4] A C2V score of ≥2 portends a high risk of stroke and usually warrants systemic anticoagulation.

BLEEDING RISK

Procedure-Related Factors

Table 4.2 provides the risk of bleeding in the absence of antithrombotics.[8]

Patient-Related Factors

In addition to the binary factor of presence versus absence of use of anticoagulant, HAS-BLED is a validated multivariable score in AF patients that was developed to determine the 1-year risk of significant bleeding (intracranial bleeding, hospitalization, hemoglobin decrease >2 grams/deciliter (g/dL), or transfusion) while on anticoagulation[9] and, compared to other bleeding scoring systems, is the best predictor of bleeding in AF patients.[10] The HAS-BLED score is calculated as a sum of points associated with the below patient attributes, each of which is assigned an equal weight of 1 point[9]:

- *H*ypertension: systolic blood pressure >160 millimeters (mm) of mercury
- *A*bnormal renal function (dialysis, status post renal transplant, or serum creatinine >2.25 milligrams [mg]/dL) or abnormal hepatic function (cirrhosis, total bilirubin >2 times the upper limit of normal [ULN]; or aspartate aminotransferase, alanine aminotransferase, or alkaline phosphatase >3 times the ULN)
- *S*troke: prior history of CVA

TABLE 4.2	Procedure-Related Hemorrhage Risk in Patients Not on Antithrombotics[8]
Procedure	**Hemorrhage Risk (%)**
Colonic polypectomy	0.07-1.7
Colon EMR of lesion >10 mm	3.7-11.3
Esophageal EMR	0.6-0.9
Duodenal EMR	6.3-12.3
Endoscopic submucosal dissection	2-6.9
ERCP with sphincterotomy	0.1-0.2
ERCP with sphincteroplasty	0.19
Ampullectomy	1-7
Esophageal dilation	0-1.7
Esophageal, duodenal, enteral stent	0.5-1
Colonic stent	0-4.5
Percutaneous endoscopic gastrostomy	≤2
EUS with FNA	0.13
EUS with brushing of pancreas cyst	0-3.3

EMR, endoscopic mucosal resection; ERCP, endoscopic retrograde cholangiopancreatography; EUS, endoscopic ultrasound; FNA, fine needle aspiration.

Reprinted by permission from Springer: Veitch AM. Endoscopy in patients on antiplatelet agents and anticoagulants. *Curr Treat Options Gastroenterol.* 2017;15(2):256-267. Copyright © 2017 Springer Science+Business Media, LLC.

- *B*leeding: prior major bleeding or other predisposition to bleeding
- *L*abile international normalized ratio (INR): unstable or high INR or INR in the therapeutic range <60% of the time
- *E*lderly: age >65 years
- *D*rug use: prior alcohol use (≥8 drinks per week), prior drug use, antiplatelet agents, or nonsteroidal anti-inflammatory drugs

Guidance regarding periprocedural antithrombotic management for low- and high-thrombotic-risk patients undergoing low- and high-risk bleeding procedures is in Table 4.3.

BRIDGING

Bridging is when a non-warfarin-based agent, often low-molecular-weight heparin (LMWH), is used while warfarin is interrupted. Patients may be bridged off and on warfarin with the goal to exchange a long duration of action anticoagulant (warfarin) for a shorter duration of action anticoagulant (LMWH) to minimize the duration of subtherapeutic anticoagulation, periprocedurally. Bridge only when patients are at high risk of thrombosis or embolism (Table 4.4).[2-4,11]

TABLE 4.3	Periprocedural Antithrombotic Management for Low- and High-Thrombotic-Risk Patients Undergoing Low- and High-Risk Bleeding Procedures[4]	
	Low-Risk Bleeding Procedure	**High-Risk Bleeding Procedure**
Low thrombotic risk	Continue antithrombotics	Hold anticoagulants. Resume warfarin on the day of procedure, resume DOAC when hemostasis is achieved.
		Continue antiplatelets except hold P2Y12 inhibitors 5-7 d (3-5 for ticagrelor). If on P2Y12 inhibitor, can change to aspirin until P2Y12 inhibitor can be resumed. If on DAPT, hold P2Y12 inhibitor for 5-7 d (3-5 for ticagrelor) and continue aspirin.
High thrombotic risk	Continue antithrombotics	Bridge. Restart warfarin on same day as procedure. Resume DOAC when hemostasis is achieved.
		Continue antiplatelets except hold P2Y12 inhibitors 5-7 d (3-5 for ticagrelor). If on P2Y12 inhibitor, can change to aspirin until P2Y12 inhibitor can be resumed. If on DAPT, hold P2Y12 inhibitor for 5-7 d (3-5 for ticagrelor) and continue aspirin.

DAPT, dual antiplatelet therapy; DOAC, direct-acting oral anticoagulant.

Reprinted from Acosta RD, Abraham NS, Chandrasekhara V, et al. The management of antithrombotic agents for patients undergoing GI endoscopy. *Gastrointest Endosc.* 2016;83(1):3-16. Copyright © 2016 Elsevier. With permission.

POLYPECTOMY

Antithrombotics are of special concern during colonoscopy with polypectomy as colonoscopy is a common GI procedure; polypectomy is often indicated, and postpolypectomy bleeding is the most common complication with a frequency of 7%.[12] Polypectomy is considered high risk for bleeding; continue aspirin if there is a high thromboembolic risk but otherwise consider interrupting aspirin therapy.[4,13] P2Y12 inhibitors should be held for 3 to 14 days prior to polypectomy or other high-risk procedures, depending on the agent used.

TABLE 4.4	Bridging Recommendations[2-4,11]
Condition	**Management**
Nonvalvular AF with C2V <2 and no other thromboembolic diagnosis (prior stroke, TIA, intracardiac thrombus, cardioembolic event)	Do not bridge
AF with any of: C2V ≥2, mechanical cardiac valve, history of CVA	Bridge
Bileaflet mechanical aortic valve replacement (AVR)	Do not bridge
Mechanical AVR + any thromboembolic diagnosis; old-generation mechanical AVR; nonbileaflet AVR; mechanical mitral valve replacement; two or more mechanical valves	Bridge
VTE within previous 3 mo or severe thrombophilia	Bridge

AF, atrial fibrillation; CVA, cerebrovascular accident; TIA, transient ischemic attack; VTE, venous thromboembolism.

From Baron TH, Kamath PS, McBane RD. Management of antithrombotic therapy in patients undergoing invasive procedures. *N Engl J Med.* 2013;368(22):2113–2124. doi:10.1056/ NEJMra1206531. Review. PMID: 23718166; Acosta RD, Abraham NS, Chandrasekhara V, et al. The management of antithrombotic agents for patients undergoing GI endoscopy. *Gastrointest Endosc.* 2016;83(1):3-16. doi:10.1016/j.gie.2015.09.035. Epub November 24, 2015. PMID: 26621548; Douketis JD, Spyropoulos AC, Spencer FA, et al. Perioperative management of antithrombotic therapy: antithrombotic therapy and prevention of thrombosis, 9th ed: American College of Chest Physicians evidence-based clinical practice guidelines. *Chest.* 2012;141(2 suppl):e326S-e350S. doi:10.1378/chest.11-2298. PMID: 22315266.

CORONARY STENTS AND DUAL ANTIPLATELET THERAPY

Dual antiplatelet therapy (DAPT) has well-proven benefits in patients undergoing PCI. DAPT usually combines aspirin with another antiplatelet agent, typically a P2Y12 inhibitor, and most commonly in the setting of PCI and may be indicated in the setting of other vascular stents or for neuroprotective reasons. The risk of DAPT is believed to be greater than either agent alone, but the risk is unclear.[1] Depending on the indication for the procedure (e.g., screening colonoscopy vs emergent endoscopic retrograde cholangiopancreatography) and the indication for the P2Y12 inhibitor, interruption may not always be possible as the American College of Cardiology and American Heart Association recommend at least 12 months of uninterrupted DAPT in patients with coronary drug-eluting stents.[14] For bare metal stents, avoid DAPT interruption for the first 30 days after PCI.[4] When DAPT interruption is required, the recommendation is to interrupt the nonaspirin antiplatelet agent, unless the cardiac issue is very recent, in which case, deferral of the procedure may be required[4] (Table 4.5).

TABLE 4.5	Periprocedural Antithrombotic Management for Select Cardiac Indications in High-Risk Procedure[3,4]	
Thrombotic Risk	**Cardiac Concern**	**Antithrombotic Management**
Low to moderate	ACS or PCI > 6 mo preceding procedure; stable coronary artery disease	Antiplatelets: continue aspirin, hold P2Y12 inhibitors 5 d in advance and resume upon adequate hemostasis. Warfarin: interrupt 5 d in advance without bridging and resume after adequate hemostasis. DOACs: interrupt 2 d in advance, if normal renal function. If impaired renal function and renally metabolized, consider holding for 3 d. Do not bridge. Resume after adequate hemostasis.
High	ACS or PCI 6 wk to 6 mo preceding procedure	Defer procedure until >6 mo from cardiac concern, if possible. If not possible: ■ Aspirin and P2Y12 inhibitor recommendations are same as for moderate to low risk. ■ Warfarin recommendations are the same as for moderate to low risk except bridging is encouraged. ■ DOACs: recommendations are the same as for moderate to low risk. ■ Consider Cardiology consultation.
Very high	ACS or PCI <6 wk preceding procedure	Defer procedure.

ACS, acute coronary syndrome; DOAC, direct-acting oral anticoagulant; PCI, percutaneous coronary intervention.

From Chan FKL, Goh KL, Reddy N, et al. Management of patients on antithrombotic agents undergoing emergency and elective endoscopy: joint Asian Pacific Association of Gastroenterology (APAGE) and Asian Pacific Society for Digestive Endoscopy (APSDE) practice guidelines. *Gut.* 2018;67(3):405-417. doi:10.1136/gutjnl-2017-315131. Epub January 13, 2018. Review. PMID: 29331946 and Acosta RD, Abraham NS, Chandrasekhara V, et al. The management of antithrombotic agents for patients undergoing GI endoscopy. *Gastrointest Endosc.* 2016;83(1):3-16. doi:10.1016/j.gie.2015.09.035. Epub November 24, 2015. PMID: 26621548.

DIRECT-ACTING ORAL ANTICOAGULANTS

Direct-acting oral anticoagulants (DOACs)[15] reach peak anticoagulant effect in 10 to 12 hours; hence, their interruption is based on this quick onset and quick offset of action (Table 4.6).[15] For most patients, regardless of renal function, interruption of the DOAC is 48 hours from the time of the procedure.

TABLE 4.6	Days of Direct-Acting Oral Anticoagulant (DOAC) Interruption by Creatinine Clearance (CrCl) in milliliters/ minutes for High-Risk Procedures[2,4]				
CrCl	Dabigatran	CrCl	Apixaban	Rivaroxaban	Edoxaban
≥80	2-3	≥60	1-2	1-2	≥1
50-79	2-3	30-59	3	3	≥1
30-49	3-4	15-29	4	4	≥1
15-29	4-6				
<15	Dabigatran contraindicated				

From Baron TH, Kamath PS, McBane RD. Management of antithrombotic therapy in patients undergoing invasive procedures. *N Engl J Med.* 2013;368(22):2113-2124. doi:10.1056/NEJMra1206531. Review. PMID: 23718166 and Acosta RD, Abraham NS, Chandrasekhara V, et al. The management of antithrombotic agents for patients undergoing GI endoscopy. *Gastrointest Endosc.* 2016;83(1):3-16. doi:10.1016/j.gie.2015.09.035. Epub November 24, 2015. PMID: 26621548.

However, dabigatran is predominantly renally excreted; >48 hours of dabigatran interruption is required for patients with renal dysfunction (Table 4.4).

REVERSAL AGENTS

Reversal agents are described in Table 4.7. Reversal of vitamin K antagonists (warfarin) deserves special consideration, given warfarin is commonly prescribed and significantly increases the bleeding risk.[16] Warfarin-related or nutrition-related prolongation of the PT/INR can be partially or wholly reversed with fresh frozen plasma (FFP) and/or vitamin K. The benefits of FFP are more immediate reversal, which is beneficial for patients with significant bleeding, and temporary duration of action, which is important if the patient needs to be anticoagulated promptly after the procedure. However, FFP is more costly, carries the risk of transfusion reaction, and results in a significant volume load that not all patients may tolerate well, depending on their comorbidities. The benefits of using vitamin K for reversal include smaller volume, longer-lasting reversal effect, and the option for oral administration. However, there is a rare risk of anaphylaxis, the reversal effect is not immediate, and significant vitamin K exposure will delay the effect of warfarin when anticoagulation is resumed. The reversal agent chosen depends on the bleeding risk of the procedure, the indication for warfarin, the urgency to resume anticoagulation, and the degree of GI bleeding, if present. Prothrombin complex concentrate is a reversal agent, which contains all four vitamin K-dependent coagulation factors (II, VII, IX, X) as well as protein C and protein S. This should be considered in the case of life-threatening bleeding in patients and/or need for urgent procedure. This is a costly reversal agent.

T A B L E 4.7	Antithrombotic Considerations for Urgent Procedures[2,4]		
Specific Drug	**Duration of Action**	**Elective Procedure**	**Reversal for Urgent Procedure**
Aspirin	7-10 d	No interruption	Consider continuing although ASGE recommends holding or giving platelets
NSAIDs	Varies	No interruption	Hold
Dipyridamole	2-3 d	Consider holding for 2 d	Hold
Cilostazol	2 d	Consider holding for 2 d	Hold
P2Y12 inhibitors	Ticagrelor 3-5 d, clopidogrel and prasugrel: 5-7 d, ticlopidine: 10-14 d	Hold for the drug's duration of action	Hold
GPIIb/IIIa inhibitors	1-2 s: tirofiban, 4 h: eptifibatide, 24 h: abciximab	Not applicable as elective procedures do not occur for these patients	Hold
PAR-1 inhibitor	5-13 d: Vorapaxar	Hold (no direct guidance but consider holding for drug's duration of action)	Hold
Vitamin K antagonist	5 d: warfarin	Hold for 5 d	Vitamin K, PCC
UFH	Intravenous: 2-6 h Subcutaneous: 12-24 h	Hold for 4-6 h	Protamine sulfate[a] 1-1.5 mg per 100 international units of heparin with frequent lab monitoring
LMWH	24 h: enoxaparin, dalteparin	Hold for 24 h	Protamine sulfate or recombinant VIIa (rVIIa)
Antithrombin-mediated factor Xa inhibition	36-48 h: fondaparinux	Hold for 36-48 h	Protamine sulfate, consider rVIIa

(continued)

TABLE 4.7	Antithrombotic Considerations for Urgent Procedures[2,4]—(Continued)		
Specific Drug	Duration of Action	Elective Procedure	Reversal for Urgent Procedure
Direct factor Xa inhibitors	For apixaban, rivaroxaban, and edoxaban, see Table 4.6	Hold as per Table 4.6	Andexanet alfa reverses 2 factor Xa inhibitors (rivaroxaban, apixaban) but not other DOACs
Direct thrombin inhibitor	For dabigatran, see Table 4.6	Hold as per Table 4.6	Idarucizumab

LMWH, low-molecular-weight heparin; NSAIDs, nonsteroidal anti-inflammatory drugs; UFH, unfractionated heparin.

[a]Allergic reaction or adverse effects related to high dose or rapid administration can occur. Although uncommon, the adverse events can be severe. This is more likely in patients with known fish allergy, status post vasectomy, or left ventricular dysfunction.

From Baron TH, Kamath PS, McBane RD. Management of antithrombotic therapy in patients undergoing invasive procedures. *N Engl J Med*. 2013;368(22):2113–24. doi:10.1056/NEJMra1206531. Review. PMID: 23718166 and Acosta RD, Abraham NS, Chandrasekhara V, et al. The management of antithrombotic agents for patients undergoing GI endoscopy. *Gastrointest Endosc*. 2016;83(1):3-16. doi:10.1016/j.gie.2015.09.035. Epub November 24, 2015. PMID: 26621548.

For guidance on metabolism-based antithrombotic management in patients undergoing elective procedures and guidance on use of reversal agents in urgent procedures, see Table 4.7.

References

1. Abu Daya H, Younan L, Sharara AI. Endoscopy in the patient on antithrombotic therapy. *Curr Opin Gastroenterol*. 2012;28(5):432-441. doi:10.1097/MOG.0b013e328355e26f. Review. PMID: 22885943.
2. Baron TH, Kamath PS, McBane RD. Management of antithrombotic therapy in patients undergoing invasive procedures. *N Engl J Med*. 2013;368(22):2113-2124. doi:10.1056/NEJMra1206531. Review. PMID: 23718166.
3. Chan FKL, Goh KL, Reddy N, et al. Management of patients on antithrombotic agents undergoing emergency and elective endoscopy: joint Asian Pacific Association of Gastroenterology (APAGE) and Asian Pacific Society for Digestive Endoscopy (APSDE) practice guidelines. *Gut*. 2018;67(3):405-417. doi:10.1136/gutjnl-2017-315131. Epub January 13, 2018. Review. PMID: 29331946.
4. Acosta RD, Abraham NS, Chandrasekhara V, et al. The management of antithrombotic agents for patients undergoing GI endoscopy. *Gastrointest Endosc*. 2016;83(1):3-16. doi:10.1016/j.gie.2015.09.035. Epub November 24, 2015. PMID: 26621548.
5. Strauss AT, James TW, Mathews SC. Fellow education improved through mobile clinical decision support application: a multi-center approach involving peri-procedural antithrombotic use. *Gastroenterology*. 2018;155(6):2014-2015. doi:10.1053/j.gastro.2018.08.034. Epub August 27, 2018. PMID: 30165048.

6. Nutalapati V, Tokala KT, Desai M, et al. Development and validation of a web-based electronic application in managing antithrombotic agents in patients undergoing GI endoscopy. *Gastrointest Endosc.* 2019;90(6):906-912. doi:10.1016/j.gie.2019.06.015. PMID: 31228431.

7. Eisen GM, Baron TH, Dominitz JA, et al. Guideline on the management of anti-coagulation and antiplatelet therapy for endoscopic procedures. *Gastrointest Endosc.* 2002;55:775-779. PMID: 12024126.

8. Veitch AM. Endoscopy in patients on antiplatelet agents and anticoagulants. *Curr Treat Options Gastroenterol.* 2017;15(2):256-267. doi:10.1007/s11938-017-0137-z. Review. PMID: 28540489.

9. Pisters R, Lane DA, Nieuwlaat R, et al. A novel user-friendly score (HAS-BLED) to assess 1-year risk of major bleeding in patients with atrial fibrillation: the Euro Heart Survey. *Chest.* 2010;138(5):1093-1100. doi:10.1378/chest.10-0134. Epub March 18, 2010. PMID: 20299623.

10. Lip GY, Frison L, Halperin JL, et al. Comparative validation of a novel risk score for predicting bleeding risk in anticoagulated patients with atrial fibrillation: the HAS-BLED (hypertension, abnormal renal/liver function, stroke, bleeding history or predisposition, Labile INR, elderly, drugs/alcohol concomitantly) score. *J Am Coll Cardiol.* 2011;57(2):173-180. doi:10.1016/j.jacc.2010.09.024. Epub November 24, 2010. PMID: 21111555.

11. Douketis JD, Spyropoulos AC, Spencer FA, et al. Perioperative management of antithrombotic therapy: antithrombotic therapy and prevention of thrombosis, 9th ed: American College of Chest Physicians evidence-based clinical practice guidelines. *Chest.* 2012;141(2 suppl):e326S-e350S. doi:10.1378/chest.11-2298. PMID: 22315266.

12. Heldwein W, Dollhopf M, Rösch T, et al. The Munich Polypectomy Study (MUPS): prospective analysis of complications and risk factors in 4000 colonic snare polypectomies. *Endoscopy.* 2005;37(11):1116-1122. doi:10.1055/s-2005-870512. PMID: 16281142.

13. Veitch AM, Vanbiervliet G, Gershlick AH, et al. Endoscopy in patients on antiplatelet or anticoagulant therapy, including direct oral anticoagulants: British Society of Gastroenterology (BSG) and European Society of Gastrointestinal Endoscopy (ESGE) guidelines. *Endoscopy.* 2016;48(4):c1. doi:10.1055/s-0042-122686. Epub 2017 Jan 23. PMID: 28114689.

14. Levine GN, Bates ER, Bittl JA, et al. 2016 ACC/AHA guideline focused update on duration of dual antiplatelet therapy in patients with coronary artery disease: a report of the American College of Cardiology/American Heart Association Task force on Clinical Practice Guidelines. *J Am Coll Cardiol.* 2016;68(10):1082-1115. doi:10.1016/j.jacc.2016.03.513. Epub March 29, 2016. PMID: 27036918.

15. Barnes GD, Ageno W, Ansell J, et al. Recommendation on the nomenclature for oral anticoagulants: communication from the SSC of the ISTH. *J Thromb Haemost.* 2015;13(6):1154-1156. doi:10.1111/jth.12969. PMID: 25880598.

16. Gerson LB, Michaels L, Ullah N, et al. Adverse events associated with anti-coagulation therapy in the periendoscopic period. *Gastrointest Endosc.* 2010;71(7):1211-1217.e2. doi:10.1016/j.gie.2009.12.054. PMID: 20598248.

PART TWO

Upper Endoscopy Procedures

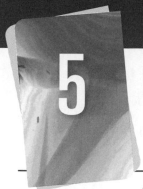

5 Esophagogastroduodenoscopy

Arpan H. Patel, MD

Upper gastrointestinal (GI) endoscopy provides a means for accurate diagnosis and therapy of upper GI diseases. The purpose of this chapter is to provide an overview of upper GI endoscopy, its clinical indications, contraindications, the procedure itself, and a summary of known adverse events. It is not intended to be a comprehensive source of instruction. Endoscopic technique and interpretation are best taught by an experienced endoscopist, supplemented by a review of recent inclusive texts[1-4] that outline technique and pathology in detail. Training guidelines have been established by professional societies.[5]

INDICATIONS
Diagnostic
1. To establish the site of upper GI bleeding
2. To visually define and/or biopsy abnormalities seen on radiological studies (ulcers, filling defects, and cancers)
3. To evaluate healing of medically treated gastric ulcers
4. To evaluate dysphagia, dyspepsia, abdominal pain, gastric outlet obstruction, chest pain after negative cardiac evaluation, and iron deficiency anemia after negative colonoscopy
5. To evaluate odynophagia
6. To determine the extent of damage after a caustic ingestion
7. To sample for infection (e.g., cytomegalovirus, *Helicobacter pylori*) or disease (e.g., graft vs. host disease, eosinophilic esophagitis)

Therapeutic
1. Esophageal, gastric, and duodenal polypectomy
2. Removal of foreign bodies
3. Disintegration of bezoars and food impactions

4. Treatment of bleeding lesions with directed thermal or injection therapy
5. Treatment of esophageal varices (banding and/or sclerotherapy)
6. Placement of guidewires or balloons for esophageal and gastric dilation
7. Placement of small-intestinal feeding tubes and percutaneous gastrostomy tubes
8. Treatment of Barrett esophagus with tissue vaporization
9. Palliation of esophageal, gastric, or duodenal tumors with stent placement
10. Facilitation of pancreatic necrosectomy after creation of a cyst gastrostomy
11. Bariatric endoscopy with suturing including outlet revision, endoscopic sleeve gastroplasty

CONTRAINDICATIONS
Absolute
1. Shock (unless used as a preoperative to guide emergent surgical therapy)
2. Acute myocardial infarction
3. Severe dyspnea with hypoxemia
4. Coma (unless patient is intubated)
5. Seizures
6. Acutely perforated ulcer or perforated esophagus
7. Atlantoaxial subluxation

Relative
1. Uncooperative patient
2. Coagulopathy (relative contraindication is with the use of thermal therapy)
   a. Prothrombin time 3 seconds over control
   b. Partial thromboplastin time (PTT) 20 seconds over control
   c. Bleeding time >10 minutes
   d. Platelet count <50,000/mm^3
3. Myocardial ischemia
4. Thoracic aortic aneurysm

PREPARATION
1. The patient should have nothing by mouth for 6 hours prior to the procedure. If this is not possible due to the need for emergent esophagogastroduodenoscopy (EGD), the stomach should be evacuated by means of an orogastric or nasogastric lavage. Intubation for airway protection should be considered in patients who are having vigorous upper GI bleeding in

which it is not possible to completely evacuate the stomach, such as in variceal bleeding and in patients with decreased consciousness.

2. Review the patient's chart, including x-rays and coagulation studies.
3. See the patient prior to the procedure. Be certain the study is indicated and that the patient understands the risks and benefits and agrees to the procedure. Obtain written informed consent from the patient or his or her legal proxy.
4. Write a preprocedure note that documents cardiovascular and airway assessment, comorbidities, and informed consent.
5. Start an intravenous (IV) line; anesthetize the patient's throat with a topical agent such as lidocaine spray, and attach the pulse oximeter. Oxygen saturation, blood pressure, and pulse rate are routinely monitored during procedures requiring conscious sedation.
6. Administer a short-acting narcotic such as fentanyl through the IV line. There should be at least a 2-minute pause in between doses given slight delay in medication effect and risk of respiratory depression with escalating narcotic dosage.
7. If needed, slowly administer midazolam (0.75 to 2 mg) intravenously until an appropriate level of sedation is reached. Watch the patient carefully for respiratory depression and give preoperative medication cautiously in elderly or malnourished patients.

EQUIPMENT

1. Endoscope of choice. A small-caliber endoscope is routinely used. The endoscope diameters for adult endoscopes typically range from 8.6 to 11 mm. Larger endoscopes with multiple channels are used when more complex therapeutic procedures are anticipated. Comparisons of the technical details of commercially available endoscopes have been published[6]
2. Fiber-optic light source or video-processing monitor depending on the type of the endoscope used
3. Video monitor for video endoscopy or a video adaptor or camera for fiber-optic imaging
4. Washing cannula and syringe, unless the endoscope is fitted with a water jet
5. Computer disc for image storage for video endoscopy or camera
6. Accessories: Biopsy forceps, cytology brush, band ligator, injection needle, snare, etc
7. Insufflation source: using CO_2 has become the ideal option although using oxygen is a reasonable option when no therapeutic intervention is being performed

PROCEDURE
Passing the Endoscope

1. Administer medication so that patient is sedated. Level of sedation will be dependent on whether the patient is receiving conscious sedation versus anesthesia assistance for monitored anesthesia care or general anesthesia.
2. Place the recumbent patient in the left lateral position with the bite block in place.
3. Hold the scope with the left hand on the controls and the right hand on the shaft at the 25- to 30-cm mark in a partially flexed (60°) configuration.
4. With the patient's neck partially flexed, pass the endoscope through the hypopharynx. Under direct visualization using light pressure, slowly guide the tip of the scope past the epiglottis to rest on the cricopharyngeus, which is located in the midline posterior to the larynx and between the pyriform sinuses, 15 to 18 cm from the incisors (Fig. 5.1). Gently insert the endoscope into the esophageal lumen during relaxation of the cricopharyngeus. If the patient is sedated using conscious sedation, this can be achieved by asking the patient to swallow. Be certain to keep the scope in the midline, out of the pyriform sinuses and posterior to the larynx.

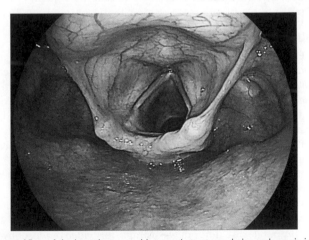

FIG. 5.1 View of the hypopharynx and laryngeal structures during endoscopic intubation. The cricopharyngeus is posterior at the 6 o'clock position. (From Kawada K, Kawano T, Sugimoto T, et al. Observation of the pharynx to the cervical esophagus using transnasal endoscopy with blue laser imaging. In: Amornyotin S, ed. *Endoscopy—Innovative Uses and Emerging Technologies.* March 23, 2015. Available at http://dx.doi.org/10.5772/60541; https://creativecommons.org/licenses/by/3.0/. Copyright © 2015 The Author(s). Licensee IntechOpen.)

5. Once the scope has passed the upper esophageal sphincter (20 cm), advance it under *direct vision* at all times and with only enough air insufflation to permit visualization.

Visualization of Esophagus, Stomach, and Duodenum

1. Advance the scope through the distal esophagus, identifying the gastroesophageal junction by the change from white- to coral-colored mucosa ("Z" line) and the lower esophageal sphincter. A hiatal hernia is present if the gastroesophageal junction and gastric folds are above the level of the diaphragm. Barrett esophagus is identified by an irregular Z line with fingers or islands of pink gastric epithelium extending into the whitish esophageal mucosa.

2. Observe the motility of the stomach, particularly the antrum, for asymmetry and fixation, as subtle invasive lesions are sometimes suspected from dampening of gastric contractions.

3. Insert the scope through the pyloric channel into the duodenal bulb, then into the second portion of the duodenum by torquing clockwise and turning the tip posteriorly (to the right). This can also be achieved by moving your left hand with the endoscope across your body to the right.

4. The duodenal bulb and pyloric channel are visualized best by slowly withdrawing the scope while rotating the tip by torquing the shaft from side to side. Pay particular attention to the superior and posterior portions of the duodenal bulb as lesions can often be missed in this area.

5. Returning to the stomach, pay special attention to the incisura and the gastroesophageal junction, visualizing both by retroflexion as well as by forward viewing. The endoscope is retroflexed by maximally turning the tip upward so that it is in a J shape. By rotating the retroflexed scope, the entire gastric cardia can be thoroughly visualized.

6. After thoroughly evaluating the stomach, by slowly withdrawing the scope while rotating the tip in a 360° fashion, remove the excess air from the stomach by suction to minimize abdominal distension.

Biopsy

1. To obtain adequate depth of sampling, gently compress the open biopsy forceps against the mucosa.

2. It is not necessary to perform a biopsy on a routine duodenal bulbar ulcer unless lymphoma is suspected or if nodularity or a mass is seen.

3. Always perform a biopsy on a gastric ulcer, unless it is a pyloric channel ulcer or prepyloric erosion that is clearly benign.

Biopsies should be performed to include the *margin* of the ulcer in all four quadrants, the base several times, and the mucosa next to the ulcer (i.e., at least six to eight biopsies). Avoid performing a biopsy in an area where there is evidence of active or recent bleeding from the ulcer (clot on the base or visible vessel).

4. In the case of ulcer disease, especially in the case of duodenal ulcers, biopsies should be taken from the antrum, incisura, body, and the fundus to assess for the presence of *H. pylori*. The biopsy may be used for a rapid urease test (Clotest) or sent for histologic assessment of the presence of *H. pylori*.

5. Esophageal biopsies can be obtained more easily by opening the biopsy forceps, withdrawing the forceps until they are close to the endoscope, turning the tip of the scope toward the mucosa, then partially deflating the lumen.

6. If the biopsy forceps do not pass through the distal channel, straighten the endoscope and try again.

Cytology

Cytologic examination of possible malignant lesions will complement biopsies by increasing the yield of positive results.

1. Obtain cytologic specimens before biopsies to diminish dilution of cells by blood. Brush suspicious areas (gastric ulcers, mucosal masses) to obtain adequate cellular material. The use of a disposable, retractable brush protected by a plastic sheath will protect the sample from being lost in the biopsy channel of the endoscope.

2. Stroke the brush over a glass slide moistened with normal saline.

3. Place the slide in a preservative in a Pap smear bottle.

4. Submucosal cytologic specimens can be obtained from mass lesions by aspiration of saline through a sclerotherapy needle inserted into the lesion.

5. Lesions to be brushed should be cleansed of surface mucus, blood, and exudate by a jet of water through the biopsy channel.

Subacute Bacterial Endocarditis Prophylaxis

Subacute bacterial endocarditis prophylaxis is not routinely recommended in routine diagnostic upper endoscopy. Limited data are available for patients with high-risk cardiac lesions such as prosthetic valves. With upper endoscopic procedures that increase the risk of bacteremia such as esophageal dilatation and sclerotherapy, routine antibiotic prophylaxis is recommended in high-risk individuals such as those with prosthetic valves.

Antibiotic prophylaxis for intermediate-risk patients should be addressed on an individual basis. Complete guidelines, including antibiotic regimens, are available from the American Society of Gastrointestinal Endoscopy.[7] These guidelines should be available in a procedure and policy manual in the procedure unit for quick reference.

MISCELLANEOUS

1. In patients with achalasia, the esophagus should be emptied of retained food prior to endoscopy with a large-diameter tube and lavage. This will permit better visualization and reduce the risk of aspiration.
2. If esophageal varices are encountered and are not clinically suspected, make sure they are *carefully* documented by multiple observers and photographs. Grading of esophageal varices provides prognostic information to the referring provider.
3. Endoscopic images should be attached to the procedure note to allow the referring physician to visualize the morphologic findings.

POSTPROCEDURE

1. Perform vital signs every 3 to 5 minutes immediately following the procedure.
2. Document the procedure with a note that includes the indications for the procedure, the details of procedure performed, medications administered, findings, and recommendations.
3. Give nothing by mouth until the gag reflex and sensation in the throat return.
4. A driver should be present prior to discharge of the patient. Detailed instructions should be given since many patients do not recall verbal discussions after sedation.

ADVERSE EVENTS

Overall rate of adverse events of the procedure and the medications are estimated at 0.13% with mortality in the range of 0.014%.[8]

1. Drug-induced
   a. Respiratory arrest (0.07%)
   b. Phlebitis
2. Perforation (0.033% to 0.1%). The most common sites are the pharynx, upper esophagus, and stomach
3. Bleeding (0.03%). This is from biopsies, dislodging clots from bleeding points, and Mallory-Weiss tears induced by retching during endoscopy

4. Aspiration (0.08%). The risk can be decreased by giving the patient nothing by mouth, lavaging patients with bleeding or achalasia, and using minimum air insufflation
5. Retropharyngeal hematomas and crush injuries
6. Infection
   a. Transient bacteremia (5%). There are approximately seven reported cases of bacterial endocarditis temporally associated with upper endoscopy.[9]
   b. There is no evidence of HIV being transmitted by properly cleaned endoscopes and equipment[10]
7. Adverse events to the endoscopist
   a. Bitten finger
   b. Herpetic conjunctivitis
   c. Because of the potential transmission of hepatitis and HIV viruses, gloves, gown, and mask should be worn at all times, and all specimens should be handled in accordance with universal precaution guidelines

2018 CPT CODES

43235—Upper gastrointestinal endoscopy including esophagus, stomach, and either the duodenum and/or jejunum as appropriate; diagnostic, with or without collection of specimen(s) by brushing or washing (separate procedure)

43236—With directed submucosal injection(s), any substance

43239—With biopsy, single or multiple

43241—With transendoscopic intraluminal tube or catheter placement

43243—With injection sclerosis of esophageal/gastric varices

43244—With band ligation of esophageal/gastric varices

43245—With dilation of gastric/duodenal stricture(s) (e.g., balloon, bougie)

43246—With directed placement of percutaneous gastrostomy tube

43247—With removal of foreign body

43248—With insertion of guidewire followed by dilation of esophagus over guidewire

43249—With transendoscopic balloon dilation of esophagus (<30 mm)

43233—With dilation of esophagus with balloon (30 mm diameter or larger) (includes fluoroscopic guidance, when performed)

43250—With removal of tumor(s), polyp(s), or other lesion(s) by hot biopsy forceps

43251—With removal of tumor(s), polyp(s), or other lesion(s) by snare technique

43254—With EMR (endoscopic mucosal resection)

43255—With control of bleeding, any method

43258—With ablation of tumor(s), polyp(s), or other lesion(s) not amenable to removal by hot biopsy forceps, bipolar cautery, or snare technique

43266—With placement of endoscopic stent (includes pre and post dilation and guidewire passage, when performed)

43270—With ablation of tumor(s), polyp(s), or other lesion(s) (includes pre and post dilation and guidewire passage, when performed)

References

1. Chandrasekhara V. *Clinical Gastrointestinal Endoscopy*. 3rd ed. Elsevier; 2018.
2. Haycock A. *Cotton and Williams' Practical Gastrointestinal Endoscopy: The Fundamentals*. 7th ed. Wiley Blackwell; 2014.
3. Wallace M. *Gastroenterological Endoscopy*. 3rd ed. Thieme; 2018.
4. Chun H. *Clinical Gastrointestinal Endoscopy: A Comprehensive Atlas*. 2nd ed. Springer; 2018.
5. Ekkelenkamp VE. Training and competence assessment in GI endoscopy: a systematic review. *Gut*. 2016;65(1):607-615.
6. Varadarajulu S, Banerjee S, Barth BA, et al. GI endoscopes. *Gastrointest Endosc*. 2011;74(1):1-6.e6.
7. Khashab MA, Chithadi KV, Acosta RD, et al. Antibiotic prophylaxis for GI endoscopy. *Gastrointest Endosc*. 2015;81(1):81-89.
8. Levy I. Complications of diagnostic colonoscopy, upper endoscopy, and enteroscopy. *Best Pract Res Clin Gastroenterol*. 2016;30(5):705-718.
9. Nelson D. Infectious disease complications of GI endoscopy: Part I, endogenous infections. *Gastrointest Endosc*. 2003;57(4):546-556.
10. Nelson D. Infectious disease complications of GI endoscopy: Part II, exogenous infections. *Gastrointest Endosc*. 2003;57(6):695-711.

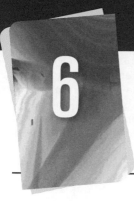

6

Dilation of the Esophagus: Wire-guided Bougie (Savary, American) and Balloon Dilators

Chanakyaram A. Reddy, MD
Joan W. Chen, MD, MS

The two most common types of esophageal dilators used in endoscopy suites are fixed-diameter push-type "bougies" and balloons. Bougie dilators apply radial and axial forces along the entire stricture length, while balloon dilators apply radial force to portions of the stricture that come into contact with the balloon.

Wire-guided, compared to non–wire-guided, dilation offers the ability to dilate difficult and convoluted strictures with some control over the path of the bougie. Both of the two available systems, the Savary-Gilliard and the American endoscopy systems, offer a wire with a spring tip for insertion into the stomach. Neither system has been demonstrated to be superior to the other with respect to safety or quality of the dilation.

There are several esophageal balloon dilators with a variety of designs, lengths, and calibers. These include single-diameter or multiple sizes that can be used over a guidewire or through-the-scope (TTS). This chapter will focus on the use of TTS balloon dilators as this method allows for dilation at multiple sizes with one instrument and is more commonly used than other types of balloon dilators in current endoscopy practices. Balloons are expanded by injection of liquid (water or radiopaque contrast to facilitate fluoroscopic visualization if needed) with use of a hand-held accessory.

Both wire-guided bougie and TTS esophageal dilators are commonly used without clear data indicating significant differences in efficacy or adverse events between the two techniques.[1] Decision-making in regards to which dilation method to use may vary based on institutional practice, operator experience, or the location and characteristics of the stricture. Balloon dilators are usually limited to short-segment, mid to distal esophageal strictures; whereas, bougie dilators can be used in long-segment and proximal strictures and in a diffusely narrowed esophagus. TTS balloon dilators require a 2.8 mm working channel and are not compatible with the majority of smaller-caliber endoscopes such as a neonatal endoscope. Furthermore, bougie dilators are reusable while majority of balloon dilators are single-use only. Lastly, TTS balloon dilators lack tactile feel that can be appreciated while using push-type bougie dilators but do offer direct endoscopic visualization of the dilation, and the use of multidiameter balloon dilators may shorten procedure time.

INDICATIONS

1. To provide relief of dysphagia in subjects with esophageal strictures secondary to most commonly acid-peptic disease or variety of other causes including eosinophilic esophagitis, caustic injury, radiation injury, pill-induced esophagitis, postendoscopic therapy, or postsurgical anastomosis scarring
2. To dilate esophageal webs or rings
3. Congenital esophageal anomalies such as tracheoesophageal fistula
4. Cricopharyngeal bar
5. Some cases of achalasia (pneumatic dilation should be used in this setting)
6. As short-term palliation in esophageal malignancy

CONDITIONS UNLIKELY TO BENEFIT FROM DILATION

1. Extrinsic malignant compression
2. Motility disorders
3. Empiric dilation for dysphagia with normal endoscopic findings[2,3]

CONTRAINDICATIONS

1. Cardiac instability, respiratory insufficiency, or other life-threatening cardiopulmonary conditions
2. Significant bleeding diathesis
3. Warfarin, heparin, or thienopyridine (e.g., clopidogrel) antiplatelet therapy
4. Lack of patient cooperation
5. An impacted food bolus (however, dilation may be performed after disimpaction)
6. Severe cervical spinal arthritis
7. Acute or incompletely healed esophageal perforation
8. Severe acute esophagitis (e.g., from untreated reflux or infection) may be a relative contraindication

PREPARATION

1. Subjects should be NPO for 6 hours prior to the examination.
2. Obtain written consent.
3. Administer a topical anesthetic for pharyngeal anesthesia.
4. Start an intravenous line for the administration of systemic sedation.

WIRE-GUIDED BOUGIE (SAVARY OR AMERICAN) DILATION

Equipment

1. Upper endoscope
2. Spring-tipped wire
3. Appropriate range of dilator sizes, generally up to 18 to 20 mm (54 to 60 French)
4. Lubricant
5. Gloves
6. Available fluoroscopy, for complex or tight strictures

Procedure

1. Perform diagnostic upper endoscopy. If the esophageal stricture is too tight to allow passage of the adult upper endoscope, a pediatric or neonatal scope may be necessary to traverse the stricture. Special note should be made of any tortuosity, diverticula, or angulation, as these conditions may increase the risk of adverse event or ineffective bougienage. The approximate minimal diameter of the stricture should be noted by comparing it to the scope tip or to an open forceps.
2. Under direct endoscopic observation, place the spring-tipped guidewire into the gastric antrum, spring tip first. In situations when the stricture is not traversable even by a small caliber endoscope, the guidewire may be placed with fluoroscopic guidance. In situations when fluoroscopy is not available and the stricture is short, the wire may be passed through the stricture as long as it does not meet resistance. For longer strictures, blind passage of the guidewire is inadvisable, and the best course would be to postpone the procedure until fluoroscopic guidance is available. With such strictures, a barium study can provide valuable information regarding stricture morphology.
3. After the guidewire is placed in the antrum, withdraw the scope slowly and advance the guidewire 5 cm through the scope for every 5 cm of scope withdrawn. In this fashion, the wire tip will remain in the antrum even after complete withdrawal of the endoscope.
4. After the endoscope has been removed from the patient, have an assistant hold the wire position firmly at the patient's mouth, then slide the scope completely off of the wire and remove the endoscope.

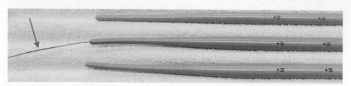

FIG. 6.1 Image of American dilators with a portion of a guidewire emerging through the center dilator. The arrow points to the guidewire marking, with each hash mark representing 20 cm. In this image, the four marks indicate 80 cm of inserted wire.

5. Note the wire position at the incisors. At least 60 to 80 cm of wire should be inside of the patient. If this is not the case, the endoscope may need to be reinserted and the wire repositioned. The wire often has markings every 20 cm (Fig. 6.1). If so, assess the wire marking at the mouth to ensure that there is no migration of the wire for the remainder of the procedure.[4]

6. Apply lubricant and pass a dilator approximately 1 to 2 mm larger than the smallest diameter of the stricture onto the wire.

7. Optimal endoscopist position is standing at the level of the head or slightly below.

8. When the dilator is just outside the patient's mouth, fix the wire in space with the left hand or by an assistant, so that proximal migration of the wire into the patient does not occur with passage of the dilator.

9. Slightly hyperextend the patient's neck to allow for smoother passage of the dilator.

10. With the wire fixed, pass the dilator smoothly, holding it in the right hand so that the resistance to the dilator is easily appreciable.

11. Pass the dilator into the patient, until all but 3 to 4 inches is in, or until anything greater than mild-moderate resistance is encountered (Fig. 6.2). If greater resistance is encountered, consider withdrawal of the dilator and exchange for a smaller caliber dilator.

12. After passage of the dilator, slowly withdraw the dilator over the guidewire to ensure that the wire tip remains in the antrum. After complete withdrawal, assess the wire placement at the mouth to confirm that the wire has not migrated.

13. Repeat steps 6 through 12 with the next sized dilator.

14. Although few data support it, most endoscopists use the "rule of threes" for dilation: Pass no more than three dilators to resistance at any given sitting. Any more than small amounts of blood on the dilator should also prompt termination of the procedure.

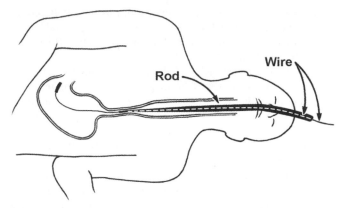

FIG. 6.2 Correct positioning for Savary dilation. Note the extension of the patient's neck, as well as the position of the wire in the antrum.

15. After three dilations, remove the last dilator and the wire together as one unit. Hub the proximal end of the spring tip to the tip of dilator while inside the gastric lumen prior to withdrawal to facilitate easier removal. Postdilation inspection of the treated stricture can be performed at the physician's digression.

TTS BALLOON DILATION
Equipment
1. Upper endoscope
2. Appropriate range of available balloon dilator sizes. Generally, TTS balloons range in sets of three sizes beginning from 6 to 8 mm up to 18 to 20 mm
3. Lubricant
4. Gloves
5. Fluoroscopy, if available, for complex or tight strictures

Procedure
1. Perform diagnostic upper endoscopy. If the esophageal stricture is too tight to allow passage of the adult upper endoscope, a pediatric or neonatal scope may be necessary to traverse the stricture. Note that TTS balloons require a 2.8 mm working channel and are not compatible with the majority of smaller caliber endoscopes. Thus, switching to a wire-guided bougie dilator might be necessary in the setting of a very tight stricture.
2. Position the endoscope distal to the stricture or in the stomach lumen.

3. Under direct endoscopic observation, pass the deflated balloon catheter through the accessory endoscope channel and adjust the endoscope and the balloon to position the balloon across the stricture.

4. Prior to the start of balloon inflation, the endoscopist should attempt to secure the balloon position to avoid migration during balloon distention. Migration can be prevented by maintaining contact with the balloon catheter and the endoscope.

5. With the use of multidiameter balloon dilators, the first dilation stage (e.g., 12 mm for the 12 to 15 mm balloon) is maintained under direct endoscopic visualization for at least a few seconds (Fig. 6.3) before the balloon is inflated stagewise to the next sizes. There is no clear data on the optimal duration of balloon inflation at each stage.

6. If needed, repeat step 5 using the next larger stage balloon.

7. Although the "rule of threes" mainly refers to bougie-type dilators, it is often extrapolated to TTS dilators. However, as endoscopic visualization of the effect of dilation is available to the endoscopist, the maximum balloon size can be determined by the endoscopist during dilation.

8. Upon completion of the dilation, ensure that the balloon is fully deflated prior to removing the balloon catheter from the accessory channel after which the endoscope can be withdrawn.

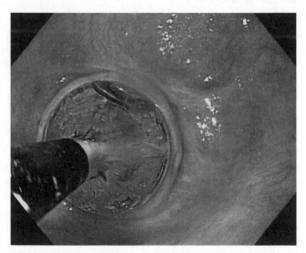

FIG. 6.3 Endoscopic image showing balloon inflation after optimal placement, providing real-time visualization of stricture dilation.

POSTPROCEDURE

1. Monitor vital signs.
2. Elevate the head of the bed to reduce aspiration risk.
3. Give clear liquids for the rest of the day.
4. Continue an acid-suppressive regimen with proton pump inhibitors for acid-peptic strictures to reduce the rate of recurrence.[5]
5. Instruct the patient to return for chest pain, fevers, shortness of breath, hematemesis, or blood per rectum with low threshold for admission and imaging (typically water-soluble contrast esophagram) to evaluate for perforation.

ADVERSE EVENTS

1. The most dreaded adverse event of dilation is esophageal perforation which occurs at a rate ranging from 0.1% to 0.4% of cases.[6]
2. Esophageal hemorrhage, less than 0.1% of cases.
3. Aspiration causing respiratory distress, less than 0.1% of cases.
4. Transient bacteremia, probably occurs commonly possibly exceeding rates of 20%. Resulting sepsis is very rare (less than 0.1%), as is infection of prosthetic heart valves (less than 0.1%).[7,8]

CPT CODES

43226—Esophagoscopy, flexible, transoral; with insertion of guidewire followed by passage of dilator(s) over guidewire
43220—Esophagoscopy, flexible, transoral; with transendoscopic balloon dilation (less than 30 mm diameter)
43213—Esophagoscopy, flexible, transoral; with dilation of esophagus, by balloon or dilator, retrograde (includes fluoroscopic guidance, when performed)

References

1. Standards of PC, Pasha SF, Acosta RD, et al. The role of endoscopy in the evaluation and management of dysphagia. *Gastrointest Endosc.* 2014;79(2): 191-201.
2. Colon VJ, Young MA, Ramirez FC. The short- and long-term efficacy of empirical esophageal dilation in patients with nonobstructive dysphagia: a prospective, randomized study. *Am J Gastroenterol.* 2000;95(4):910-913.
3. Scolapio JS, Gostout CJ, Schroeder KW, et al. Dysphagia without endoscopically evident disease: to dilate or not? *Am J Gastroenterol.* 2001;96(2):327-330.
4. Fleischer DE, Benjamin SB, Cattau EL Jr, et al. A marked guide wire facilitates esophageal dilatation. *Am J Gastroenterol.* 1989;84(4):359-361.
5. Swarbrick ET, Gough AL, Foster CS, et al. Prevention of recurrence of esophageal stricture, a comparison of lansoprazole and high-dose ranitidine. *Eur J Gastroenterol Hepatol.* 1996;8(5):431-438.

6. Hernandez LV, Jacobsen JW, Harris MS. Comparison among the perforation rates of Maloney, balloon, and savary dilation of esophageal strictures. *Gastrointest Endosc.* 2003;58(4):640-642.

7. Chan MF. Complications of upper gastrointestinal endoscopy. *Gastrointest Endosc Clin North Am.* 1996;6(2):287-303.

8. Zubarik R, Eisen G, Mastropietro C, et al. Prospective analysis of complications 30 days after outpatient upper endoscopy. *Am J Gastroenterol.* 1999;94(6):1539-1545.

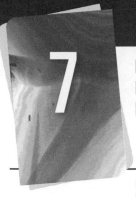

7

Feeding Tubes (Nasogastric, Nasoduodenal, and Nasojejunal)

Dhyanesh A. Patel, MD
Keith L. Obstein, MD, MPH, FASGE, FACG, AGAF

Nasoenteral feeding is an effective means of providing temporary nutrition for the majority of patients who are unable to eat due to medical or psychological comorbidities. Multiple studies in different patient populations have shown that use of enteral nutrition when compared to parenteral nutrition is associated with decreased infectious complications, cost, and hospital length of stay.[1-3] Bedside nasoenteric tube placement is the most common technique used in the hospital setting and can be placed by a nurse, midlevel provider, or physician. Large bore tubes (14 to 18 French) can also be used for suctioning and should primarily be reserved for nasogastric (NG) placement, while small-bore tubes (8 to 12 French) can be used for nasoduodenal or nasojejunal feeding. Postpyloric feeding may be preferred in patients who are critically ill, as it has been shown to reduce the rate of pneumonia by 30% when compared to gastric feeding.[4,5] Furthermore, early enteral nutrition should be considered within 24 to 48 hours in critically ill patients (if there is no contraindication)—as, when compared to withholding or delayed enteral nutrition, it has been shown to reduce mortality (RR = 0.70; 95% CI, 0.49-1.00; P = .05) and infectious morbidity (RR = 0.74; 95% CI, 0.58-0.93; P = .01).[5] In patients with severe acute pancreatitis, NG feeding has been recently shown to be noninferior to nasojejunal feeding, and thus the choice of access should be based on institutional resources (i.e., the ease and feasibility of placing small bowel enteral access devices).[6] Furthermore, feeding tolerance with either gastric or postpyloric nasoenteral access should be continually assessed to reduce the risk of adverse events.

INDICATIONS

1. Patient is unwilling or unable to maintain adequate nutrition with oral feeding alone
2. Consider postpyloric feeding (nasoduodenal or nasojejunal) in patients with:
   a. Critical illness
   b. Abnormal gastric motility
   c. History of pulmonary aspiration
   d. History of significant gastroesophageal reflux

CONTRAINDICATIONS

1. Absolute
   a. Gastrointestinal tract mechanical obstruction (esophageal, gastric, pyloric, small bowel, or colonic). If foregut obstruction, can consider placement past the obstruction if feasible
   b. Severe maxillofacial trauma and/or basilar skull fracture (avoid transnasal tube placement)
2. Relative
   a. Short bowel syndrome
   b. Malabsorption
   c. Severe uncontrolled coagulopathy
   d. Large esophageal varices (avoid large bore tube placement)
   e. Recent esophageal surgery or perforation (carbon dioxide [CO_2] should be used in these cases for insufflation)

PRECAUTIONS/PREPARATION

1. Be careful when placing nasoenteral tubes in patients with altered mental status, depressed sensorium, or endotracheal tubes who are unable to swallow on request; as the risk of inadvertent placement into the trachea is reported to be 1.3% (with potential risk of bronchopulmonary injury).[7] Below are potential methods to reduce this risk:
   a. Clinical clues are helpful, but lack adequate sensitivity:
      i. Observe patient for cough, hoarseness, or cyanosis
      ii. Can consider placing the external end of the tube under water to observe for air bubbles
   b. Consider placement using radiographic guidance or direct visualization:
      i. Fluoroscopic guidance
      ii. Endoscopic guidance
      iii. Two-step radiographic guidance: Pass the tube to 30 cm from the nares and obtain a portable chest radiograph and advance the tube only if it is midline

2. Always read the package insert for the feeding tube to be used and examine the tube for defects prior to placement. Review the schematic on the package of the tube for its dimensions.

3. Assess patient for any history of nasal or sinus surgeries and use the most patent nostril. If able, ask the patient to breathe with closure of each individual nostril and ask the patient for preference of which nostril to use.

4. Patient positioning is important and, if able, upright or left lateral positions are helpful in reducing risk of aspiration compared to the supine position.

5. Give nothing by mouth for at least 4 hours and preferably for 6 hours (unless NG access is urgently indicated in patients with severe nausea/vomiting in whom, access is needed for decompression of the gastrointestinal tract).

6. Always review the indications, procedure, risks, benefits, and alternatives with patient (if able) prior to placement of naso-enteral access. Document informed consent based on institutional practice.

7. Always wear gloves and protective eyewear (universal precautions).

BEDSIDE PLACEMENT

1. Choose the diameter of the tube based on the indication. If the patient needs decompression of the gastrointestinal tract, use a large bore tube (14 to 18 French, Fig. 7.1). If the primary indication is enteral feeding or postpyloric placement, use a small-bore tube (8 to 12 French, Fig. 7.2). For adults, 10 French outer diameter provides a good balance between patient comfort and reducing the likelihood of clogging. If the patient is unable to swallow on request or has an endotracheal tube, choose the feeding tube with a tip that is equal to or greater than 5 mm in width.

2. In patients that need both gastric decompression and jejunal feeding, a combined nasojejunal feeding tube with gastric decompression tube can be used.

3. Choose weighted or unweighted feeding tube based on availability. It should be noted that contrary to expectation, unweighted enteral tubes are more likely to pass spontaneously from the stomach to the duodenum to achieve post-pyloric placement.[8]

4. Tubes coated with hydromer water-activated lubricant in the lumen and on the tip should be submerged in water and flushed with a 20-mL syringe of water to activate the hydromer lubricant.

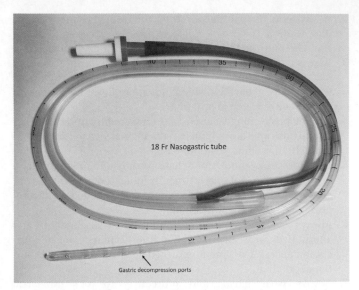

FIG. 7.1 18 Fr Nasogastric tube with gastric decompression ports marked.

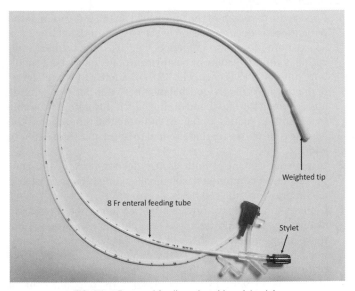

FIG. 7.2 8 Fr enteral feeding tube with weighted tip.

TABLE 7.1	Approximate Distance From Nasal Opening to Varying Locations of the Foregut in an Average Adult Without Any Significant Looping of the Tube
Marks on the Tube (cm)	**Location in the Foregut**
25	Upper esophagus
45	Gastroesophageal junction
65	Pylorus
100	Beyond the ligament of Treitz

Nasogastric Tube Placement

1. Using the NG tube, measure and mark the distance from the entrance to the patient's nose to the level just below the diaphragm. Table 7.1 shows the approximate distance from nasal opening to varying locations of the foregut in an average adult without any significant looping of the tube.

2. Place lubricating jelly or 2% lidocaine jelly (can also act as a local anesthetic) into the chosen nostril and also on the NG tube. If available, cetacaine (benzocaine or tetracaine) spray can also be sprayed in the posterior oropharynx for local anesthesia if no contraindications, but it can be rarely associated with a small risk (0.035%) for acquired methemoglobinemia.[9]

3. With the patient in the appropriate position (preferably sitting upright with head flexed forward), carefully place the NG tube into the nostril, directing it straight back toward the occiput.

4. Once the tip reaches the posterior pharyngeal wall, slight resistance may be felt. Do not advance the tube if significant resistance is felt, which may suggest malposition of the tube, obstruction within the nose, or potential pressure of the tube against the cribriform plate.

5. Have the patient sip water through a straw if possible and then gently advance the tube forward (might feel a subtle pull on the tube suggestive of opening of the upper esophageal sphincter and esophageal peristalsis). Continue to advance the tube slowly as able (should be minimal to no resistance) to the measured distance (previously marked location on the NG tube).

6. If patient is unable to swallow, monitor carefully for spontaneous swallows (subtle pull on the tube) and then advance slowly. This is the most uncomfortable and riskiest part of the procedure as the tube may enter the trachea. Patients who are intubated with a cuffed endotracheal tube are at higher risk of potential tracheal intubation with the tube and as previously noted, should be monitored carefully for coughing or

cyanosis; however, these clinical signs are not reliable and the most important marker may actually be resistance to advancing the tube. If significant resistance is felt, tube should be retracted and other modalities (fluoroscopic or endoscopic guidance) should be used to avoid potential adverse event (bronchopulmonary injury).

7. Once confident that the tip of the tube is in the stomach (advanced to the previously measured distance), the following maneuvers to assess placement may be utilized:

   a. Auscultation over the upper abdomen as air is insufflated into the tube.

   b. Aspiration of fluid that is unequivocally gastric (pH < 4).

   c. Every patient should have an *abdominal radiograph to confirm placement in the stomach prior to initiation of tube feeding*, as the above bedside maneuvers are not reliable.[10] If a single-view X-ray is indeterminate, can perform PA and lateral film.

Nasoduodenal or Nasojejunal Placement

1. In addition to above steps, once tip of the tube is in the stomach, consider turning the patient to the right lateral position (if able) and then infuse 500 mL of air down the tube. Next, slowly advance the tube to the 75-cm mark and secure the tube. Obtain an abdominal radiograph to confirm postpyloric placement.

2. If jejunal access is desired, tape the tube to the face with approximately 20 to 30 cm of slack to allow the tube to advance on its own by peristalsis to the 95 to 105 cm mark. Obtain an abdominal radiograph at 12-hour intervals to check for progression of the tube into the jejunum and advance the tube based on the results of the imaging.

3. Use of pharmacologic agents can be considered (metoclopramide 10 mg IV bolus or erythromycin 250 mg IV over 15 minutes) to assist in postpyloric placement of the tube if there are no medical contraindications; however, evidence behind the efficacy of these agents for this indication has been mixed with a recent systematic review concluding no benefit when compared to placebo.[11]

4. If available at the hospital, an electromagnetic placement device (EPMD) such as CORTRAK (Avanos Medical, Inc., Alpharetta, GA, USA) can be used to potentially increase the yield of nasoduodenal or nasojejunal placement without need for radiography or endoscopy. This technology has been approved by the US Food and Drug Administration and uses an electromagnetic signal from the distal tip of the tube to create an image on a receiver that allows live detection of tube

passage through the esophagus, stomach, and into the small intestine.[12] Unfortunately, a recent review of adverse events related to this technology found 54 adverse events between January 1, 2006, and February 29, 2016, with most events (98%) involving tube placement into the lungs with some resulting in death.[13] These events may have been from inadequate training and interpretation of the EMPD bedside tracings.[13] Therefore, use of this technology should be reserved for providers with specialized training and experience to ensure competency and reduce the risk of an adverse event/life-threatening complication.

5. Once tube placement is confirmed radiographically, remove the stiff stylet. If unable to blindly place nasoduodenal or nasojejunal access at bedside, consider fluoroscopic or endoscopic methods as noted below.

Fluoroscopic/Radiographic Placement

1. Consult radiology for assistance in fluoroscopic-guided placement. In critically ill patients, placement can be done at bedside using portable C-arm fluoroscopy and a compatible bed. Depending on institutional resources and availability, fluoroscopic placement may be preferred over endoscopic placement in order to avoid the risk of sedation (as the success rate of fluoroscopic nasoduodenal and nasojejunal tube placement is 90% to 100%).[14-16]

Endoscopic Placement (Without Guidewire)

1. Prepare the patient as usual for upper endoscopy including informed consent.

2. If available, tie suture material (e.g., 3.0 prolene suture) around the tube near the tip and 5, 10, and 15 cm distal to the tip, leaving the ends of the suture material 2 cm long.

3. Insert the upper endoscope into the posterior pharynx and hold position with adequate visualization of the larynx, vocal cords, and esophageal inlet as noted in Fig. 7.1. Pass the feeding tube through the naris in the pharynx and observe the tip of the tube enter the esophagus on endoscopy, then advance the endoscope into the stomach along with the feeding tube.

4. Use endoscopic forceps through the working channel to grasp the suture material at the tip of the tube and guide it through the pylorus into the duodenum. Sequentially grasp the more distal sutures and push the feeding tube as far/deep into the small intestine as possible until resistance is met. Some providers also use a hemostatic clip to affix the tube in position in the small bowel by clipping the distal suture to the bowel wall.

5. Ensure no loop is formed in the stomach. If present, reduce the looping of the tube in the stomach prior to removal of the endoscope. Slowly withdraw the endoscope with a rotating and "jiggling" motion while monitoring the feeding tube to ensure that it is not being dragged out with the endoscope.

6. Confirm appropriate tube placement with an abdominal radiograph (*before* initiation of tube feeding and/or administration of medications) and then remove the stylet.

Endoscopic Placement (With Guidewire, Video 7.1)

1. Obtain a nasoenteric tube designed for insertion over a guidewire and read the package instructions for manufacturer specific considerations.

2. Use an ultraslim endoscope with a diameter of <5 to 6 mm to perform upper endoscopy through the nose. Advance the tip of the small-diameter endoscope as far as possible into the small bowel. This can be achieved with aspirating air from the stomach (to ensure that it is completely decompressed) before intubating the duodenum and using external abdominal pressure to reduce the loop in the stomach.

3. Use the wire packaged with the over-the-wire tube or use a long (450 cm) guidewire. We prefer the guidewire due to its longer length and flexibility that allow for deeper cannulation of the small bowel. Pass the wire through the working channel of the endoscope and advance it slowly into the small bowel. If significant resistance is met, retract the wire, and then slowly advance again. Fluoroscopic guidance during this part of the procedure can be helpful to verify deep cannulation of the jejunum and avoidance of looping; however, it is not essential.

4. Remove the endoscope slowly while advancing the guidewire through the working channel to avoid moving the tip of the wire (i.e., remove the endoscope while leaving the guidewire in position in the small intestine). Once the endoscope is in the stomach, ensure that there is no large loop in the stomach (straight path from the GE junction to the pylorus). This is essential, as a large loop in the stomach will cause the tube to retract back and coil in the stomach.

5. Use the desired tube (single-lumen nasoenteric tube) or a double-lumen gastric decompression and jejunal feeding tube (Fig. 7.3), and flush the tube with 20 mL of water to active the lubricant.

6. With the help of members of the endoscopy team (i.e., technician, nurse, etc.), hold the wire at the patient's nose and hold the distal end of the wire firmly at a point on a fixed object in a straight line from the patient's nose (to avoid withdrawal). After

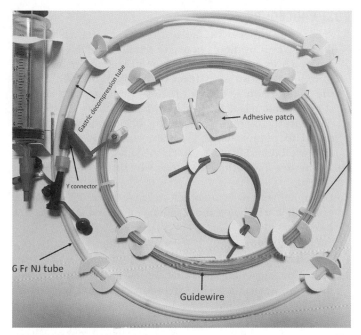

FIG. 7.3 Nasojejunal feeding tube (16 Fr) with a gastric decompression tube (9 Fr).

applying lubrication to the outside of the selected tube, pass the nasoenteric tube over the wire. Once the tube is near the naris, advance the tube slowly into the patient (while ensuring that the distal end of the tube is fixed in a straight line) to at least 100 to 110 cm and preferably 120 cm or more (to ensure that it is beyond the ligament of Trietz). If available, fluoroscopic guidance can be used as the tube is advanced into the patient to ensure that it is not looped or in a detrimental position. As an additional pearl, once approximately 40 cm of the tube is in the patient, the ultraslim endoscope can be passed alongside the tube to allow for direct visualization of the tube as it is advanced further over the wire and through the pylorus to assess/adjust for any looping. The endoscope is then withdrawn while the wire and tube remain in place to prevent tube dislodgement. If available, fluoroscopic guidance can again be used to ensure that the tube is not looped or in a detrimental position.

7. Once the tube is at the desired insertion distance, carefully remove the guidewire (although not necessary, this too can be performed under fluoroscopic guidance to ensure that the tube does not move from the intended position).

8. Confirm placement of the tube with an abdominal radiograph prior to use.

POST PROCEDURE

1. Secure the tube to the nose using tape or a nasal bridle device. Nasal bridle devices are readily available and consist of a 5-French tube that is looped around the nasal septum, and the two ends from each nostril are tied around the feeding tube to secure the tube. A recent meta-analysis showed that nasal bridles are more effective at securing nasoenteric tubes and preventing dislodgement than traditional use of tape alone.[17] Magnetic nasal bridal systems are also available (Fig. 7.4). Check the schematic on the package for the size of the bridal to ensure that it will fit the tube placed.

2. Use a pen with permanent ink to mark the tube at the nasal exit, which can be used as guidance if the tube loosens and begins to slide out.

ADVERSE EVENTS

1. In general, most nonprocedural adverse events of nasoenteral tubes are associated with long-term use. Thus, most nasoenteric tubes are only recommended for temporary enteral feeding for 4 to 6 weeks or less.[18]

2. Inadvertent placement into the tracheobronchial tree: This is the most dreaded adverse event of small-bore feeding tubes with blind insertion and carries an overall rate of

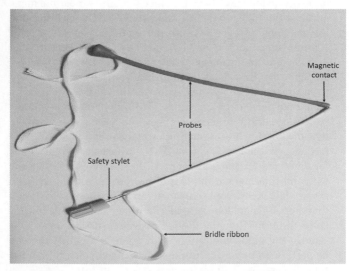

FIG. 7.4 Magnetic tube retaining system 12 Fr (bridle); AMT Bridle System, AMT Inc., Ohio, USA.

1.9% with a cumulative mortality approaching 20% due to tracheobronchial injury.[19] The risk is greatest in patients who are unable to swallow on request during the procedure (altered mental status, depressed sensorium, endotracheal tube in place).

3. Epistaxis (1.8%) or sinusitis (7.7% with extended placement).[20,21] Risk factors include preexisting nasal pathology, history of sinus surgeries, and severe coagulopathy.

4. Aspiration pneumonia (25% to 40% with long-term use in critically ill patients).[22] It is difficult to estimate a true cause and effect relationship as most patients that are critically ill are also at high risk for ventilator-associated pneumonia. Postpyloric feeding tube placement should be considered in critically ill patients to reduce the risk (as noted previously).

5. Perforation of the gastrointestinal tract is a rare complication (primarily reported in case reports) and usually occurs at the level of cricopharyngeus (due to esophageal narrowing and lack of longitudinal esophageal muscle fibers at this level).[23]

6. Penetration of the brain by the tip of a small-bore feeding tube is also reported in multiple case studies and primarily in patients with history of craniofacial trauma.[24]

7. Inadvertent withdrawal of the tube back into the stomach or completely out of the patient. This risk can be reduced by using a nasal bridle device to secure the tube as noted above.

8. The tube can become clogged. Use of a large diameter tube, flushing the tube with 50 mL of water after each use, and using liquid medications (when feasible) instead of crushed medications can reduce this risk. If the tube becomes clogged, gently place 60 mL of lukewarm water into the tube (do not force the water into the tube), clamp the tube for 20 minutes, and then reassess to determine success. Water is superior when compared to carbonated beverages; *do not use meat tenderizer*.[25,26] If water does not work, alkalinized pancreatic enzyme suspension mixed with bicarbonate can be used.[27] Lastly, if available, an endoscopic cytology brush can be used to mechanically declog the tube (ultrasmall-diameter brushes are available); however, care should be taken to avoid insertion against significant resistance due to risk of perforating the tube.

9. Tube feeding–associated diarrhea can occur. This is more likely with use of bolus feedings into the small bowel due to dumping syndrome. Antidiarrheal medications and changes in tube feeding formula(s) can be used in this scenario to see if they improve patient tolerance/symptoms.

CPT CODES

43753—NG/OG tube placement by physician

43752—NG/OG tube placement by physician and fluoroscopic guidance

44500—Nasoenteric tube placement

74340—Nasoenteric tube placement with radiological supervision and interpretation

43241—Upper GI endoscopy; diagnostic with transendoscopic intraluminal tube or catheter placement

References

1. Elke G, van Zanten AR, Lemieux M, et al. Enteral versus parenteral nutrition in critically ill patients: an updated systematic review and meta-analysis of randomized controlled trials. *Crit Care.* 2016;20(1):117.
2. Quan H, Wang X, Guo C. A meta-analysis of enteral nutrition and total parenteral nutrition in patients with acute pancreatitis. *Gastroenterol Res Pract.* 2011;2011:698248.
3. Seres DS, Valcarcel M, Guillaume A. Advantages of enteral nutrition over parenteral nutrition. *Therap Adv Gastroenterol.* 2013;6(2):157-167.
4. Alkhawaja S, Martin C, Butler RJ, et al. Post-pyloric versus gastric tube feeding for preventing pneumonia and improving nutritional outcomes in critically ill adults. *Cochrane Database Sys Rev.* 2015;(8):CD008875.
5. McClave SA, Taylor BE, Martindale RG, et al. Guidelines for the provision and assessment of nutrition support therapy in the adult critically ill patient: Society of Critical Care Medicine (SCCM) and American Society for Parenteral and Enteral Nutrition (A.S.P.E.N.). *JPEN J Parenter Enteral Nutr.* 2016;40(2):159-211.
6. Chang YS, Fu HQ, Xiao YM, et al. Nasogastric or nasojejunal feeding in predicted severe acute pancreatitis: a meta-analysis. *Crit Care.* 2013;17(3):R118.
7. McWey RE, Curry NS, Schabel SI, et al. Complications of nasoenteric feeding tubes. *Am J Surg.* 1988;155(2):253-257.
8. Lord LM, Weiser-Maimone A, Pulhamus M, et al. Comparison of weighted vs unweighted enteral feeding tubes for efficacy of transpyloric intubation. *JPEN J Parenter Enteral Nutr.* 1993;17(3):271-273.
9. Chowdhary S, Bukoye B, Bhansali AM, et al. Risk of topical anesthetic-induced methemoglobinemia: a 10-year retrospective case-control study. *JAMA Intern Med.* 2013;173(9):771-776.
10. Bennetzen LV, Hakonsen SJ, Svenningsen H, et al. Diagnostic accuracy of methods used to verify nasogastric tube position in mechanically ventilated adult patients: a systematic review. *JBI Database Syst Rev Implement Rep.* 2015;13(1):188-223.
11. Silva CC, Bennett C, Saconato H, et al. Metoclopramide for post-pyloric placement of naso-enteral feeding tubes. *Cochrane Database Syst Rev.* 2015;1:CD003353.
12. Powers J, Luebbehusen M, Spitzer T, et al. Verification of an electromagnetic placement device compared with abdominal radiograph to predict accuracy of feeding tube placement. *JPEN J Parenter Enteral Nutr.* 2011;35(4):535-539.
13. Bourgault AM, Aguirre L, Ibrahim J. Cortrak-assisted feeding tube insertion: a Comprehensive review of adverse events in the MAUDE Database. *Am J Crit Care.* 2017;26(2):149-156.
14. Baskin WN, Johanson JF. An improved approach to delivery of enteral nutrition in the intensive care unit. *Gastrointest Endosc.* 1995;42(2):161-165.

15. Ott DJ, Mattox HE, Gelfand DW, et al. Enteral feeding tubes: placement by using fluoroscopy and endoscopy. *AJR Am Journal Roentgenology.* 1991;157(4):769-771.

16. Park JH, Song HY, Min SH, et al. A novel method of punctured Miller-Abbott tube placement using a guidewire under fluoroscopic guidance. *AJR Am J Roentgenol.* 2012;198(3):W274-W278.

17. Bechtold ML, Nguyen DL, Palmer LB, et al. Nasal bridles for securing naso-enteric tubes: a meta-analysis. *Nutr Clin Pract.* 2014;29(5):667-671.

18. DeLegge MH. Enteral access–the foundation of feeding. *JPEN J Parenter Enteral Nutr.* 2001;25(2 suppl):S8-S13.

19. Sparks DA, Chase DM, Coughlin LM, et al. Pulmonary complications of 9931 narrow-bore nasoenteric tubes during blind placement: a critical review. *JPEN J Parenter Enteral Nutr.* 2011;35(5):625-629.

20. Patrick PG, Marulendra S, Kirby DF, et al. Endoscopic nasogastric-jejunal feeding tube placement in critically ill patients. *Gastrointest Endosc.* 1997;45(1):72-76.

21. George DL, Falk PS, Umberto Meduri G, et al. Nosocomial sinusitis in patients in the medical intensive care unit: a prospective epidemiological study. *Clin Infect Dis.* 1998;27(3):463-470.

22. McClave SA, DeMeo MT, DeLegge MH, et al. North American summit on aspiration in the critically ill patient: consensus statement. *JPEN J Parenter Enteral Nutr.* 2002;26(6 suppl):S80-S85.

23. Prabhakaran S, Doraiswamy VA, Nagaraja V, et al. Nasoenteric tube compli-cations. *Scand J Surg.* 2012;101(3):147-155.

24. Psarras K, Lalountas MA, Symeonidis NG, et al. Inadvertent insertion of a nasogastric tube into the brain: case report and review of the literature. *Clin Imaging.* 2012;36(5):587-590.

25. Metheny N, Eisenberg P, McSweeney M. Effect of feeding tube properties and three irrigants on clogging rates. *Nurs Res.* 1988;37(3):165-169.

26. Bankhead R, Boullata J, Brantley S, et al. Enteral nutrition practice recom-mendations. *JPEN J Parenter Enteral Nutr.* 2009;33(2):122-167.

27. Marcuard SP, Stegall KL, Trogdon S. Clearing obstructed feeding tubes. *JPEN J Parenter Enteral Nutr.* 1989;13(1):81-83.

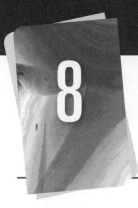

8

Percutaneous Endoscopic Gastrostomy (PEG), Percutaneous Endoscopic Gastrostomy and Jejunostomy (PEGJ), and Direct Percutaneous Endoscopic Jejunostomy (DPEJ)

Endashaw Omer, MD
Stephen McClave, MD

The primary indication for enteral feeding is the provision of nutritional support to meet metabolic requirements for patients with inadequate oral intake. Gastric feeding is the most common type of enteral feeding. The goal of enteral nutrition is to prevent loss of weight, correct nutritional deficiencies, rehydrate, promote the growth of children with the potential for growth retardation, and improve the quality of life.[1,2]

Percutaneous endoscopic gastrostomy (PEG) was first introduced in 1980 by the application of endoscopy to insert a feeding tube into the stomach.[3] However, gastric feeding via PEG is not suitable for all patients, especially those whose gastric function is impaired (i.e., gastroparesis) or those who are at risk of aspiration. In these cases, delivery of nutrients directly to the small intestine is a preferred approach.[4-6]

Endoscopic placement of jejunal feeding tubes can be achieved either indirectly, by passing a feeding tube through a PEG tube or existing PEG tract (PEGJ), or directly, by puncturing the small bowel by direct percutaneous endoscopic jejunostomy (DPEJ). The latter overcomes the tendency for frequent tube clogging or obstruction of the narrow lumen of the jejunal extension tube of the PEGJ, providing a more secure and sustained feeding approach. In cases of severe gastroparesis or partial gastric outlet obstruction, the use of DPEJ with a concurrent PEG for venting purposes or converting a PEG tube to PEGJ is recommended. The latter has a gastric port which is used for venting and/or medications and a jejunal port for feeding.[7,8]

INDICATIONS

1. Prediction or evidence of inadequate oral intake quantitatively or qualitatively to maintain nutrition for more than 4 weeks.
2. Inability to stabilize or improve nutritional status with the use of oral supplements and/or tips provided by a speech pathologist to improve swallowing.

3. Expectation that the PEG feeding will maintain or improve the quality of life.
4. Palliative drainage of secretions in gastrointestinal obstruction or chronic gastroparesis.

CONTRAINDICATIONS

1. Coagulopathy (INR > 1.7, PTT > 50)
2. Platelets < 50,000
3. Interposed organ (liver, colon).
4. Severe peritoneal carcinomatosis
5. Severe noncirrhotic ascites
6. Cirrhotic ascites
7. Peritonitis
8. Anorexia nervosa
9. Severe psychosis
10. Gastric tumor infiltration at the potential site for PEG
11. Peritoneal dialysis

ETHICAL ISSUES

Ethical issues surrounding end-of-life PEG placement can be complicated. Patient *autonomy* is the most important factor that drives the decision-making process. The patient's own goals of care define the need for PEG, assuming the likelihood that the feeding tube placement will meet those goals. Any sense of *futility* on the part of the physician based on perceived short postprocedure patient longevity should not be factored in, as this sets up a clash of values (patient versus physician appreciation of benefit). The principle of *justice* should be protected, as a patient should never find out that the decision to withhold PEG placement was based on a poor evaluation by some scoring system or committee.[9,10]

PREPARATION FOR ALL PERCUTANEOUS ENTERAL ACCESS TECHNIQUES

1. The patient should be NPO for at least 4 hours.
2. Antibiotic prophylaxis: Antibiotics administered within several hours of the procedure reduce the risk of postprocedural infection at the PEG/DPEJ site. A first-generation cephalosporin is appropriate coverage in a non-PCN allergic patient. Patients who may already be receiving broad-spectrum antibiotics do not need additional prophylactic antibiotics.[11]
3. Adequate platelets and clotting parameters are necessary for safe PEG/DPEJ placement. Patients who have had normal labs within a recent period of time, have not had clinical changes,

and have no history of bleeding do not necessarily need lab work done specifically for PEG placement. The international normalized ratio (INR) should be < 1.5 and the platelet count should be > 50,000.

4. Correct coagulopathy.
5. Two physicians (scope and skin persons) are needed for most of the procedures.
6. Place patient in supine position on endoscopy table.

PEG (PERCUTANEOUS ENDOSCOPIC GASTROSTOMY): PONSKY PULL AND SACKS-VINE PUSH TECHNIQUE

Equipment

Upper endoscope, commercially available PEG kit (available in sizes 16 FR to 24 FR, all are designed to be removed by traction method), abdominal binder for patients who are anticipated to inadvertently pull out their PEG tubes.

Procedural Steps

1. Delineate landmarks on the anterior abdominal wall. Using an indelible marker, mark the coastal margin and midline. Percuss both RUQ and LUQ to evaluate for low lying left lobe of the liver and enlarged spleen.
2. Pass the scope in the standard fashion through the mouth into the stomach. Dim room lights to allow transillumination of the endoscope light. Insufflate the stomach while the skin person applies pressure on area of transillumination with a fingertip looking for area of specific focal indentation of anterior gastric wall. Preferred location is on the patient's right side of midline, close to the umbilicus. This ensures the shortest most perpendicular distance from skin to stomach and positions the stoma in the antrum or distal body. Such placement facilitates conversion of PEG to PEGJ if the need arises. Mark the identified site.
3. The selected site should be away from the xiphoid process or ribs by at least 2 cm to avoid damage to nerves and vasculature beneath the ribs and to prevent pain if the tube abuts bony tissue. Avoid incisional scars from previous abdominal surgery if possible, as adhered loops of bowel may be present at these sites which might get inadvertently punctured during PEG placement.
4. Disinfect the site of PEG placement with chlorhexidine or povidone-iodine (betadine).
5. Place sterile drape over the site.
6. Anesthetize the site with lidocaine—create a wheal by intradermal injection.

7. Foutch safe-tract technique.[12] This additional step is done to confirm that there is no intervening loop of bowel. After puncturing the skin with a needle and syringe containing 2 to 3 mL of saline or lidocaine, aspirate while simultaneously advancing the needle into the stomach. As soon as the tip of the needle passes into the gastric lumen (seen on endoscopy), bubbles should appear in the syringe. This helps ensure the absence of an intervening loop of bowel. If bubbles are seen before the needle tip appears in the stomach, the needle has likely traversed through an intervening loop of bowel, and a separate site should be selected.

8. Make a superficial horizontal incision (about 1 cm long) using the scalpel enclosed in the PEG kit.

9. A catheter (plastic sheath) with indwelling trocar is inserted in a thrusting motion through the incision to create the fistula tract through the abdominal wall and anterior gastric wall. The scope person passes a snare through the scope into the stomach.

10. The scope person snares the trocar and sheath within the gastric lumen. The skin person removes the metal part of the trocar leaving the outer plastic sheath (sealing the trocar with his/her finger to maintain insufflation of the stomach).

11. Pass a single-stranded guidewire (Sacks-Vine technique) or double-stranded vinyl string loop (Ponsky technique) through the trocar. The scope person opens the snare, sliding off the catheter onto the guidewire or string (Fig. 8.1A).

12. The skin person feeds the wire/string, while the scope person withdraws the scope and wire/string together (Fig. 8.1B). At this point, the guidewire/string enters the skin, passes through the anterior gastric wall, and exits the mouth.

13. Two techniques

    A. **Push technique (Sacks-Vine)** uses a PEG tube with a long plastic leader. It is passed over the guidewire which is held taut by the skin person. As the tip of the leader tube emerges out through the incision site, it is grabbed and pulled by applying counter pressure to the abdomen.

    B. **Pull technique (Ponsky)** uses a double-stranded loop of a vinyl string. The PEG tube has a separate string loop at its end. Attach the string exiting the mouth to the loop of the PEG tube in a luggage tag fashion. The skin person pulls the PEG tube through the mouth, down the esophagus, and out through the gastric wall via the skin incision site (Fig. 8.1C).

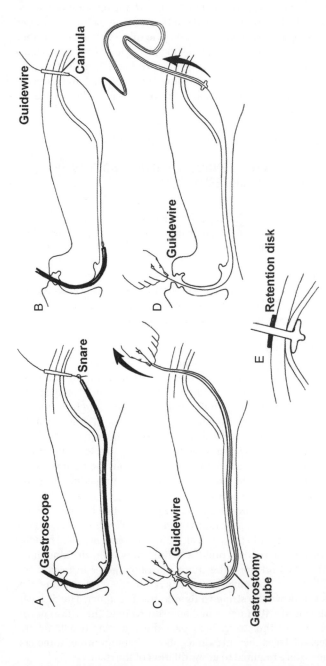

FIG. 8.1 A–E Correct placement of a PEG tube using the pull technique.

14. The scope person may follow the PEG tube with the endoscope by snaring the internal bolster OR re-introducing the scope after the PEG tube is pulled out through the gastric wall. Under direct endoscopic visualization, the tube is pulled out further until the internal bolster is snugged against (but not indenting) the mucosa on the anterior gastric wall[13] (Fig. 8.1D).
15. The stem length on the feeding tube is noted and external bolster placed down against the skin over one layer of gauze (Fig. 8.1E).
16. Place the nursing clip on the tube.
17. Cut at desired length and put on the cap.

PEG (PERCUTANEOUS ENDOSCOPIC GASTROSTOMY): RUSSEL INTRODUCER TECHNIQUE

Indications

Large exophytic oropharyngeal or esophageal cancer, recent oropharyngeal mucosal incisions from head and neck surgery, tight esophageal stricture.[14]

Equipment

Upper endoscope (regular or neonatal scope), 22 gauge spinal needle, PEG Kit, multiple T-fasteners, a one-piece device with multiple dilating segments of increasing size.

Procedural Steps

1. Prepare the abdomen in similar fashion as PEG.
2. Upon transillumination, identify an area on the anterior abdominal wall (by passing the 22 gauge spinal needle proximal to the antrum), to determine a large enough circumferential area within the stomach to allow for placement of the T-fasteners around the intended site of the trocar.
3. Make an incision after anesthetizing the site. Pass the trocar.
4. Introduce a guidewire through the trocar, secure it with the snare, and hold in place throughout the procedure to maintain intraluminal access.
5. T-fastener placement: Use the 22 gauge spinal needle to determine site and angle prior to placement of each T-fastener. Pass the T-fastener in the same angle as the spinal needle. Then flip down the blue flap, pull the string away from the blue outer cannula, and press the inner plastic catheter to release the T-fastener. The inner cannula is removed and the sliding disk is slid down the string to tighten the T-fastener. The disk can be closed with fingers or hemostat to hold the T-fastener in place. Cut the string. Next pass the sounding needle for the second T-fastener and do as above. A minimum of three fasteners are required to allow dilation of the tract.

6. Remove the trocar leaving the wire in the stomach.
7. Pass the one-piece dilating apparatus over the guidewire into the stomach. Pass the first gray catheter, then the second over the first. A back and forth motion is required as the dilator passes through the abdominal and gastric wall in order to dilate the tract. Each are visualized endoscopically as the dilators reach the gastric lumen.
8. Pass all five dilating segments of increasing size in the same manner. After pushing the last dilating segment into position (which is actually the outer peel-away sheath), the end can be twisted to remove the inner dilators leaving the last peel-away sheath in place.
9. Pass an 18 or 20 FR gastrostomy tube.
10. Inflate the balloon and peel-away the outer sheath.
11. Secure the external bolster under a single layer of gauze.

Postprocedure Care

1. Feeding can be safely administered 4 hours after an uncomplicated procedure.
2. Keep the external bolster firmly against the skin for 3 to 4 days, then loosen it by ½ to 1 cm to allow room for movement and prevent buried bumper syndrome.
3. In the first few days following placement, the PEG site should be examined at least once per day for erythema, drainage, induration, and other skin problems. Expect to see a small amount of clear drainage in the first few weeks following insertion.
4. Ensure that the site remains dry by changing layer of gauze once or twice a day as needed.
5. After the fourth postprocedure day, the site may be cleansed using a mild, pH-balanced soap, commercial cleanser, or 0.9% sodium chloride. Use a cotton-tipped applicator to clean close to the tube to remove crusts or drainage.
6. After maturation of the stomal tract (usually by 7 to 10 days), the gauze can be eliminated.

Complications[15]

1. Those associated with upper endoscopy (see Chapter 5)
2. Oversedation
3. Aspiration
4. Bleeding
5. PEG site infection
6. Inadvertent piercing of the colon or adjacent loop of small bowel causing subsequent fistula formation
7. Inadvertent removal of the PEG tube
8. Buried bumper syndrome

9. Migration of the internal bolster (usually a balloon system) causing gastric outlet obstruction
10. Gastric ulcer

JEJUNAL FEEDING

Indications

1. Gastric outlet obstruction or gastroparesis.
2. High risk of aspiration of gastric contents.
3. Previous gastric resection or gastric bypass, where PEG placement may not be feasible.
4. Intrathoracic stomach in those patients requiring enteral access.

Contraindications

The contraindications for jejunal feeding are the same as those outlined for PEG placement.

TWO-PIECE PEGJ: KIRBY TECHNIQUE[15]

The Two-Piece PEGJ can be performed by either the Kirby or Johlin techniques. In both, the jejunal extension can be placed through a newly placed PEG or an existing PEG (with mature tract).

Equipment

Pediatric colonoscope, PEG kit (if not already placed), long 320 cm biopsy forceps, long 480 cm 0.035 inch guidewire, scissors, and an air valve (fashioned from the cap of a separate feeding tube).

Procedural Steps

1. If an initial PEG tube has not been placed, it should be placed as described above.
2. Cut the PEG tube to about 10 to 12 cm and place the air valve in the open end of the PEG tube (to keep the stomach well distended during endoscopy).
3. The scope person passes the scope into the stomach and the long forceps are passed through the working channel of the scope.
4. The skin person passes guidewire through the air valve and PEG into the stomach.
5. The scope person grabs the soft part of the guidewire with the forceps and drags the wire deep into the small bowel (proximal jejunum). The wire may be pulled slightly into the channel for better visualization.
6. The biopsy forceps are passed further out into the jejunum, holding the end of the guidewire in place.

7. The scope is withdrawn back to the stomach using the keyhole technique (i.e., the scope is pulled out about 5 cm and then pushed 1 to 2 cm back in, which helps keep the bowel from telescoping off the end of the endoscope and causing rapid displacement of the guidewire tip proximally).

8. When the scope is brought back to the proximal stomach, the scope person confirms that the guidewire goes straight from the PEG stomal tract to the pylorus. Any loop present should be reduced.

9. At this point, the guidewire is seen coming into the stomach through the PEG internal bolster and going straight to the pylorus and small bowel, parallel to the long biopsy forceps.

10. Remove the air valve.

11. Advance the jejunal extension tube with the stylet in over the guidewire slowly into the small bowel without forming a loop in the stomach.

12. Free the forceps gently and pull it out.

13. The proximal end of the jejunal extension tube (which has ports for jejunal feeding and gastric decompression) should be completely inserted into the end of the PEG tube.

14. Withdraw the scope.

15. Flush the tube. Similar to a new PEG placement, the jejunal port may be used for feeding in 4 hours (or immediately if placed through an existing PEG).

TWO-PIECE PEGJ: JOHLIN TECHNIQUE[16]

This particular technique for a two-piece PEGJ ensures the deepest placement of the guidewire, reducing the risk of the jejunal extension tube from falling back into the stomach.

Equipment
Pediatric colonoscope, snare, 480 cm 0.035 inch guidewire, scissors, hemostat, improvised air valve, PEG kit with jejunal extension tube.

Procedural Steps
1. If an initial PEG tube has not been placed, it should be placed as described above.

2. Cut the PEG tube to 10 to 12 cm.

3. Place the improvised air valve on the end of the PEG and pass the snare through the valve into the stomach.

4. Introduce the scope through the mouth and pass down into the stomach.

5. Pass the scope carefully through the open snare, before passing further down through the pylorus into the small bowel. Close and open the snare. A spongy sensation with closure

of the snare confirms that the scope has actually passed through the snare. Open the snare completely and continue to advance the scope into proximal jejunum.

6. Pass the guidewire through the working channel of the scope and out further if possible into the small bowel. The scope is then withdrawn back to the proximal stomach using the key-hole technique as described previously in the Kirby technique.

7. Once in the stomach, the scope is positioned above the PEG so that the guidewire exiting the operating channel of the scope can be seen passing through the snare and down through the pylorus into the small bowel.

8. Pull the open snare out through the PEG until a loop of the guidewire is visualized outside the PEG.

9. The scope person pulls on the wire as it exits the working channel of the scope, to help determine which side of the guidewire loop is passing up through the scope and which side is passing down into the small bowel. As the skin person holds the loop apart with two hands, movement on one side of the wire loop indicates that side which is passing up through the scope. This side is then pulled out through the PEG, leaving the other side of the loop in place (corresponding to the end of the guidewire passed through the PEG that is positioned deep into the small bowel).

10. A kink is usually formed in the guidewire during this process, which should be straightened with a hemostat.

11. Remove the air valve.

12. Advance the jejunal extension tube (with stylet or stiffener in place) over the guidewire. The guidewire is held at a fixed point while the skin person slowly passes the jejunal extension tube over the guidewire. Endoscopically, the jejunal tube is visualized to traverse the antrum over the guidewire into the small bowel without making a loop.

13. The end of the jejunal tube (again with ports for jejunal feeding and gastric decompression) is inserted into the end of the PEG tube.

14. Pull out the guidewire and stiffener (stylet) of the jejunal extension tube.

15. Flush the tube. The jejunal port may be used for feeding in 4 hours (or immediately if an existing PEG with mature tract was involved).

ONE-PIECE PEGJ

The one-piece PEGJ is best for patients who have an existing PEG tube with mature tract, but have been unable to tolerate gastric feeding. The larger diameter of this tube helps keep it in position in the small bowel and ensures jejunal access for feeding while providing gastric decompression via the gastric ports if needed to reduce aspiration.[17,18]

Equipment Required
Neonatal (ultrathin) 5.9 mm scope, 480 cm 0.035 inch guidewire, 45-cm-long 18 or 22 FR PEGJ tube kit, and silicone lubricating oil.

Procedural Steps
1. Remove the existing PEG tube, either manually by traction or endoscopically.
2. Pass the neonatal scope through the mature PEG tract directly through the pylorus into the small bowel without forming a loop in the stomach. Advance the scope as far down into the small bowel beyond the ligament of Treitz as possible.
3. Advance the guidewire further out into the jejunum.
4. Withdraw the scope off the guidewire using the key-hole technique, leaving the wire deep within the small intestine.
5. The scope person then passes the scope through the mouth into the stomach, in order to visualize the wire passing straight from the stoma through the pylorus into the small bowel without forming a loop in the stomach. Any loop of the guidewire in the stomach should be reduced at this time prior to passing the tube over the wire.
6. Apply the silicone lubricating oil liberally over the wire. Flush the jejunal port of the tube with water to activate the luminal hydrophilic lubricant.
7. With the wire held at a fixed point, the PEGJ tube is passed over the guidewire. Endoscopically, the tube should be visualized to traverse the antrum, passing through the pylorus into the small bowel without making a loop.
8. Pull out the guidewire.
9. Inflate the balloon.
10. Flush both gastric and jejunal ports.
11. Pull down the external bolster and note the stem length.
12. The tube can be used immediately for feeding.

DPEJ (DIRECT PERCUTANEOUS ENDOSCOPIC JEJUNOSTOMY)
Placement of the DPEJ is the best endoscopic procedure to ensure a more permanent and durable jejunal access.[19,20]

Equipment
Pediatric colonoscope, 14 FR (or max 16 Fr) Ponsky-style PEG feeding tube kit, snare, 22 gauge spinal needle.

Procedural Steps

1. Mark anatomic landmarks (coastal margin, iliac crest on both sides); percuss right and left upper quadrant to ensure that there is no evidence for low lying left lobe of liver.

2. Disinfect large area of the abdomen with povidone-iodine or chlorhexidine. Drape the area below the iliac crest to avoid obscuring anatomic landmarks.

3. The scope person passes the scope into the stomach without insufflating air, places the snare in working channel of the scope, and waits until the skin person is ready with a 22 gauge sounding needle and a lidocaine needle/syringe for skin anesthesia. As the scope is passed through the pylorus and subsequently traverses the ligament of Treitz, the transillumination function is turned on. When transillumination is seen, the skin person palpates the area watching for maximal point of indentation endoscopically. It is important to recognize that the small bowel is not as easy to trans-illuminate and that the area may not be localized in the left upper quadrant.

4. Under direct endoscopic visualization, the 22 gauge sounding needle is passed into the small bowel through the skin at the point of transillumination and indentation. Several attempts may be required before the needle is seen in the lumen of the small bowel. A different angle of the sounding needle should be used at each attempt. Once visualized, the scope person grabs the sounding needle with a snare. This temporarily fixes and secures the relevant jejunal loop to the abdomen wall.

5. Inject lidocaine to anesthetize the skin immediately adjacent to the spinal needle.

6. Perform the Foutch safe-tract maneuver as described above, to ensure there is no intervening loop of bowel.

7. Make a small punctate incision with a scalpel. Pass the trocar with its plastic sheath by a thrusting motion through the incision parallel to and in the same angle as the sounding needle.

8. The scope person opens the snare and transfers from the sounding needle to the trocar. The skin person removes the sounding needle.

9. The inner metal cannula of the trocar is removed, and the blue double-stranded vinyl guidewire is passed into the jejunum.

10. The scope person opens the snare, slides off the trocar, and onto the double-stranded vinyl string.

11. The scope person withdraws the scope with the guidewire out through the mouth. The plastic sheath of the trocar is then removed.

12. The loop at the end of a Ponsky-style (pull) 14 Fr Ponsky is connected to the double-stranded vinyl guidewire loop using a luggage tag connection.

13. The skin person gently pulls the vinyl guidewire dragging the tube down through the esophagus and stomach into the small bowel.

14. The endoscope is reintroduced into the bowel using the snare to grab the internal bolster. By pulling the scope into the small bowel, the tension of external bolster can be set accurately while visualizing the internal bolster up against the intestinal mucosa.

15. Secure the external bolster and note the stem length. Keep the external bolster firmly against the skin for 3 to 4 days, before loosening by ½ to 1 cm to allow room for movement and prevent buried bumper syndrome.

16. Initiate tube feeding in 4 hours.

17. Postprocedure care is the same as described above for the PEG technique.

References

1. Blumenstein I, Shastri SY, Stein J. Gastroenteric tube feeding: techniques, problems and solutions. *World J Gastroenterol.* 2014;20(26):8505-8524.

2. McClave SA, Taylor BE, Martindale RG, et al. Guidelines for the provision and assessment of nutrition support therapy in the adult critically ill patient: society of Critical Care Medicine (SCCM) and American Society for Parenteral and Enteral Nutrition (A.S.P.E.N.). *J Parenter Enteral Nutr.* 2016;40(2):159-211.

3. Gauderer MW, Ponsky JL, Izant RJ. Gastrostomy without laparotomy: a percutaneous endoscopic technique. *J Pediatr Surg.* 1980;15:872-875.

4. Mathus-Vliegen LM, Koning H. Percutaneous endoscopic gastrostomy and gastrojejunostomy: a critical reappraisal of patient selection, tube function and the feasibility of nutritional support during extended follow-up. *Gastrointest Endosc.* 1999;50(6):746-754.

5. Windsor AC, Kanwar S, Li AG, et al. Compared with parenteral nutrition, enteral feeding attenuates the acute phase response and improves disease severity in acute pancreatitis. *Gut.* 1998;42:431-435.

6. Panagiotakis PH, DiSario JA, et al. DPEJ tube placement prevents aspiration pneumonia in high-risk patients. *Nutr Clin Pract.* 2008;23(2):172-175.

7. Zopf Y, Rabe C, Bruckmoser T, et al. Percutaneous endoscopic jejunostomy and jejunal extension tube through percutaneous endoscopic gastrostomy: a retrospective analysis of success, complications and outcomes. *Digestion.* 2009;79:92-97.

8. Fan A, Baron T, Rumalla A, et al. Comparison of direct percutaneous endoscopic jejunostomy and PEG with jejunal extension. *Gastrointest Endosc.* 2002;56:890-894.

9. Angus F, Burakoff R. The percutaneous endoscopic gastrostomy tube. Medical and ethical issues in placement. *Am J Gastroenterol.* 2003;98:272-277.

10. Lynch MC. Is tube feeding futile in advanced dementia? *Linacre Q.* 2016;83;(3):283-307.

11. Sharma VK, Howden CW. Meta-analysis of randomized, controlled trials of antibiotic prophylaxis before percutaneous endoscopic gastrostomy. *Am J Gastroenterol.* 2000;95:3133-3136.

12. Foutch PG, Talbert GA, Waring JP, et al. Percutaneous endoscopic gastrostomy in patients with prior abdominal surgery: virtues of the safe tract. *Am J Gastroenterol.* 1988;83(2):147-150.

13. Sartori S, Trevisani L, Nielsen I, et al. Percutaneous endoscopic gastrostomy placement using the pull-through or push-through techniques: is the second pass of the gastroscope necessary?. *Endoscopy.* 1996;28:686-688.

14. Russell TR, Brotman M, Norris F. Percutaneous gastrostomy. A new simplified and cost-effective technique. *Am J Surg.* 1984;148:132-137.

15. Kirby DF, Delegge MH, Fleming CR. American Gastroenterological Association technical review on tube feeding for enteral nutrition. *Gastroenterology.* 1995;108:1282-1301.

16. Leichus L, Patel R, Johlin F. Percutaneous endoscopic gastrostomy/jejunostomy (PEG/PEJ) tube placement: a novel approach. *Gastrointest Endosc.* 1997;45:79-81.

17. Adler DG, Gostout CJ, Baron TH. Percutaneous transgastric placement of jejunal feeding tubes with an ultrathin endoscope. *Gastrointest Endosc.* 2002;55:106-110.

18. DeLegge MH, Kirby DF Jr. Percutaneous endoscopic gastrojejunostomy: a dual center safety and efficacy trial. *JPEN J Parenter Enteral Nutr.* 1995;19(3):239-243.

19. Todd BH. Direct percutaneous endoscopic jejunostomy. *Am J Gastroenterol.* 2006;101(7):1407-1409.

20. Varadarajulu S, Delegge MH. Use of a 19-gauge injection needle as a guide for direct percutaneous endoscopic jejunostomy tube placement. *Gastrointest Endosc.* 2003;57:942-945.

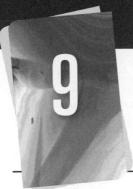

9

Ablation Therapy for Barrett Esophagus

Allon Kahn, MD
Cadman L. Leggett, MD

Ablation therapy for Barrett esophagus (BE) consists of the application of thermal energy (radiofrequency ablation), a cryogen (cryoablation), or a photosensitizer (photodynamic therapy) to induce superficial tissue injury and necrosis. Radiofrequency ablation (RFA) and cryoablation are safe, effective, and durable modalities that are considered the current standard of care in ablation therapy. It is important that patients with BE treated with ablation therapy be enrolled in a comprehensive surveillance program.

INDICATIONS

Ablation therapy is often used in combination with endoscopic resection in patients with BE with high-grade dysplasia or intramucosal adenocarcinoma. Patients with BE and low-grade may be considered for ablation therapy when the diagnosis is confirmed by a pathologist with expertise in BE and in cases of multifocal and/or recurrent low-grade dysplasia.

CONTRAINDICATIONS

Absolute

1. Known esophageal perforation or deep mucosal disruption
2. Inability to place ventilation tubing for active ventilation[a]
3. Esophageal varices in the region of targeted ablation

Relative

1. Significantly large hiatal hernia with intrathoracic stomach[a]
2. Known distal stricture or obstruction that may interfere with ventilation[a]

---

[a]Contraindications primarily relate to the spray cryotherapy modality, given the use of active instillation of cryogen and the need for placement and use of ventilation tubing to prevent gaseous distention.

3. Prior history of gastric bypass surgery[a]
4. Prior radiation therapy to the esophagus
5. Ulceration or mucosal break (including pretreatment biopsy)
6. Eosinophilic esophagitis
7. Prior history of Heller myotomy or peroral endoscopic myotomy

PREPARATION

1. The patient must be instructed to fast overnight prior to the procedure, in order to ensure clearance of gastric contents. This is important both to minimize risk for aspiration and to ensure adequate function of ventilation tubing with cryotherapy.
2. Informed consent must be obtained prior to beginning the procedure. Possible adverse events and complications should be explained to the patient in sufficient detail.
3. Deep sedation or general anesthesia is commonly employed due to the length of the procedure and associated pain.
4. Antiplatelet therapy and/or anticoagulation should be held prior to the procedure if clinically appropriate

RADIOFREQUENCY ABLATION

RFA is a bipolar thermal ablative modality that requires contact between an electrode array and the esophagus. Circumferential RFA is performed in patients with a BE segment >2 cm in length, while focal RFA is performed to treat shorter segments or as follow-up to circumferential ablation. Fig. 9.1 highlights the steps involved in RFA.

EQUIPMENT

1. Upper endoscope with working channel ≥2.8 mm, light source, and image processor
2. Patient monitoring equipment (e.g., blood pressure cuff, pulse oximeter, capnography) as dictated by the degree and manner of sedation/anesthesia
3. Personal protective equipment (e.g., gloves, face mask/shield, gown)
4. Barrx flex energy generator, connector and footswitch
   a. Barrx RFA catheters: Fig. 9.2 summarizes the various catheters used for RFA
   b. Barrx RFA cleaning cap
   c. RFA endoscopic guidewire or Savary guidewire
   d. Wet gauze
   e. 1% N-acetylcysteine solution

---

[a]Contraindications primarily relate to the spray cryotherapy modality, given the use of active instillation of cryogen and the need for placement and use of ventilation tubing to prevent gaseous distention.

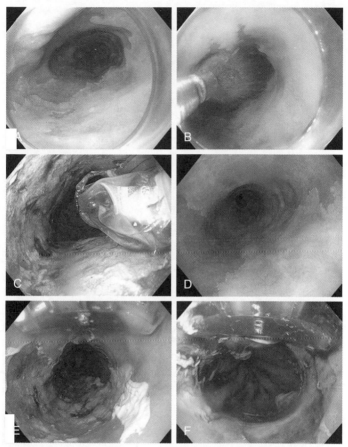

FIG. 9.1 A long-segment of Barrett esophagus (BE) is inspected under (A) high-definition white light endoscopy and narrow band imaging. B, The esophagus is irrigated with 1% N-acetylcysteine solution prior to (C) circumferential radiofrequency ablation (RFA) using the Barrx 360 express balloon catheter. On follow-up surveillance endoscopy, (D) residual islands of BE are identified. E, Focal RFA using the Barrx 90 catheter is performed over the BE islands and (F) circumferentially across the gastroesophageal junction.

PROCEDURE

Prior to performing ablation therapy, the BE segment should be carefully examined under high-definition white-light endoscopy and narrow band imaging with attention to areas of mucosal irregularity that may require endoscopic resection. If endoscopic resection is performed, it is best to postpone ablation therapy in order to avoid a higher rate of complications including perforation, bleeding, and stenosis. Endoscopic landmarks including

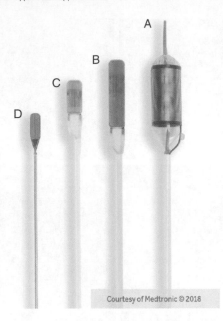

Courtesy of Medtronic © 2018

	Electrode Length (mm)	Electrode Width (mm)	Ablation Protocol	Energy Setting	Figure
Circumferential Ablation					
BARRX 360 express	40	Circumferential	1-clean-1	10 J/cm^2	A
Focal Ablation					
BARRX Ultra Long	40	13	1-clean-1		B
BARRX 90	20	13	2-clean-2	12 J/cm^2	C
BARRX 60	15	10	2-clean-2		-
Touch-up Ablation					
BARRX Endoscopic Catheter	15.7	7.5	2-clean-2	12 J/cm^2	D

FIG. 9.2 Radiofrequency Ablation Catheters. (Used with permission from Medtronic © 2018.)

the gastroesophageal junction and squamocolumnar junction should be located and measured in centimeters from the incisors. The maximal and circumferential extent of the BE segment should be recorded along with the location of any BE islands.

Circumferential RFA With Barrx 360 Express RFA Balloon Catheter

1. Irrigate the esophagus with 1% N-acetylcysteine solution and suction contents.
2. Place guidewire through the endoscope's instrument channel and into the gastric body; remove endoscope leaving guidewire in place.
3. Pass the Barrx 360 express RFA balloon catheter over the guidewire and into the esophagus.
4. Reintroduce the endoscope alongside the RFA catheter for direct visualization with the tip of the endoscope proximal to the balloon.
5. Align the proximal edge of the balloon electrode 1 cm above the top of the BE segment. Confirm generator displays default energy-density setting of 10 J/cm^2.
6. Inflate the balloon using the gray pedal on footswitch. Once the balloon is fully inflated, hold down the suction button and press the blue pedal on footswitch to deliver ablation energy one time.
7. Move the endoscope along with the catheter distally 4 cm and align the proximal end of the electrodes with the distal end of previous ablation zone. Repeat this step until ablation overlaps with the gastroesophageal junction.
8. Deflate the balloon and disconnect the catheter. Rotate catheter clockwise to re-wrap the electrode array on the balloon. Withdraw the endoscope along with the catheter and wire.
9. Place the Barrx RFA cleaning cap on the distal end of the endoscope. Reintroduce the endoscope and remove the coagulated tissue with tip of cap.
10. Clean the ablation catheter by inflating the balloon (outside of the patient) and using a wet gauze. Deflate balloon in preparation for ablation.
11. Repeat ablation process (steps 2-10). Prior to reintroduction of the Barrx 360 express RFA balloon catheter, manually wrap the electrode to reduce overall balloon diameter.

Focal RFA With Barrx 90, 60, and Ultra Long RFA Catheters

1. Irrigate the esophagus with 1% N-acetylcysteine solution and suction contents.
2. Wet and slide the catheter strap (Barrx 90 or 60 catheters) on the distal end of the endoscope until the tip of the endoscope is aligned with the distal end of the strap. For the ultra long RFA catheter, use alcohol to swab the inside of the catheter strap prior to placement.
3. Rotate the catheter so that it appears at the 12- or 6-o'clock position in the endoscopy monitor.

4. Gently advance the endoscope through the oropharynx with the electrode array facing the tongue.

5. Once in the esophagus, connect the ablation catheter to the output cable. Check that the energy generator is set to 12 J/cm^2.

6. Working proximal to distal, rotate and position the ablation catheter so that the targeted BE tissue is at 12 o'clock in the endoscopic view. Once the catheter is positioned over the desired treatment area, deflect the endoscope upward to assure good contact with the mucosal surface.

7. Press the blue pedal on footswitch to deliver energy. Keep the ablation catheter in place until the generator displays "Catheter Ready." Press the blue pedal to deliver a second ablation treatment. (Do not apply a second ablation with the Barrx ultra long RFA focal catheter.)

8. Treatment of the gastroesophageal junction should be performed circumferentially. To do so, position the tip of the catheter proximal to the top of the gastric folds, deflect the catheter upward, perform ablation (step 7), rotate the endoscope to cover an area adjacent to the ablation site, and repeat ablation until circumferential treatment is achieved.

9. When tissue ablation is complete, use the catheter tip to remove all coagulated tissue with a gentle proximal to distal motion.

10. Disconnect the ablation catheter from the output cable. Remove the endoscope and ablation catheter. Clean the electrode surface with a wet gauze.

11. Repeat ablation (steps 4-10) over previously treated areas.

Touchup RFA With Barrx Channel RFA Endoscopic Catheter

1. Place the Barrx RFA cleaning cap on the distal end of the endoscope.

2. Irrigate the esophagus with 1% N-acetylcysteine solution and suction contents.

3. Place the introducer into the instrument channel of the endoscope.

4. Insert the tip of the ablation catheter into the introducer with the electrode surface facing outward.

5. Remove the introducer from the biopsy port by sliding it along the catheter shaft.

6. Rotate the catheter electrode by applying torque to the catheter shaft.

7. Position the catheter in direct contact with the treatment area by deflecting the endoscope. Ensure that the default energy setting is 12 J/cm^2. Depress blue pedal on the footswitch to deliver energy. Deliver two doses of ablative energy to the targeted area before moving to the next target.

8. Remove the catheter from the endoscope and clean the electrode surface with a wet gauze.
9. Use the cleaning cap to remove all coagulum from ablated areas.
10. Reintroduce the catheter into the endoscope and repeat ablation to treated areas (steps 3-10).

CRYOTHERAPY ABLATION

Several cryogen delivery devices are available, including spray catheters and balloon-based systems. The most commonly utilized cryogens are liquid formulations of nitrogen and nitrous oxide. A liquid carbon dioxide–based spray delivery system (Polar Wand) is no longer in production. Unlike RFA, cryoablation is considered a noncontact ablation modality. Fig. 9.3 highlights the steps involved in liquid nitrogen spray cryotherapy.

EQUIPMENT

1. Upper endoscope with working channel ≥2.8 mm, light source, and image processor
2. Patient monitoring equipment (e.g., blood pressure cuff, pulse oximeter, capnography) as dictated by the degree and manner of sedation/anesthesia
3. Personal protective equipment (e.g., gloves, face mask/shield, gown)
4. Cryotherapy delivery device (spray catheter or balloon catheter)
5. Cryotherapy console/delivery system
   a. truFreeze spray cryotherapy—console, cryogen delivery catheter, foot pedal system, endoscope cap
   b. C2 CryoBalloon—foot pedal, controller, nitrous oxide cartridges, balloon catheter
6. Guidewire (i.e., jagwire, spring-tip piano wire)

PROCEDURE

(Please refer to section above regarding endoscopic examination prior to performing ablation therapy.)

Liquid Nitrogen Spray Cryotherapy (CSA truFreeze)

1. Establish a dry endoscope and instrument channel. Any liquid present on the endoscope or within the instrument channel will freeze and may interfere with adequate cryogen delivery or visualization. Thoroughly dry the working end of the endoscope in particular. To clear fluid from the instrument channel, a 60 mL syringe filled with air can be instilled rapidly.

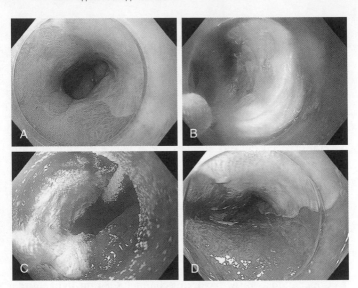

FIG. 9.3 An area of long-segment Barrett esophagus was selected for spray cryotherapy. The area is depicted under (A) high-definition white-light endoscopy. B, The cap is attached, and cryogen delivery catheter is seen emerging from the endoscope working channel on the lower left. The cryogen is delivered until a freezing effect is observed, as depicted. Also note the foggy appearance of the image in tile B due to frosting on the camera lens, which is typical in spray cryotherapy. Cryogen is delivered until the timer expires. C, After a round of freezing, ice crystals are seen forming on the mucosa. D, Once thawing is complete, the image clarity is restored and mucosal hyperemia is seen as a consequence of tissue freezing.

2. Do not use the endoscope suction or lens cleaning function during the cryotherapy procedure. Both of these functions will interfere with adequate cryogen delivery and lessen the effectiveness of cryoablation.
3. Place plastic cap on distal end of the endoscope. The cap has alignment markers at 12 o'clock proximally and 3 o'clock distally to facilitate appropriate positioning.
4. Place guidewire through the instrument channel and into the gastric body. Withdraw the endoscope and note the position of the guidewire, ensuring not to displace it proximally.
5. Thread the ventilation tubing onto the guidewire and position the tubing in the gastric body. Graduated markings are present on the ventilation tubing to facilitate proper positioning. Remove the guidewire once the tubing is adequately positioned.
6. Secure the ventilation tubing to the patient's bed or pillow with tape to avoid kinking or movement during the

procedure. It is extremely important to secure the tubing in a position that will allow for adequate flow during the entire procedure and to regularly check its patency throughout the process.

7. Remove the cryogen delivery catheter from its packaging. Scan the RFID tag on the catheter pouch against the yellow sticker on the scan pad on the right side of the truFreeze console and press the "Scan" button. A "beep" will be heard, indicating that the system has initiated the precooling process.

8. A spring introducer is provided in the equipment kit. Place this introducer into the biopsy cap.

9. Insert the endoscope back to the desired location of treatment and insert the cryogen delivery catheter into the instrument channel of the endoscope. While doing so, turn on the "Defrost" function to remove any residual fluid from the channel.

10. Position the catheter approximately 2 cm beyond the distal end of the endoscope.

11. Press and release the "Suction" pedal to begin active ventilation.

12. Set the timer on the truFreeze console to the appropriate interval based on the endoscopist's assessment of needed duration of each freeze cycle. In ablation of BE, freezing is typically applied in 20-second cycles, two to three times per tissue area.

13. Once precooling has completed, position the endoscope 2 to 3 cm from the target area for ablation. Be sure not to touch the catheter to the tissue during the ablation procedure.

14. Engage and hold the "Cryogen" foot pedal to begin the freezing process. Once the tissue begins to display evidence of freezing, communicate to the endoscopic technician to begin the timer.

15. Use a washcloth or gauze pad to handle the endoscope with your right hand, as it may become dangerously cold to the touch throughout the procedure.

16. Using the left-hand rotation and control body wheels, gently maneuver the endoscope back and forth in a painting motion across the intended treatment area to provide uniform freezing. Be aware that the level of freezing may leave the endoscope susceptible to damage. Aggressive torquing of the endoscope is discouraged.

17. When the set time expires, the console will emit a series of loud beeps.

18. Disengage the "Cryogen" foot pedal to cease the flow of cryogen.

19. The lens may have a film of frozen fluid over it. Wait for this to naturally thaw and do not attempt to use fluid or section to clear the film. Allow the tissue to thaw.

20. Between and during each cycle of treatment, ensure that the patient's abdomen is closely monitored by the endoscopy staff. Any evidence of abdominal distention or firmness should trigger immediate cessation of cryogen flow and close examination of the ventilation tubing for kink or obstruction to flow.

21. Repeat treatment until all intended targets have been adequately treated.

22. Press the release the "Suction" pedal to turn off active ventilation.

23. Engage the "Defrost" function and repeat until the cryogen delivery catheter can be easily removed from the instrument channel.

24. Examine the treated area for evidence of postablation changes, such as hyperemia and superficial mucosal bleeding.

25. Remove the endoscope and ventilation tubing.

Liquid Nitrous Oxide Balloon Cryotherapy (C2 CryoBalloon)

1. Perform an adequate endoscopic examination to visualize the structure(s) you are planning to ablate and make appropriate measurements of endoscopic landmarks.

2. Position the foot pedal in the desired location.

3. Remove the controller and cartridges from the provided kit.

4. Plug the interconnect cable from the foot pedal to the controller.

5. Insert a cartridge into the controller and screw the controller cap onto the controlled to unseal the cartridge.

6. Remove the catheter balloon probe from the packaging. The probe itself is housed in a protective sheath. Insert the probe and sheath into the biopsy cap. Thread the probe into the instrument channel until it emerges from the working end of the endoscope into endoscopic view.

7. Withdraw the protective sheath from the biopsy cap and slide back onto the catheter.

8. With the endoscope facing the esophageal lumen, advance the balloon probe until the black catheter is visible proximal to the balloon. Insert the catheter connector into the controller body.

9. Select the desired timer for each freeze cycle. Typically, each freeze cycle will last 10 seconds.

10. Once the cartridge pressure is adequate, the blue "Ready" icon will illuminate.

11. Quickly press and release the inflation pedal to inflate the balloon. No sizing is required, as the balloon will automatically inflate to the diameter of the esophagus.

12. Pull the inflated balloon gently against the endoscope tip to allow for visualization inside the balloon.

13. To visualize the region currently targeted by the ablation catheter, quickly press and release the ablation trigger for 1 second to create a "puff" of cryogen.

14. Position the balloon probe proximally or distally to reach the desired location. The balloon may deflate during this process and can be inflated as noted above.

15. To rotate the ablation catheter within the balloon, rotate the handle of the controller clockwise or counterclockwise and closely observe the probe within the balloon. The side holes should be visible and can be used to gauge the position.

16. Once the proper location is reached, depress and hold the ablation trigger. Once the prespecified treatment cycle duration has been reached, cryogen flow will cease.

17. Repeat treatment until all intended targets have been adequately treated. Only one treatment cycle is typically needed per focal site. Any "skipped" areas between ablation sites can be ablated with a shorter, 5-second cycle. Each cartridge will allow for approximately three 10-second treatments, allowing for several preablation "test puffs" to confirm placement. Replace cartridges as needed to treat the entire target zone.

18. Examine the treated area for evidence of postablation changes, such as hyperemia and superficial mucosal bleeding.

19. Press and hold the "Deflate" button and withdraw the balloon probe catheter, then the endoscope. If resistance is met, the probe and catheter can be withdrawn as a unit.

POSTPROCEDURE

1. The patient should be monitored in the recovery unit until they have fully recovered from sedation. Pertinent findings and procedural details should be shared with the patient.

2. Instructions should be given to the patient regarding possible complications, such as postprocedural pain or bleeding.

3. Patients are instructed to maintain a liquid diet for 24 hours.

4. Patients can be provided with viscous lidocaine solution and/ or liquid acetaminophen with codeine for postprocedure pain control.

ADVERSE EVENTS

1. Adverse events inherent to a diagnostic upper endoscopy including bleeding and perforation.
2. Patient may experience chest pain, dysphagia, and odynophagia for 3 to 4 days following ablation therapy. These symptoms are more common following RFA compared to cryoablation.
3. Gastric perforation is a rare but serious adverse event of cryotherapy. It occurs exclusively in the spray cryotherapy modality, where adequate ventilation is needed to prevent buildup of the instilled gas product.
4. The most common delayed complication is the development of esophageal stricture requiring endoscopic dilation. This has been reported in 3% to 13% of patients.

CPT CODES

43229—Esophagoscopy, flexible, transoral; with ablation of tumor(s), polyp(s), or other lesion(s) (includes pre- and postdilation and guidewire passage, when performed)

43270—Esophagogastroduodenoscopy, flexible, transoral; with ablation of tumor(s), polyp(s), or other lesion(s) (includes pre- and postdilation and guidewire passage, when performed)

43499—Unlisted procedure, esophagus—requires supporting documentation outlining the precise procedural details and resources required

Bibliography

1. Shaheen NJ, Falk GW, Iyer PG, Gerson L. ACG clinical guideline: diagnosis and management of Barrett's esophagus. *Am J Gastroenterol.* 2016;111(1):30-50.
2. Shajan P, Monkemuller K. Ablative endoscopic therapies for Barrett's esophagus-related neoplasia. *Gastroenterol Clin N Am.* 2015;44:337-353.
3. CSA Medical Inc. *TruFreeze System Rapid AV spray Kit - Instructions for Use.* Lexington, Massachusetts; 2017.
4. C2 Therapeutics Inc. *C2 Cryoballoon Ablation System – Instruction Manual.* Redwood City, California; 2017.
5. Parsi MA, Trindade AJ, Bhutani MS, et al. Cryotherapy in gastrointestinal endoscopy. *VideoGIE.* 2017;2(5):89-95.

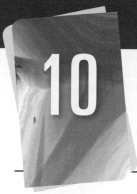

10 Endoscopic Mucosal Resection of Esophageal Lesions

Sumit Singla, MD

Cyrus Piraka, MD

Endoscopic mucosal resection (EMR) typically refers to the removal of flat or sessile lesions of the upper GI tract, although it is often used to describe a type of endoscopic resection of the mucosal layer of any part of the bowel with the use of submucosal lifting and snare resection of tissue. EMR is a well-established diagnostic and therapeutic modality for the management of esophageal lesions. This review will assist in understanding the applicable disease states, technique, and safety of this procedure in the upper GI tract and specifically in the esophagus.

DISEASE STATE

1. Barrett esophagus
   a. Intramucosal adenocarcinoma
   b. High-grade dysplasia
   c. Low-grade dysplasia
2. Squamous cell carcinoma
3. Other differentiated or undifferentiated lesions in the superficial or deep mucosa or shallow submucosa

TECHNIQUE

1. Careful examination
   a. Understand the indication for the procedure and perform a high-quality examination. This should include the use of an attached clear plastic cap and high-definition white light. Evolving technologies, such as the use of chromoendoscopy, confocal endomicroscopy, optical coherence tomography, and magnification endoscopy (not currently available in the United States), may improve the fidelity of this examination. Chromoendoscopy with Lugol iodine may aid in defining the presence and extent of squamous cell cancer (where dysplastic tissue is unstained). Part of

the rationale for performing a high-quality endoscopic examination is to exclude the presence of deeply invasive malignancy. This may also be performed in conjunction with endoscopic ultrasound (EUS) and other newer modalities to exclude malignancy.

b. The most common indication for EMR is removal of dysplastic/neoplastic lesions associated with Barrett esophagus. EUS is generally regarded as the gold standard for accurate staging of cancer associated with Barrett esophagus via TNM classification.[1,2] However, distinguishing between high-grade dysplasia, cancer confined to the superficial and deep mucosa (T1a) and cancer invading into submucosa (T1b) can be challenging and may overstage or less likely understage the lesion.[3,4] Clinical evidence and expert opinion have validated the central role of EMR in the removal of tissue and in providing the most accurate staging of early esophageal malignancy (see Fig. 10.1).

c. According to the Japanese Society for Gastroenterological Endoscopy criteria for EMR of early endoluminal cancers, early esophageal cancers are amenable to EMR if they meet the following criteria:

   i. Are less than 2 cm

   ii. Involve less than 1/3 of the esophageal wall

   iii. Are confined to the esophageal mucosa (stage T1a)

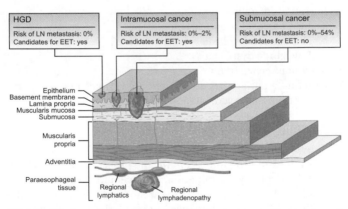

FIG. 10.1 Staging animation depicting depth of lesions amenable to endoscopic eradication therapy (EET), including endoscopic mucosal resection (EMR). HGT, high-grade dysplasia; LN, lymph node. (Adapted from Komanduri S, Muthuswamy VR, Wani S. Controversies in endoscopic eradication therapy for Barrett's esophagus. *Gastroenterology*. 2018;154(7):1861-1875. Copyright © 2018 American Gastroenterological Association. With permission.)

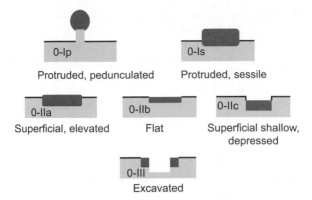

FIG. 10.2 Paris classification of neoplastic lesions within the digestive tract. (From Schlemper RJ, Hirata I, Dixon MF. The macroscopic classification of early neoplasia of the digestive tract. *Endoscopy*. 2002;34(2):163-168. Copyright © 2002 Georg Thieme Verlag KG.)

2. While European and American guidelines do not specifically address lesion size and circumference that would preclude resection, most expert centers currently attempt EMR even with larger lesions. The majority of studies demonstrating safety and efficacy do not specify a distinct size criteria at which resection should be deferred[5,6]
3. Description of the lesion (Fig. 10.2)
   a. Japanese Society for Gastrointestinal Endoscopy
      i. Type I lesions are protuberant
         • Ip—pedunculated
         • Ips/sp—subpedunculated
         • Is—sessile
      ii. Type II lesions are flat
         • IIa—superficial elevated
         • IIb—flat
         • IIc—flat depressed
         • IIc + IIa lesions—elevated area within a depressed lesion
         • IIa + IIc lesions—depressed area within an elevated lesion
      iii. Type III lesions are ulcerated
      iv. Type IV lesions are laterally spreading
   b. Paris system[1]
      i. Type 0-I lesions are polypoid
         • Type 0-Ip—protruded, pedunculated
         • Type 0-Is—protruded, sessile

      ii. Type 0-II lesions are nonpolypoid
- Type 0-IIa—slightly elevated
- Type 0-IIb—flat
- Type 0-IIc—slightly depressed

      iii. Type 0-III lesions are excavated

4. Ligation EMR

  a. Equipment

     i. High-definition endoscope with attached clear distal attachment
- Commercially available EMR kits can be affixed to standard and therapeutic upper endoscopes

     ii. Band-EMR kit (tailored to gastroscope size—standard or therapeutic)

     iii. Injection needle (optional)

     iv. Injectate solution
- Varies based on center
- At most centers, consists of dilute epinephrine with methylene blue or indigo carmine

  b. Technique (Fig. 10.3)

     i. Perform detailed endoscopic evaluation to develop a resection plan
- Assess and document location, morphology, borders, and size of lesion
- Consider marking planned resection margins with snare tip coagulation
- Plan piecemeal versus en bloc resection—the latter approach is preferred if cancer is suspected within a focal lesion, although wide margins should be obtained in this case as well

     ii. Attach ligator to working channel (technique will vary depending on kit used)

     iii. Inject desired lifting solution into submucosa (if applicable, a smaller needle may be required when using a standard gastroscope)

     iv. Carefully suction desired tissue into the cap

     v. Deploy band over tissue

     vi. Pass snare through working channel

     vii. Maneuver snare around lesion to the base of pseudopolyp
- Closure of the snare completely below the band is preferred, though placement above the band is acceptable
- With slight torque toward the lumen, consider opening and closing the snare slightly to release any captured muscularis propria

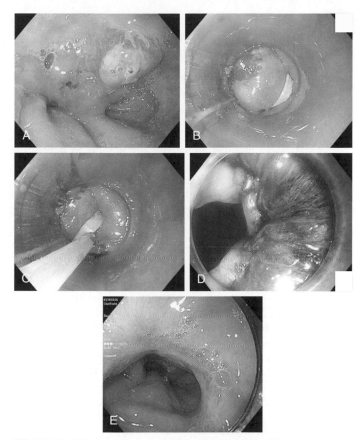

FIG. 10.3 Band ligation endoscopic mucosal resection (A) Polypoid lesion arising from Barrett esophagus, noted with HD white light. B, Following injection and band deployment. C, Snare maneuvered beneath band. D, Following resection with extension of margins. Final pathology consistent with moderately differentiated intramucosal adenocarcinoma with negative deep and lateral margins, without evidence of angiolymphatic invasion. E, Scar at the site of EMR noted during 3-month follow-up esophagogastroduodenoscopy (EGD). The remainder of the Barrett segment has been ablated.

    viii. Apply current to resect tissue
- Various current specifications have been utilized to resect tissue—in our practice, we utilize Endocut 3-1-3
    ix. Suction specimen into cap and remove tissue with the scope or push into stomach for later retrieval
    x. Repeat process until resection of desired tissue is achieved, taking care to have enough overlap of resection pieces to avoid bridges of unresected tissue

5. Cap EMR
   a. Equipment
      i. High-definition endoscope with attached clear distal attachment
     ii. Commercially available kit containing a clear plastic cap and a special crescent-shaped snare
   iii. Injection needle
    iv. Injectate (see above)
   b. Technique
      i. Perform detailed endoscopic evaluation to develop a resection plan
     ii. Mark periphery of planned resection site with cautery from tip of snare, if desired
   iii. Inject lifting solution into the submucosa
    iv. Position snare within the rim of the cap by deflecting scope into the wall of bowel such as gastric mucosa with slight suction
     v. Suction the injected area into the cap
    vi. Tighten snare around pseudopolyp
   vii. Push entrapped tissue outside of cap with snare still closed firmly
   viii. Apply current to resect tissue
    ix. Suction specimen into cap and remove tissue with the scope or drop it in the stomach for later retrieval
     x. Repeat process until complete resection of desired tissue is achieved, taking care to have enough overlap of resection pieces to avoid bridges of unresected tissue
6. Comparison of techniques
   a. Generally, the two techniques are considered equivalent, and choice is dependent upon personal expertise and experience
   b. The snares used in cap EMR tend to lose their function after one to two uses and need to be replaced while the snares used for ligation EMR are more durable; although for larger lesions, multiple banding kits may be required
   c. The largest study comparing the two techniques noted that they were similar with respect to thickness of lesions. Cap-EMR specimens were larger, which is generally not clinically relevant with piecemeal resection techniques, although may be relevant for a larger focal lesion to aid in achieving en bloc resection with negative margins. Ligation EMR may be faster and more cost-effective and is generally preferred for resection of Barrett with dysplasia and early esophageal malignancy[7]

RISKS

1. Stricture formation
   a. The reported frequency of strictures varies considerably. An ASGE technical review reported the incidence as 6% to 88%.[6]
   b. Symptomatic stricture formation has been noted in approximately 25% of all patients undergoing EMR for dysplastic Barrett, in a large retrospective study. Resection of >50% circumference was strongly associated with stricture formation. Number of specimens, number of EMR sessions, and long-term tobacco use are also factors that may relatively increase the rates of stricture formation.[8]
   c. Post-EMR strictures are responsive to balloon or Savary dilation.

2. Bleeding
   a. Bleeding following esophageal EMR is uncommon. In the largest single study on safety of EMR, significant bleeding requiring treatment, hospitalization, or transfusion approximately 1.2%.[5] However, endoscopists in this study deployed clips at time of EMR at their discretion, and this percentage may therefore understate the true frequency

3. Perforation
   a. Considered a low-frequency event and occurs in approximately 0.5% of cases, when performed by experienced endoscopists.[5]
   b. Perforation rates up to 5% have been described during the performance of the first 120 EMR cases performed by a novice interventional endoscopist, suggesting a steep learning curve.[9]
   c. Perforation is more endoscopically treatable when recognized immediately with the availability of newer endoscopic closure devices, such as the over-the-scope clip and endoscopic suturing, as well as easy-to-use fully covered esophageal stents

4. Anesthesia complication
   a. Similar to rates of anesthesia adverse events for other indications. Many centers utilize endotracheal intubation for esophageal EMR.

5. Altered diet
   a. Most centers recommend sequential advancement of diet. The exact protocol varies among institutions, with most centers advocating for a liquid diet, followed by soft foods, followed by resumption of a general diet over the course of several days.

6. Chest pain
   a. The reported frequency of post-EMR chest pain varies, as does the definition. Most centers refer to a rate of up to 50%.
7. Altered medication regimen
   a. Patients are generally instructed to continue their twice-daily proton pump inhibitor (PPI) and use Carafate four times daily for 2 weeks.[8]
   b. Most centers recommend avoidance of nonsteroidal anti-inflammatory agents, antiplatelet medications, and anticoagulants for 1 to 2 weeks, unless patients at high risk for vascular event.[5,8]
   c. The administration of rectal NSAIDs, liquid acetaminophen, viscous lidocaine, and limited supplies of Tylenol with codeine has been recommended at various centers to treat post-EMR chest pain.
   d. For cases where a large area of resection is performed, particularly >50% and up to 100% circumference, some centers advocate the use of topical steroids to reduce the risk of stricture formation.

SUCCESS RATES

Numerous studies have reported the long-term success of EMR for treatment of Barrett with dysplasia, often in conjunction with post-EMR radiofrequency ablation, as upward of 95%.[10,11]

CONCLUSION

EMR is a well-described, safe, and effective strategy for removing malignant or premalignant tissue from the esophagus. Specifically, recent literature has established its utility as a diagnostic and therapeutic modality in patients with dysplastic Barrett esophagus.

References

1. Rosch T. Endosonographic staging of esophageal cancer: a review of literature results. *Gastrointest Endosc Clin N Am*. 1995;5:537-547.
2. Kelly S, Harris KM, Berry E, et al. A systematic review of the staging performance of endoscopic ultrasound in gastro-oesophageal carcinoma. *Gut*. 2001;49:534-539.
3. Chak A, Canto M, Stevens PD, et al. Clinical applications of a new through-the-scope ultrasound probe: prospective comparison with an ultrasound endoscope. *Gastrointest Endosc*. 1997;45:291-295.
4. Larghi A, Lightdale C, Memeo L, et al. EUS followed by EMR for staging of high-grade dysplasia and early cancer in Barrett's esophagus. *Gastrointest Endosc*. 2005;62(1):16-23.
5. Tomizawa Y, Iyer PG, Wong Kee Song LM, et al. Safety of endoscopic mucosal resection for Barrett's esophagus. *Am J Gastroenterol*. 2013;108:1440-1447.

6. Hwang JH, Konda V, Abu Dayyeh BK, et al. Endoscopic mucosal resection. *Gastrointest Endosc*. 2015;82(2):215-226.

7. Pouw RE, van Vilsteren FG, Peters FP, et al. Randomized trial on endoscopic resection-cap versus multiband mucosectomy for piecemeal endoscopic resection of early Barrett's neoplasia. *Gastrointest Endosc*. 2011;74:35-43.

8. Lewis JJ, Rubenstein J, Singal A, Elmunzer BJ, Kwon RS, Piraka CR. Factors associated with esophageal stricture formation after endoscopic mucosal resection for neoplastic Barrett's esophagus. *Gastrointest Endosc*. 2011;74(4):753-760.

9. Van Vilsteren FG, Pouw RE, Herrero LA, et al. Learning to perform endoscopic resection of esophageal neoplasia is associated with significant complications even within a structured training program. *Endoscopy*. 2012;44:4-12.

10. Chadwick G, Groene O, Markar SR, et al. Systematic review comparing radiofrequency ablation and complete endoscopic resection in treating dysplastic Barrett's esophagus: a critical assessment of histologic outcomes and adverse events. *Gastrointest Endosc*. 2014;79(5):718.

11. Pech O, May A, Manner H, et al. Long-term efficacy and safety of endoscopic resection for patients with mucosal adenocarcinoma of the esophagus. *Gastroenterology*. 2014;146:652 660.

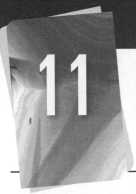

11

Endoscopic Management of Foreign Bodies of the Upper Gastrointestinal Tract

Dustin A. Carlson, MD

Ingestion of foreign bodies or food impaction is a common cause of gastrointestinal emergency.[1] The majority of foreign bodies pass spontaneously through the alimentary tract, but endoscopic intervention is required in 10% to 20% of cases. Generally, food bolus disimpaction or foreign body retrieval by endoscopic means is successful in over 90% of cases with surgical intervention being potentially required if an object fails to progress over several days or symptoms of obstruction or perforation develop.[2,3] While foreign body ingestion carries substantial morbidity, the rate of fatality is low.[1,2,4,5]

Foreign body ingestions occur more commonly in the pediatric than adult population, with the peak incidence between 6 months and 6 years.[5] In adults, foreign body ingestion may occur more frequently among patients with psychiatric disorders, mental impairment, alcohol intoxication, or those seeking secondary gain with access to a medical facility. Food bolus impaction is most often observed in those with underlying esophageal pathology, such as peptic strictures or eosinophilic esophagitis (EoE).

INDICATIONS FOR ENDOSCOPY

Indications for endoscopic intervention, as well as timing of intervention, are dependent on both the nature of the object, its particular location within the GI tract, and the patient's clinical status.[1] Risks of aspiration and GI perforation are the primary factors related to recommendations regarding endoscopic intervention with ingested foreign bodies and are focuses of the initial evaluation (e.g., assessment of airway, ventilatory status, and evaluation for possible perforation, such as peritoneal signs or subcutaneous crepitus in the thorax or neck). In general, foreign objects requiring removal include any item lodged in the esophagus and items within upper endoscopic reach (i.e., in the stomach or proximal duodenum) that are sharp, long (>6 cm), magnets, or batteries.[1]

Emergent

1. Esophageal obstruction with any object (recognized by inability to tolerate oral secretions)
2. Sharp object in the esophagus
3. Disk battery in the esophagus

Urgent (i.e., Within 24 Hours)

1. Esophageal impaction not meeting criteria for emergent endoscopy as above (i.e., incomplete obstruction of a non-sharp, non–disk battery foreign body)
   a. All esophageal foreign bodies should be removed prior to 24 hours from occurrence
2. Sharp object within stomach or proximal duodenum that can be safely removed
3. Objects >6 cm in length at or above the proximal duodenum
4. Magnets within endoscopic reach

Routine

1. Objects in stomach >2.5 cm in diameter
2. Disk and cylindrical batteries within the stomach when signs/symptoms of gastric mucosal injury are present or without sign of GI injury if not expelled from the stomach within 48 hours
3. Blunt objects that fail to pass out of stomach within 3 to 4 weeks

CONTRAINDICATIONS FOR ENDOSCOPIC INTERVENTION

Absolute

1. Evidence of free mediastinal or peritoneal air
2. Narcotic packets. Endoscopic recovery should not be attempted due to the risk of rupture, as leakage of contents can be fatal
3. Same as standard upper endoscopy

Relative

1. Upper esophageal stricture
2. Zenker diverticulum
3. Postligament of Treitz position of foreign body (as the majority of these will pass spontaneously)
4. Same as standard upper endoscopy

Special Considerations

1. High esophageal impaction
2. Esophageal impaction of prolonged or unknown duration (prolonged impaction may result in tissue necrosis, increasing the risk of major adverse events)

- In both instances consider anesthesiology +/− surgical consultation. General endotracheal anesthesia is helpful for airway protection in these cases, or when overall risk of aspiration is deemed to be high (e.g., large amounts of food within the esophagus).
- Laryngoscopy or rigid esophagoscopy is the preferred method for impacted sharp objects at the level of the cricopharyngeus.[1,6]

PREPARATION
Historical Considerations

1. Assess circumstances (e.g., object, timing) of suspected ingestion.
2. Obtain a replica of a foreign body for inspection if it is a non-food object.
3. Determine the presence of known esophageal pathology (anatomic or dysmotility).
4. Characterize prior symptoms of dysphagia or a history of any previous food impaction.
5. Determine the presence of any neurologic impairment (e.g., cerebrovascular accident, multiple sclerosis) that may increase risk of aspiration.

Physical Examination

1. Assess ventilation, airway compromise, and risk of aspiration.
2. Assess swelling, tenderness, or crepitus in the neck region and thorax to assess for esophageal perforation.
3. Assess the abdomen for evidence of peritonitis or small bowel obstruction.

Anatomic Considerations

1. Impaction or obstruction most often occurs at areas of acute angulations or physiologic narrowing.
   a. Cricopharyngeus muscle
   b. Aortic arch
   c. Esophagogastric junction
   d. Pylorus
   e. Ligament of Treitz
   f. Ileocecal valve

Radiologic Considerations

1. Exclude perforation by assessing for the presence of mediastinal, subdiaphragmatic, or subcutaneous air.
2. Identify and localize the object with radiographs.

3. Only radiopaque objects may be visualized, e.g., metal objects and steak bones
   a. Commonly encountered objects that are radiolucent (and thus will unlikely be observed on radiography) include chicken bones, most fish bones (depends on type of fish), wood (e.g., toothpicks), plastic, and most glass.
4. Biplane radiographs will commonly be sufficient to localize and identify objects.
   a. Computed tomography (CT) scans may also be useful if a radiopaque item cannot be identified or localized on biplane radiographs.
5. Oral-contrast radiography should not be routinely performed due to the risk of aspiration and because coating of the foreign body and mucosal lining often compromises subsequent endoscopy.
6. Nonvisualized objects are frequently encountered and still warrant endoscopic evaluation.

Pharmacologic Considerations

1. Medication (e.g., glucagon 1 mg intravenously) to relax the esophagus and allow spontaneous passage of a food bolus can be considered in the setting of an esophageal food impaction.[3,7] The favorable safety profile of glucagon supports an attempt; however, its use should not delay endoscopic intervention in emergent settings.
2. Proteolytic enzymes (e.g., papain) should **NOT** be used because it has been associated with hypernatremia, erosion, and esophageal perforation.

EQUIPMENT

1. Endoscopes
   a. Standard or therapeutic
      i. Single channel, larger diameter channel
      ii. Dual channel, instances when two devices may be required to manipulate the object
2. Retrieval devices[8]
   - Most retrieval devices can be used with a standard 2.8 mm channel, though a therapeutic channel (3.7 mm) is required for some.
   - Selection of retrieval device is generally based on the size and shape of object to be retrieved. Consider simulation (see below) to dictate.
   - Endoscopic retrieval devices are available from multiple manufactures; the following list includes representative products and manufacturers, but is not intended to be comprehensive.

   a. Forceps:
- **i.** Rat tooth (available in multiple sizes from multiple manufacturers)
- **ii.** Alligator jaw (available in multiple sizes from multiple manufacturers)
- **iii.** Raptor (US Endoscopy, Mentor, OH, USA)
- **iv.** Shark tooth (Olympus; Center Valley, PA, USA)
- **v.** V-shaped (Olympus)
- **vi.** Rubber tip (Olympus)

   b. Loop snares (available in multiple sizes from multiple manufacturers)

   c. Roth Net retrieval devices (US Endoscopy)

   d. Graspers (2 to 5 prong; available in multiple sizes from multiple manufacturers)

   e. Retrieval baskets (available in multiple sizes from multiple manufacturers)

   f. Clear plastic cap

3. Foreign Body Hood Protector (Avanos Medical, Inc, Alpharetta, Georgia, USA)

4. Overtubes (US Endoscopy).

   a. Esophageal and gastric lengths which allow for the following:
- **i.** Airway protection during withdrawal of foreign body
- **ii.** Multiple passes for piecemeal extraction
- **iii.** Protection of esophageal mucosa during retrieval of sharp objects

5. Suction equipment

   a. One wall-unit suction canister each for the endoscope and patient

PROCEDURE

Simulation

1. Perform a "dry run" by simulating the extraction prior to endoscope insertion.

2. Using a replica of the foreign body (if available), experiment with various devices and grasping methods to determine the optimal approach.

Intubation

1. Assure proper functioning of suction equipment.

2. Place the patient in the left lateral position with either head-of-bed elevation to 30° to 45° or reverse Trendelenburg position.

3. Advance the endoscope into the hypopharynx, and note possible obstruction at the level of the cricopharyngeus, which might require endotracheal intubation or laryngoscopy for extraction.

4. As the patient swallows, gently insert the endoscope into the esophageal lumen during relaxation of the cricopharyngeus.
5. Once the endoscope has passed the upper esophageal sphincter, advance it under direct vision with minimal air insufflation until the foreign body/food impaction is reached. Direct visualization is necessary at all times in order to avoid inadvertently striking the object, resulting in further impaction or penetration into the mucosal wall.

Overtube Insertion

1. Overtubes should be backloaded onto the endoscope and then advanced forward after esophageal intubation.
2. As a result of inherent stiffness and diameter discrepancy (compared to the gastroscope), attempts to advance the overtube (especially the esophageal length) beyond the hypopharyngeal shelf may be met with resistance and have even resulted in perforation.
   a. Note: The outer diameter of the overtube, which is > 19 mm, should be taken into account before attempted passage, particularly in the case of an identified or suspected diffuse (or proximal), narrow-caliber esophagus as in EoE or radiation-induced strictures.
   b. Softening the overtube by running it under warm water can be helpful to reduce the stiffness element.
   c. Applying endoscopic lubricant to the inner, taper-end portion of the overtube assembly may aid positioning of the endoscope. To do so, the overtube assembly can be disassembled, lubricated, and then reassembled before loading on to the endoscope.

The endoscopic equipment used to remove upper intestinal foreign bodies varies by the type of object and is discussed in further detail below.

Esophageal Food Impaction

1. Fluid lavage should be utilized sparingly or avoided to prevent aspiration, especially with large amounts of retained food debris or high-grade esophageal obstruction. An air-filled syringe to clear debris from the suction channel should be utilized instead.
2. Push-technique: Although early recommendations were leery of pushing an endoscopic bolus into the stomach due to a risk of perforation, advancing an endoscopic bolus into the stomach with gently applied pressure has been safely reported in multiple series.[1,2,9,10] An attempt to advance the endoscope around the food impaction to evaluate the underlying esophageal pathology remains the generally preferred initial step. While placing excessive pressure on a

food bolus should still be avoided to minimize the risk of perforation, advancing an esophageal bolus into the stomach negates the alternative of retrieval, which requires passage of the bolus over the airway and a theoretic opportunity for aspiration.

3. If retrograde removal of the food bolus appears to be necessary, then one of the following approaches should be pursued:
   a. Place an esophageal-length overtube to protect the airway and to facilitate piecemeal extraction.
   b. Consider requesting endotracheal intubation to provide airway protection during withdrawal of the foreign body.
   c. Use of pronged grasper, toothed-forceps, or snare may be useful for retrieval of solid food boluses (e.g., meat).
   d. Use of an endoscopic cap or retrieval net to collect food particles in somewhat enclosed collections.

4. Esophageal dilation after disimpaction may be considered if there are no obvious contraindications. However, if significant mucosal irritation is present, such as after a prolonged food impaction event, dilation should be avoided due to the associated increased risk of perforation.
   a. If dilation is not performed, an early follow-up endoscopy (e.g., 1 to 2 weeks) should be coordinated to repeat endoscopy for dilation to minimize subsequent events, with dietary caution recommended in the interim.

5. Esophageal biopsies to aid establishment of a diagnosis of EoE should also be considered immediately following esophageal disimpaction.

Blunt Objects

Blunt objects should be removed with devices that are best suited for the shape of the object. Simulation with a replica object (when available) and device(s) outside the body is helpful to determine the best approach.

1. Extraction of coins can be accomplished with any number of devices, including grasping forceps (e.g., rat tooth), a Roth Net, retrieval baskets, or loop snares.

2. Disk batteries, as well as smooth rounded objects, are effectively removed using the Roth Net.[11]

3. Blunt, long (>6 cm) objects (e.g., toothbrushes, spoons) can be grasped with a snare close to the cephalad end of the object such that it will align itself with the long axis of the esophagus during withdrawal. Other options include the following:
   a. Use of a gastric length overtube followed by withdrawal of the entire apparatus.
   b. Double-wire loop-snare technique with a dual-channel therapeutic endoscope to manage the orientation of the object during withdrawal.

4. Objects within the esophagus that cannot be secured may be advanced into the stomach to facilitate a position that may allow for easier grasping.
5. Consider use of an overtube to provide airway protection in the event the foreign body is dislodged during withdrawal through the hypopharynx.

Sharp Objects

1. Determine the optimal device for grasping the object and the optimal orientation to allow for removal.
   a. Polypectomy snares may be preferred for removal of both toothpicks and tacks, although grasping forceps and retrieval basket are also successful.[11]
2. Use maneuvers or equipment intended to minimize mucosal trauma during extraction.
   a. Distend the esophagus with full insufflation to minimize mucosal contact.
   b. Always orient the object with the pointed end or sharp edge trailing during extraction.
   c. Protector hood: The hood maintains its inverted position during insertion of the endoscope; during withdrawal the bell portion then flips back to its original shape enclosing the sharp object within the hood protector.
   d. Use an overtube to protect the esophageal mucosa and to provide airway protection in the event the foreign body is dislodged during withdrawal of the hypopharynx.
   e. A technique to grasp a safety pin with forceps and subsequently close with a snare has been described.[12]

POSTPROCEDURE

1. Monitor the patient for signs or symptoms of perforation following the intervention for an acceptable recovery period.
2. Perform immediate contrast study (with gastrografin) if there is clinical suspicion of perforation, especially if the extraction was difficult or complicated.
3. Restrict diet to liquids or pureed foods when appropriate depending on the amount of intervention and the timing of the next intervention.
4. Determine disposition and an appropriate follow-up plan, such as repeat endoscopy for dilation of identified esophageal pathology.

ADVERSE EVENTS

1. Failure rate is generally considered to be very low, approximate 1% to 4%.[1,2,9]
2. Rigid endoscopy was associated with a higher adverse event rate than flexible endoscopy.[6]

3. Reported adverse event rates from endoscopy for ingested foreign body range are low, generally <0.5% risk.[2,3,9,10]

4. Specific adverse events associated with endoscopic disimpaction/retrieval may include mucosal laceration, hemorrhage, aspiration, mediastinitis, perforation, death.

5. No adverse events have been specifically attributable to retrieval devices, although bleeding and perforation have been reported with overtube insertion.

CPT CODES ASSOCIATED WITH ENDOSCOPIC FOREIGN BODY REMOVAL

43215—Esophagoscopy, **flexible**, transoral; with removal of foreign body(s)

43194—Esophagoscopy, **rigid**, transoral; foreign body removal

43247—Esophagogastroduodenoscopy, flexible, transoral; with removal of foreign body(s)

44363—Small intestinal endoscopy, enteroscopy beyond second portion of duodenum, not including ileum; with removal of foreign body

References

1. ASGE Standards of Practice Committee, Ikenberry SO, Jue TL, Anderson MA, et al. Management of ingested foreign bodies and food impactions. *Gastrointest Endosc.* 2011;73(6):1085-1091.

2. Webb WA. Management of foreign bodies of the upper gastrointestinal tract: update. *Gastrointest Endosc.* 1995;41(1):39-51.

3. Haas J, Leo J, Vakil N. Glucagon is a safe and inexpensive initial strategy in esophageal food bolus impaction. *Dig Dis Sci.* 2016;61(3):841-845.

4. Velitchkov NG, Grigorov GI, Losanoff JE, et al. Ingested foreign bodies of the gastrointestinal tract: retrospective analysis of 542 cases. *World J Surg.* 1996;20(8):1001-1005.

5. Cheng W, Tam PK. Foreign-body ingestion in children: experience with 1,265 cases. *J Pediatr Surg.* 1999;34(10):1472-1476.

6. Gmeiner D, von Rahden BH, Meco C, et al. Flexible versus rigid endoscopy for treatment of foreign body impaction in the esophagus. *Surg Endosc.* 2007;21(11):2026-2029.

7. Tibbling L, Bjorkhoel A, Jansson E, et al. Effect of spasmolytic drugs on esophageal foreign bodies. *Dysphagia.* 1995;10(2):126-127.

8. Asge Technology C, Diehl DL, Adler DG, et al. Endoscopic retrieval devices. *Gastrointest Endosc.* 2009;69(6):997-1003.

9. Vicari JJ, Johanson JF, Frakes JT. Outcomes of acute esophageal food impaction: success of the push technique. *Gastrointest Endosc.* 2001;53(2):178-181.

10. Longstreth GF, Longstreth KJ, Yao JF. Esophageal food impaction: epidemiology and therapy. A retrospective, observational study. *Gastrointest Endosc.* 2001;53(2):193-198.

11. Faigel DO, Stotland BR, Kochman ML, et al. Device choice and experience level in endoscopic foreign object retrieval: an in vivo study. *Gastrointest Endosc.* 1997;45(6):490-492.

12. Karjoo M, A-Kader H. A novel technique for closing and removing an open safety pin from the stomach. *Gastrointest Endosc.* 2003;57(4):627-629.

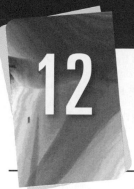

12

Pneumatic Dilation for Achalasia

Anna Tavakkoli, MD, MSc

Achalasia is a primary esophageal motility disorder that is characterized by a loss of inhibitory neurons in the esophagus with subsequent tonic contraction of the lower esophageal sphincter (LES) and loss of esophageal peristalsis.[1,2]Although achalasia is a rare disorder, with an incidence of 1:100,000, recent reports suggest a two- to fourfold increase in incidence due to unclear reasons.[1-5] Typically, achalasia is idiopathic without a clear inciting cause. However, achalasia can be termed secondary achalasia or pseudoachalasia if a defined etiology causing achalasia is found.[6] Causes of secondary achalasia range from neoplastic disorders, infiltrative disorders such as amyloidosis, Chagas disease, or circulating antibodies, such as with small-cell lung cancer.[1,6]

Patients with achalasia typically present with dysphagia to liquids and solids and regurgitation of undigested foods.[1,7] Since patients often present with dysphagia, an upper endoscopy, endoscopic ultrasound, and/or a barium esophagram are obtained to rule out a mechanical or infiltrative process. Endoscopic findings that are suggestive of achalasia include mega esophagus or significant dilation of the esophagus, presence of stasis-type mucosal changes, and in some cases, a subjective feeling of difficulty passing the endoscope through the LES.[1,7] Barium esophagram will often show a dilated esophagus with an air-fluid level and narrowing at the gastroesophageal junction (GEJ), typically described as a "bird-beak" appearance.[1,3,7] However, neither endoscopy nor barium esophagram can make a definitive diagnosis of achalasia, and esophageal manometry is considered the gold standard for diagnosis.

Based on the Chicago Classification of esophageal motility disorders, there are three types of achalasia: (1) type 1, characterized by an elevated median integrative relaxation pressure (IRP) with 100% failed peristalsis; (2) type 2, characterized by an elevated median IRP with 100% failed peristalsis and intermittent pan-esophageal pressurization, involving greater than or equal to 20% of swallows; (3) type 3, characterized by an elevated median IRP, premature/spastic contractions involving greater than or equal to 20% of swallows, and no normal peristalsis.[8] There are times where the results of esophageal impedance do not clearly indicate that a patient has achalasia. In those settings, the use of a functional lumen imaging probe (FLIP, Crospon, Galway, Ireland) can be performed. FLIP allows direct measurement of GEJ distensibility and diameter and can serve as a complementary test to aid in the diagnosis of achalasia.[1,8]

Treatment of achalasia aims at disrupting the hypertonic LES and include medical therapy, botulinum toxin, pneumatic dilation, per-oral endoscopic myotomy (POEM), and Heller myotomy. Since POEM offers achalasia patients a chance at durable symptom control, pneumatic dilation is typically used if a patient is not a candidate for POEM or the patient prefers dilation over POEM. Although patients often require multiple dilations with progressively larger balloons, it serves as an option for treatment of achalasia.

CONTRAINDICATIONS

1. Relative contraindications
   a. Poor cardiopulmonary status or comorbid illnesses preventing surgery: Some literature describes this as an absolute contraindication given the inability to undergo surgery if esophageal perforation occurs.[9] However, given limited treatment options of achalasia in the setting of poor cardiopulmonary status, an informed discussion with the patient of the risks, benefits, alternatives to treatment, and plan for management of potential adverse events makes pneumatic dilation for treatment of achalasia in these patients an option.[9]
   b. Use of anticoagulation: Pneumatic dilation while on anticoagulation is contraindicated. However, if the patient holds their anticoagulation for the appropriate duration of time, pneumatic dilation can be performed safely.

   The literature also describes a relative contraindication of pneumatic dilation among patients with an epiphrenic diverticulum or large hiatal hernia.[9] Performing pneumatic dilation in the setting of a prior Heller myotomy is not a contraindication but may require a larger balloon and multiple sessions for treatment due to scar tissue.

PREPROCEDURAL PLANNING

1. Informed consent and discussion of risks: It is important to meet with patients, either in the endoscopy unit or in a clinic setting, to discuss the risks and benefits of pneumatic dilation. Specifically, pneumatic dilation is associated with a higher

risk of perforation, anywhere between 1.5% and 5%, as compared to standard esophageal dilation. The variation in risk of perforation often depends on the size of balloon chosen for the pneumatic dilation. Furthermore, patients should be aware that they will likely require more than one pneumatic dilation for control of their symptoms and that there is a chance for decreased response, especially among patients who are older than 40 years, male gender, have a dilated esophagus, or have achalasia type III.[1,2]

2. Balloon size: The RigiFlex balloons (Boston Scientific, Marlborough, MA), which are used for pneumatic dilation, comes in sizes of 30, 35, and 40 mm (Fig. 12.1). Although data show that there is greater clinical improvement with the use of larger sized balloons, The European Achalasia Trial has shown that upfront dilation with a large pneumatic balloon is associated with an increased risk of perforation.[10,11] The trial, which compared pneumatic dilation versus laparoscopic Heller myotomy for idiopathic achalasia, initially used a 35 mm balloon for the first dilation and they found that perforation occurred in 4 of the 13 patients.[11] The protocol for the trial was then changed so that all patients started with a 30 mm balloon and received subsequent dilation with a 35 mm

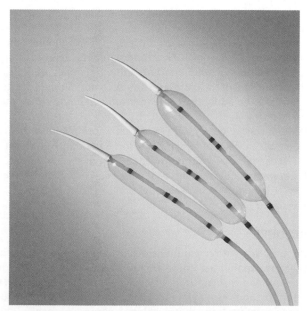

FIG. 12.1 RigiFlex pneumatic balloon dilations. (Permission for use granted by Boston Scientific Corporation.)

balloon 1 to 3 weeks later.[11] If patients were still symptomatic, a third pneumatic dilation using a 40 mm balloon was used. With this protocol, the study found a 90% 1-year success rate, 86% 2-year success rate, and 82% 5-year success rate, which was similar to Heller myotomy.[11] This study did have a 4% perforation rate and subsequent trials have used a less aggressive protocol, which typically involves starting with a 30 mm dilating balloon and repeating dilation with a 35 mm balloon only if patients remain symptomatic, with an observed perforation rate of 2%.[1,10,11] Whichever approach is taken, most providers choose to start with a 30 mm balloon to decrease the risk of perforation among these patients.

3. Preprocedural fasting: Generally, a 12-hour fast is adequate for patients prior to pneumatic dilation. However, patients with mega esophagus may require several days of clear liquids due to esophageal stasis of food and liquids. The number of days required for a clear liquid fast varies, but can be anywhere between 3 and 7 days, depending on the severity of the patient's disease.

EQUIPMENT

1. Pneumatic balloons and sphygmomanometer: As previously mentioned, the RigiFlex balloons (Boston Scientific, Marlborough, MA) are the most commonly used balloons. These balloons are a graded, polyethylene balloon system mounted on a flexible catheter and designed to go over a wire (as opposed to through the scope). The balloon comes in three sizes: 30, 35, and 40 mm and while it is not radiopaque, it has radiopaque markers that define the upper, middle, and distal borders of the balloon. The sphygmomanometer is used to inflate the balloons to the appropriate pounds per square inch (PSI).

2. Wire: Either a Savary wire or a long, more pliable wire (such as a 0.035 × 450 cm Jagwire (Boston Scientific, Marlborough, MA)) can be used for the procedure.

3. Radiopaque marker, such as a paper clip or a penny, to mark the GE junction on fluoroscopy.

4. Lubricant Jelly.

PROCEDURE

1. Pneumatic dilation should be performed in a room with fluoroscopy capabilities. There are reports of performing the dilation under direct endoscopic visualization. However, given the often tortuous esophagus that these patients have, the procedure is best performed under fluoroscopic guidance.

2. Given the size of the pneumatic balloon dilators and the risk of aspiration among these patients, these procedures are typically completed with monitored anesthesia care (MAC) or general anesthesia with endotracheal tube. The decision between MAC or general anesthesia is typically made after a discussion with the anesthesiologist.

3. After the patient is sedated and placed on the fluoroscopy table in the left lateral position, a complete endoscopy is performed. It is possible that the esophagus has food and/or fluid. Careful attention should be placed to try to aspirate and/or remove any food prior to pneumatic dilation to prevent aspiration when the patient is in recovery.

4. After the endoscopy is performed, the scope is positioned at the GE junction. The radiopaque marker (i.e., paper clip or penny) is then placed either on the patient or on the fluoroscopy monitor to mark the position of the GEJ. This will allow for appropriate positioning of the pneumatic balloon during the dilation.

5. Once the GEJ is marked, the scope is advanced to the stomach antrum, where the wire is placed, and the scope is then removed.

6. Once the scope is removed, the RigiFlex balloon is lubricated and placed over the wire. If there is difficulty passing the balloon over the wire, the head can be tilted backward, which can straighten the posterior pharynx and allow for smooth intubation of the esophagus.

7. The RigiFlex balloon is then advanced to the position of the radiopaque marker, which is at the GEJ. The balloon can then be advanced 2 to 3 cm past the GEJ to allow for proper dilation across the GEJ.

8. Gradual inflation of the balloon with the sphygmomanometer is then performed. Inflation of the balloon with the sphygmomanometer can sometimes be difficult. The RigiFlex balloon typically indicates the PSI needed for inflation (typically between 7 PSI and 12 PSI) and once the desired PSI is achieved, it should be held for 30 to 60 seconds.

9. After dilation is performed, the wire and balloon are then removed. Although not required, a postdilation endoscopic examination can help to determine whether a successful dilation occurred and rule out any possible adverse event, such as perforation.

POSTPROCEDURE

1. Monitoring: Routine monitoring of the patient should occur after the procedure. This typically involves staying in the recovery unit for 30 to 60 minutes or until awake. Ideally, the head of the bed should be slightly elevated to reduce aspiration

risk. Routine esophagram or x-ray after pneumatic dilation is not necessary and is recommended only if the clinical picture is concerning for a perforation.

2. Adverse events: The most serious adverse event is perforation and the risk of perforation can vary based on the size of the balloon used for the initial dilation (30 versus 35 mm). However, even when a 30 mm balloon is chosen for the initial dilation, the risk of perforation is upward of 5%. If there is concern for perforation, obtaining an esophagram to characterize the perforation would be the initial step. Often, these perforations can be treated with esophageal stenting.[12] If esophageal stenting is pursued, the patient should have a repeat esophagram 1 to 2 days later to confirm the perforation has been treated with the stent.[12] Patients are typically discharged on antibiotics and either nasogastric tube feeds or a soft diet.

PNEUMATIC DILATION WITH ESOFLIP

Pneumatic dilation with a 30 mm balloon can now be performed without fluoroscopy using FLIP technology (FLIP, Crospon, Galway, Ireland). esoFLIP integrates FLIP technology to dilate the GEJ in patients with achalasia and can provide data on recoil of the esophagus during the procedure. Although the largest balloon size available with esoFLIP is 30 mm, it provides an alternative option for providers and patients who want to avoid fluoroscopy.

References

1. Chandrasekhara V, Elmunzer BJ, Khashab M, et al. *Clinical Gastrointestinal Endoscopy*. New York: Elsevier; 2018.
2. Boeckxstaens GE, Zaninotto G, Richter JE. Achalasia. *Lancet*. 2014;383:83-93.
3. Pandolfino JE, Gawron AJ, MSCI. JAMA patient patient: achalasia. *J Am Med Assoc*. 2015;313(18):1876.
4. Samo S, Carlson DA, Gregory DL, et al. Incidence and prevalence of achalasia in central Chicago, 2004-2014, since the widespread use of high-resolution manometry. *Clin Gastroenterol Hepatol*. 2017;15:366-373.
5. Duffield JA, Hamer PW, Heddle R, et al. Incidence of achalasia in south Australia based on esophageal manometry findings. *Clin Gastroenterol Hepatol*. 2017;15:360-365.
6. Kahrilas PJ, Kishk SM, Helm JF, et al. Comparison of pseudoachalasia and achalasia. *Am J Med*. 1987;82:439-446.
7. Vaezi MF, Pandolfino JE, Vela MF. ACG clinical guideline: diagnosis and management of achalasia. *Am J Gastroenterol*. 2013;108:1238-1249; quiz 1250.
8. Kahrilas PJ, Bredenoord AJ, Fox M, et al. The Chicago Classification of esophageal motility disorders, v3.0. *Neurogastroenterol Motil*. 2015;27:160-174.
9. Richter JE. Achalasia – an update. *J Neurogastroenterol Motil*. 2010;16:232-242.
10. Moonen A, Annese V, Belmans A, et al. Long-term results of the European achalasia trial: a multicentre randomised controlled trial comparing pneumatic dilation versus laparoscopic Heller myotomy. *Gut*. 2016;65:732-739.

11. Boeckxstaens GE, Annese V, Varannes des SB, et al. Pneumatic dilation versus laparoscopic Heller's myotomy for idiopathic achalasia. *N Engl J Med.* 2011;364:1807-1816.
12. Elhanafi S, Othman M, Sunny J, et al. Esophageal perforation post pneumatic dilatation for achalasia managed by esophageal stenting. *Am J Case Rep.* 2013;14:532-535.

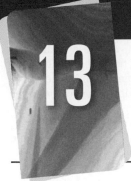

13

Placement of Esophageal Self-Expandable Metal Stents

Anna Tavakkoli, MD, MSc
Ryan Law, DO

Esophageal self-expandable metal stent (SEMS) use continues to evolve. Over the last several years increasing applications have arisen for use in patients with benign disease, and technical improvements in stent design and materials have streamlined use. Several FDA-approved SEMS are currently available; however, the only FDA-approved indication for use is palliation of malignant dysphagia. All other indications are considered off-label use. Each currently available stent has unique features, such as antimigration properties, improved fluoroscopic visualization, through-the-scope placement, and non-foreshortening during deployment.[1] SEMS are typically divided into fully covered (FCSEMS), partially covered (PCSEMS), and uncovered.[2] Partially covered stents have the proximal and distal flange uncovered with the midbody of the stent covered. The type of SEMS needs to be carefully considered for each clinical scenario though stent placement and functionality are largely similar.

INDICATIONS

1. To relieve dysphagia produced by neoplastic strictures of the esophagus.
2. To relieve dysphagia in chronic nonneoplastic strictures that have not responded to routine dilation.[3-5]
3. To seal esophageal fistulas (tracheoesophageal or bronchoesophageal), leaks or perforations.[6]
4. To provide tamponade during acute refractory esophageal variceal bleeding.[7,8]

CONTRAINDICATIONS

1. Those associated with upper endoscopy (see Chapter 5).
2. Compression of the trachea by esophageal cancer. This is a relative contraindication as bronchoscopy may be required to assess the airway prior to stent placement.

3. The use of concurrent external radiotherapy, as a bridge to surgery, or prior to chemoradiotherapy.[2] These treatments have reasonable success in decreasing tumor bulk and allowing palliation of dysphagia, thus a stent may not be necessary.
4. Lesions that require stent placement within 2 cm of the upper esophageal sphincter.
5. Severe cardiac and/or respiratory disorder.
6. Bleeding diathesis or anticipated need for chronic anticoagulation.
7. Limited life expectancy.

PREPARATION

1. Fast the patient for at least 8 hours prior to the procedure.
2. Obtain informed consent from the patient or patient representative, outlining the possible procedural adverse events as well as alternative methods of treatment.
3. Assess the patient's airway by bronchoscopy in situations where an esophageal mass involves the airway, or the patient is exhibiting signs of pulmonary compromise.
4. Administer a topical anesthetic for pharyngeal anesthesia.
5. Start an intravenous line for administration of systemic sedation.
6. Obtain oral suction in the case of retained fluid or inability to clear secretions during the procedure.

EQUIPMENT

1. Upper endoscope
2. 450 cm, 0.035 inch guidewire or Savary wire
3. Biliary extraction balloon catheter
4. Fluoroscopy. However, in the hands of experienced endoscopists, stents can be placed safely without fluoroscopy[2,9]
5. Esophageal SEMS (available in lengths ranging from 6 to 15 cm)
6. Water-soluble contrast
7. Radio-opaque marker to mark proximal and distal end of the esophageal stricture
8. Leaded aprons for radiation safety
9. Radiation dosage badges for personnel
10. Lubricant
11. Gloves

PROCEDURE

1. Assessment and marking of the lesion. Perform a diagnostic upper endoscopy to assess lesion location and characteristics to determine the appropriate SEMS. If an obstructive lesion does not allow the passage of a standard adult endoscope,

a neonatal gastroscope can be used to traverse the stenosis. Alternatively, a guidewire and extraction balloon catheter can be passed across the lesion. The balloon can then be inflated and withdrawn until resistance is met, thereby defining the distal extent of the stricture. Balloon dilation of an esophageal stenosis can be performed to allow gastroscope passage; however, this may increase the risk of adverse events, particularly in malignant strictures. Since SEMS are placed under fluoroscopy, the proximal and distal extent (if possible) of the lesion should be marked with radio-opaque markers. We recommend placement of taped paperclips on the patient's skin to identify these landmarks. Alternatively, if the C-arm is not moved, the clips can be placed on the fluoroscopy screen.

2. Choosing the correct SEMS. Ideally, the correct esophageal SEMS should aim to allow for a minimum of 2 cm on both the proximal and distal extent of the straddled lesion after stent foreshortening (if applicable).[1] The endoscopist should be familiar with the concept of foreshortening. Foreshortening occurs with braided/woven SEMS during deployment and expansion whereby the constrained stent length is up to 40% longer than the fully deployed length.[1] Laser-cut, non-foreshortening SEMS are available.

3. Placement of the stent delivery system. After marking the tumor, the endoscope is advanced into the stomach or proximal duodenum, and a long guidewire is passed and coiled in place. The endoscope is then withdrawn from the esophagus, leaving the guidewire in place (Fig. 13.1A). The patient's neck should be hyperextended (as possible) to allow for easy insertion of the stent delivery catheter. If the patient is intubated, and there is difficulty passing the stent delivery catheter, consider temporarily deflating the cuff on the endotracheal tube, which can often assist in passage. The stent introducer is then placed over the guidewire. Using the fluoroscopic markers for the proximal and distal ends of the stricture, position the fluoroscopic markers on the stent to allow for at least 2 cm on the proximal and distal end of the stricture. Alternatively, the endoscope can be replaced alongside the stent introducer to confirm positioning during deployment. Though there are individual differences based on the manufacturer, stent delivery systems usually entail a folded wire mesh stent that is compressed over a semirigid plastic catheter that can be introduced over a wire. The stent can be released from its compressed state by either withdrawing a plastic sheath housing the stent through various proprietary deployment mechanisms (Fig. 13.1B). The stent itself should be visible on fluoroscopy and should overlap both the proximal and distal markers of the tumor.

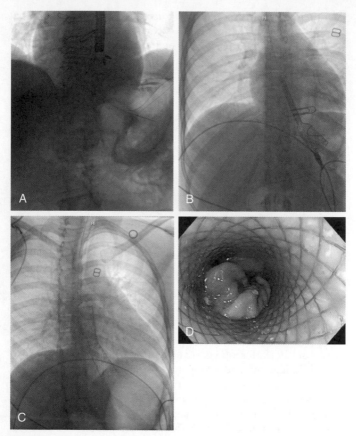

FIG. 13.1 A, Correct wire placement prior to stent placement (A) followed by initiation of the undeployed stent through lesion (B). The stent is then fully deployed (C) and the stent lumen inspected prior to procedure termination (D).

4. Stent deployment. After catheter positioning, the stent is then deployed distal to proximal, with the endoscopist continually monitoring deployment under fluoroscopy and/or endoscopy. When using woven stents, vigilant monitoring of stent deployment and expansion is necessary. Woven stents exhibit foreshortening (as mentioned above) which requires constant back tension on the delivery catheter during deployment to ensure correct placement. For many currently available stents, adjustments can be made to the stent position until a specified portion of the stent is deployed (i.e., point of no return); however, at that point the stent can no longer be reconstrained by the stent delivery system.

5. Withdrawal of the stent delivery system. Once the stent is fully deployed (Fig. 13.1C), the delivery system and guidewire can be removed. In cases with very tight strictures, care must be taken during removal of the delivery catheter. Fluoroscopic and/or endoscopic monitoring of the stent while removing the delivery system will minimize the risk of stent displacement (Fig. 13.1D). Rarely, the catheter tip can catch at the stricture, thereby increasing the risk for stent dislodgement.

POSTPROCEDURE

1. Vital signs should be monitored after the procedure. Depending on the stricture, some patients may have pain after the stent placement.
2. The head of the bed should be elevated and consider starting proton pump inhibitor if the stent crosses the gastroesophageal junction as patients will be at risk for reflux.
3. The patient should be instructed on care of the stent, mainly regarding dietary discretion. Patients should avoid difficult-to-digest and high-residue foods and lying supine or bending over after eating. Consideration should be given to sleeping with the head of the bed elevated.
4. The patient should return if there is rapid onset of dysphagia, hematemesis, melena, dyspnea, or marked chest pain.

ADVERSE EVENTS

It is important for the endoscopist to be aware of stent-related adverse events, including pain, bleeding, migration of the stents, perforations, or the onset of esophageal fistula with an overall mortality rate of 2.2%.[10] These adverse events can occur early (within 1 week) or late (after 1 week).[1,10-12]

1. Chest pain (5% with severe pain)
2. Perforation (5%)[13]
3. Bleeding (3% to 5%)
4. Tumor ingrowth (4%)
5. Gastroesophageal reflux (1% severe reflux)
6. Compromise of the respiratory system (0.1%)
7. Aspiration (5%)
8. Stent migration (20%): stent migration occurs in about 20% of patient and can often occur with noncircumferential esophageal tumors or if the caliber of the stent is too small.[1] A migrated stent can be difficult to remove endoscopically depending on the patients anatomy. Suturing of the stent in place can reduce stent migration.[14]

9. Esophageal fistula formation (5%): Fistula can be esophago-respiratory fistula or fistula between the aorta, mediastinum, or pleura.[1] These fistula form due to infiltration of the tumor or effects from radiation therapy. In cases of esophagorespiratory fistula, an uncovered esophageal stent is recommended, but bronchoscopy prior to second stent placement is recommended for placement of a tracheal stent. Tracheal stents may be needed prior to esophageal stenting of esophagorespiratory fistula to avoid acute respiratory failure.[15]

References

1. Chandrasekhara V, Elmunzer BJ, Khashab M, et al. *Clinical Gastrointestinal Endoscopy* . Philadelphia, PA: Elsevier; 2018.
2. Spaander MCW, Baron TH, Siersema PD, et al. Esophageal stenting for benign and malignant disease: European Society of Gastrointestinal Endoscopy (ESGE) clinical guideline. *Endoscopy*. 2016;48:939-948.
3. Fuccio L, Hassan C, Frazzoni L, et al. Clinical outcomes following stent placement in refractory benign esophageal stricture: a systematic review and meta-analysis. *Endoscopy*. 2016;48:141-148.
4. Repici A, Small AJ, Mendelson A, et al. Natural history and management of refractory benign esophageal strictures. *Gastrointest Endosc*. 2016;84:222-228.
5. Hirdes MMC, Siersema PD, van Boeckel PGA, et al. Single and sequential biodegradable stent placement for refractory benign esophageal strictures: a prospective follow-up study. *Endoscopy*. 2012;44:649-654.
6. Bethge N, Sommer A, Vakil N. Treatment of esophageal fistulas with a new polyurethane-covered, self-expanding mesh stent: a prospective study. *Am J Gastroenterol*. 1995;90:2143-2146.
7. Escorsell À, Pavel O, Cárdenas A, et al. Esophageal balloon tamponade versus esophageal stent in controlling acute refractory variceal bleeding: a multicenter randomized, controlled trial. *Hepatology*. 2016;63:1957-1967.
8. Escorsell À, Bosch J. Self-expandable metal stents in the treatment of acute esophageal variceal bleeding. *Gastroenterol Res Pract*. 2011;2011:910986-6.
9. Austin AS, Khan Z, Cole AT, et al. Placement of esophageal self-expanding metallic stents without fluoroscopy. *Yale Model Gov Eur*. 2001;54:357-359.
10. Simmons DT, Baron TH. Endoluminal palliation. *Gastrointest Endosc Clin N Am*. 2005;15:467-484, viii.
11. Homs MYV, Steyerberg EW, Eijkenboom WMH, et al. Single-dose brachytherapy versus metal stent placement for the palliation of dysphagia from oesophageal cancer: multicentre randomised trial. *Lancet*. 2004;364:1497-1504.
12. van Heel NCM, Haringsma J, Spaander MCW, et al. Short-term esophageal stenting in the management of benign perforations. *Am J Gastroenterol*. 2010;105:1515-1520.
13. Baron TH. Minimizing endoscopic complications: endoluminal stents. *Gastrointest Endosc Clin N Am*. 2007;17:83-104, vii.
14. Law R, Prabhu A, Fujii-Lau L, et al. Stent migration following endoscopic suture fixation of esophageal self-expandable metal stents: a systematic review and meta-analysis. *Surg Endosc*. 2018;32:675-681.
15. May A, Ell C. Palliative treatment of malignant esophagorespiratory fistulas with Gianturco-Z stents. A prospective clinical trial and review of the literature on covered metal stents. *Am J Gastroenterol*. 1998;93:532-535.

PART THREE

Small Bowel Endoscopy Procedures

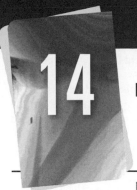

14

Push Enteroscopy

Michael D. Rice, MD
Andrew J. Read, MD

The small bowel is a difficult terrain to endoscopically examine due to its length, distensibility, and tortuosity. The length of the small bowel is highly variable and averages between 20 and 23 feet in the adult.[1-3] Small intestinal length is correlated with the height of the subject, and this variation may have an impact on enteroscopic procedural success.[4,5] Beyond the ligament of Treitz, the small bowel becomes freely mobile along the mesentery. This topography, along with the small bowel's active motility, poses challenges to the endoscopist seeking to navigate the depths of the small intestine.

For years, the available endoscopic tools limited small bowel evaluation to only its most proximal and distal segments. The large majority of the small bowel remained out of reach. In 1977, the Sonde enteroscope was introduced.[6] This long flexible fiberoptic enteroscope was inserted nasally and passively propelled by intestinal peristalsis to the terminal ileum. From there, the endoscopist was able to examine the small bowel during withdrawal. The procedure was time consuming, uncomfortable for patients, and did not permit biopsy or therapeutic maneuvers. At this time, Sonde enteroscopy is of historical interest only and no longer has a role in the evaluation of small bowel disorders.

In the early 1980s, a colonoscope was used to access the jejunum from an oral approach, allowing for biopsies and other therapeutic interventions.[7] Subsequently, dedicated push enteroscopes were developed, which permitted per-oral endoscopic access deeper into the winding and distensible small bowel.[8] The midjejunum (150 cm beyond the pylorus) could now be reached. This depth of insertion could modestly be extended with use of an overtube, although the diagnostic yield remains similar.[9-12] Push enteroscopy afforded the ability to perform diagnostic and therapeutic maneuvers available to the endoscopist via traditional esophagogastroduodenoscopy and colonoscopy. Push enteroscopy increased the diagnostic yield for occult bleeding to at least 38%.[13]

Intraoperative endoscopy (IOE) has permitted access to the small bowel via a per-oral, per-rectal, or a surgical enterostomy approach. In this setting, an endoscopist works with a surgeon who subsequently telescopes the small bowel over the endoscope. Intraoperative enteroscopy permits examination of the entire length of the small bowel in over 90% of cases and has a diagnostic yield for bleeding of approximately 79%.[14-16] It had previously been considered the gold standard for the diagnosis and management of small bowel conditions until recent years.

The noninvasive examination of the small bowel was revolutionized with the launch of video capsule endoscopy in 2001 following FDA approval.[17] Small bowel findings identified on video capsule endoscopy, distal to the reach of push enteroscopy, could be more readily reached following the introduction of the double-balloon enteroscope in 2004.[18,19] These new developments have increased the breadth of available tools in the endoscopic armamentarium to explore and treat small bowel disorders.

Despite these advances in endoscopic technology, the small bowel remains a challenging territory to endoscopically examine. Even though deeper insertion is possible with other tools, many small bowel pathologic findings are present within the proximal small bowel (duodenum to midjejunum) and remain within reach of push enteroscopy.[20] This chapter will focus on push enteroscopy evaluation of the small bowel.

PUSH ENTEROSCOPY

Indications

1. Diagnosis and/or therapy for suspected proximal small bowel bleeding
2. Overt gastrointestinal bleeding with a negative upper endoscopy and colonoscopy
3. Occult gastrointestinal bleeding or iron-deficiency anemia with a negative upper endoscopy and colonoscopy
4. Radiographic abnormalities found in the proximal and/or mid–small bowel
5. Evaluation of patients with polyposis syndrome
6. Placement of a percutaneous jejunostomy tube
7. Retrieval of foreign bodies
8. Access to altered anatomy (e.g., Whipple, Roux-en-Y gastric bypass, etc.)
9. Diagnosis and/or therapy for video capsule endoscopy findings in the proximal and/or mid–small bowel

Contraindications (Similar to Those of Upper Endoscopy)

Absolute

1. Bowel perforation, known or suspected
2. Bowel obstruction, known or suspected
3. Severe respiratory distress (unless the patient is on mechanical ventilation)
4. Atlanto-axial subluxation
5. Hemodynamic instability
6. Inability to provide adequate sedation

Relative

1. Uncooperative patient
2. Acute myocardial infarction
3. Small bowel ileus
4. Coagulopathy
   a. Elevated international normalized ratio (INR) > 1.5
   b. Partial thromboplastin time (PTT) 20 seconds over control
   c. Bleeding time > 10 minutes
   d. Platelet count < 50,000/mm^3

Equipment

1. A dedicated push enteroscope is available from various manufacturers, ranging in length from 200 to 250 cm, with an external diameter of 10.5 to 11.7 mm.[15] When a dedicated enteroscope is not available, a pediatric colonoscope may be substituted. Dedicated overtubes are also available for push enteroscopes[12]
2. Light source and video system
3. Air and water supply. Carbon dioxide insufflation may improve tolerability, where available[21]
4. Surgical lubricating jelly, gloves, eye protection, gown, shoe covers, and washcloth or gauze
5. 60-mL syringe for flushes, biopsy forceps, electrocautery equipment (argon plasma coagulation [APC], where available, if bleeding is an indication), epinephrine injection, glucagon
6. Continuous electrocardiogram, pulse oximetry monitoring, and consideration of continuous waveform capnography monitoring (especially if deeper sedation is planned, e.g., with propofol)[22]

Preparation (Similar to Upper Endoscopy)

1. Have the patient fast, a minimum of 2 hours from clear liquid ingestion and 6 hours from a light meal.[22]
2. Diagnostic push enteroscopy is considered a low-risk endoscopy procedure from a bleeding standpoint. However, if therapeutic interventions are planned, then it is important to

discontinue anticoagulation or dual antiplatelet therapy per periprocedural anticoagulation guidelines and in consultation with a patient's cardiologist or hematologist, where applicable.[23]

3. Informed consent should be performed in writing prior to initiation of the procedure.

4. Place an intravenous line for administration of sedation.

5. Antibiotic indications are the same as for upper endoscopy and are not routinely indicated.[24]

6. Sedation medications: typically, a combination of midazolam and fentanyl for moderate sedation.[22] Alternatively, where available, monitored anesthesia care with deeper sedation may be advantageous, given a typically longer procedure than standard upper endoscopy and increased stimulation with deeper small bowel insertion.

7. Position the patient in the left lateral decubitus position, as in standard upper endoscopy. Place a bite guard to protect the scope and patient's teeth.

8. If overtube use is planned, this should be back-loaded on the scope prior to insertion.[12]

Procedure

1. Gently flex the patient's head anteriorly toward the chest prior to insertion of the enteroscope. Under direct endoscopic visualization, pass the enteroscope over the patient's tongue and across the epiglottis to the cricopharyngeus muscle. With gentle pressure, traverse the upper esophageal sphincter and closely examine the esophagus and stomach.

2. It is essential to perform a careful diagnostic examination of the esophagus and stomach, including a retroflexed view of the cardia and fundus, prior to advancing the enteroscope into the small bowel. Once advanced into the small bowel, the enteroscope will invariably loop within the stomach and may cause superficial mucosal injury or "scope trauma," which may be difficult to differentiate between an underlying gastropathy or erosion if the mucosa had not been examined first. Pay particular attention to the presence of varices, Cameron's erosions, or ulcers and the presence of gastric antral vascular ectasia, as these diagnoses are often overlooked but may explain iron-deficiency anemia or melena.

3. Use of an overtube may reduce significant gastric looping and potentially allow for deeper small bowel insertion but with minimal incremental diagnostic yield.[9-12] If using an overtube, it is imperative to inspect for any esophageal strictures or varices that may be present prior to passage of an

overtube. If there is any concern that the overtube cannot safely be advanced, then the scope can be withdrawn, the overtube removed, and the scope reinserted without an overtube to complete the examination.

4. Prior to entering the small intestine, it is often helpful to attempt to shorten or straighten the enteroscope, which can be accomplished by desufflation or suctioning air from the stomach and pulling back with the enteroscope.

5. Once in the duodenum, the enteroscope should be slowly advanced, with keeping the scope tip centered within the lumen. Unlike colonoscopy, there is often significantly more visualized motility and thus successful enteroscopy is a much more dynamic process. A gastric loop will form almost immediately, which can often be reduced with gentle advancement and slight withdrawal. Gentle insufflation is necessary for adequate visualization but avoid excess insufflation which, as in colonoscopy, will make insertion more difficult and make the patient uncomfortable. When available, the use of carbon dioxide insufflation instead of room air may improve patient comfort during and after the procedure.[21]

6. Inspection of the mucosa should be done during intubation as well as during withdrawal of the endoscope. Small bowel pathology often lurks behind folds.

7. Intravenous (IV) glucagon (0.5 to 1 mg) may be given to reduce small bowel motility and improve mucosal examination. However, the timing of administration should be carefully selected, since IV glucagon has a very short half-life.

8. Working channels are present for diagnostic biopsies and therapeutic hemostasis. Cautery should be performed at lower energy settings because of the thinner wall of the small intestine. APC can be used for noncontact treatment of small bowel angioectasias.

9. Gastric and small bowel loops may cause difficulty in passing instruments through the channel. Early insertion of the biopsy forceps or heater probe into the scope prior to intubation of the small bowel may prevent this situation. In addition, "shortening" of the enteroscope prior to passing instruments may also help. Shortening occurs by pulling the enteroscope back and thus removing redundant loops while maintaining deep intubation.

10. Estimating the true depth of insertion is difficult because of looping, which occurs in the small bowel and stomach. If no pathology is found on this examination and there is concern for more distal small bowel pathology, a submucosal tattoo

can be placed to mark the distal extent of the examination, which provides a reference point for future video capsule endoscopy or device-assisted enteroscopy.

11. Average procedure time should be longer than a routine upper endoscopy and is dependent on the presence of interventions.

12. Diagnostic yield is dependent on the indication for the procedure. Push enteroscopy has a yield of approximately 40% to 60% for obscure gastrointestinal bleeding, 41% to 78% for abnormal radiographic studies, 6% to 42% for iron-deficiency anemia, and 0% to 45% for chronic diarrhea. Chronic abdominal pain and nonspecific anemia have yields of ≤ 25%.[25]

Adverse Events[13,25-29]

1. Discomfort
2. Bleeding (<1%)
3. Perforation (<1%)
4. Aspiration
5. Medication reactions
6. Mucosal damage
7. Oversedation
8. Hypotension
9. Tachycardia
10. Procedure intolerance
11. Hypoxia
12. Drug reaction
13. Major adverse events, which include perforation, bleeding, infection, and significant cardiovascular collapse such as arrhythmias and shock, may occur in 0.64% to 1% of procedures
14. Other adverse events reported in the literature, such as mucosal stripping, acute pancreatitis, and pharyngeal tears, are very rare and have been related to the use of the stiffening overtube

INTRAOPERATIVE ENTEROSCOPY

Historically, intraoperative enteroscopy has been the most complete method of evaluating the small intestine. All patients undergoing this procedure should have had an extensive negative standard workup, including a negative push enteroscopy and capsule endoscopy. Now, with deep enteroscopy using device-assisted enteroscopy (single- and double-balloon enteroscopy or spiral enteroscopy), intraoperative enteroscopy is used less frequently.[14] Nevertheless, in selected circumstances, it remains an important tool.

Procedure

1. An open laparotomy is the most common surgical procedure, and the surgeon should perform a meticulous inspection of the entire gastrointestinal tract at that time. If gross inspection does not localize a lesion, a total small bowel enteroscopy is performed in a darkened room to better define vascular lesions through transillumination of the bowel by the enteroscope light source.

2. A standard push enteroscope is often the best instrument for this procedure. The enteroscope is commonly introduced by the mouth (as in standard push enteroscopy technique) but can also be introduced via a surgical enterotomy or from the anus.[14] Carbon dioxide insufflation is preferred. Once in the stomach, the surgeon slowly guides the bowel over the scope. An assistant isolates a 15-cm segment of the bowel and pinches the distal portion, trapping air within the segment and allowing careful mucosal inspection by the gastroenterologist without overdistention (air trapping technique).

3. Use of longer enteroscopes may allow for complete visualization of the entire small bowel from oral intubation. If length or extensive air trapping hampers complete visualization of the small bowel from the oral route, retrograde views of the distal ileum via anal intubation should be performed.

4. Unlike standard endoscopy procedures, careful mucosal examination is performed during intubation because trauma (tactile and endoscopic) will be induced during endoscope insertion and bowel manipulation. Regions of iatrogenic trauma should not be mistaken for the etiology of the bleeding during withdrawal of the endoscope.

5. Adverse events are significant with overall morbidity of 18% (most adverse event of postoperative ileus) and overall mortality of 5% (often secondary to GI bleeding recurrence or sepsis).[14] Interpretation of these statistics is difficult, however, as there may be some selection bias among patients undergoing IOE, as they have already demonstrated themselves to have bleeding not identified by more traditional testing.

6. Diagnostic yields for diagnosing small bowel bleeding are approximately 79%.[14,16] However, given the associated morbidity and mortality and potential alternate diagnostic tools available, intraoperative enteroscopy should be used in only highly selected cases.

CPT CODES[15]

44360—Small intestinal endoscopy, enteroscopy beyond second portion of duodenum, not including ileum; diagnostic, with or without collection of specimen(s) by brushing or washing (separate procedure)

44361—Small intestinal endoscopy, enteroscopy beyond second portion of duodenum, not including ileum; with biopsy, single or multiple

44363—Small intestinal endoscopy, enteroscopy beyond second portion of duodenum, not including ileum; with removal of foreign body

44364—Small intestinal endoscopy, enteroscopy beyond second portion of duodenum, not including ileum; with removal of tumor(s), polyp(s), or other lesion(s) by snare technique

44365—Small intestinal endoscopy, enteroscopy beyond second portion of duodenum, not including ileum; with removal of tumor(s), polyp(s), or other lesion(s) by hot biopsy forceps or bipolar cautery

44366—Small intestinal endoscopy, enteroscopy beyond second portion of duodenum, not including ileum; with control of bleeding, any method

44369—Small intestinal endoscopy, enteroscopy beyond second portion of duodenum, not including ileum; with ablation of tumor(s), polyp(s), or other lesion(s) not amenable to removal by hot biopsy forceps, bipolar cautery, or snare technique

44370—Small intestinal endoscopy, enteroscopy beyond second portion of duodenum, not including ileum; with transendoscopic stent placement (includes predilation)

44372—Small intestinal endoscopy, enteroscopy beyond second portion of duodenum, not including ileum; with placement of percutaneous jejunostomy tube

44373—Small intestinal endoscopy, enteroscopy beyond second portion of duodenum, not including ileum; with conversion of percutaneous gastrostomy tube to percutaneous jejunostomy tube

44380—Ileoscopy, through stoma; diagnostic, with or without collection of specimen(s) by brushing or washing (separate procedure)

44382—Ileoscopy, through stoma; with biopsy, single or multiple

References

1. Fanucci A, Cerro P, Fraracci L, Ietto F. Small bowel length measured by radiography. *Gastrointest Radiol.* 1984;9(4):349-351.
2. Nightingale JM, Bartram CI, Lennard-Jones JE. Length of residual small bowel after partial resection: correlation between radiographic and surgical measurements. *Gastrointest Radiol.* 1991;16(4):305-306.
3. Treves F. Lectures on the anatomy of the intestinal canal and peritoneum in man. *Br Med J.* 1885;1(1262):470-474.
4. Underhill BM. Intestinal length in man. *Br Med J.* 1955;2(4950):1243-1246.
5. Raines D, Arbour A, Thompson HW, Figueroa-Bodine J, Joseph S. Variation in small bowel length: factor in achieving total enteroscopy? *Dig Endosc.* 2015;27(1):67-72.

6. Tada M, Akasaka Y, Misaki F, Kwaie K. Clinical evaluation of a sonde-type small intestinal fiberscope. *Endoscopy.* 1977;9(1):33-38.

7. Parker HW, Agayoff JD. Enteroscopy and small bowel biopsy utilizing a peroral colonoscope. *Gastrointest Endosc.* 1983;29(2):139-140.

8. Davies GR, Benson MJ, Gertner DJ, Van Someren RM, Rampton DS, Swain CP. Diagnostic and therapeutic push type enteroscopy in clinical use. *Gut.* 1995;37(3):346-352.

9. Keizman D, Brill S, Umansky M, et al. Diagnostic yield of routine push enteroscopy with a graded-stiffness enteroscope without overtube. *Gastrointest Endosc.* 2003;57(7):877-881.

10. Benz C, Jakobs R, Riemann JF. Do we need the overtube for push-enteroscopy? *Endoscopy.* 2001;33(8):658-661.

11. Taylor AC, Chen RY, Desmond PV. Use of an overtube for enteroscopy–does it increase depth of insertion? A prospective study of enteroscopy with and without an overtube. *Endoscopy.* 2001;33(3):227-230.

12. Tierney WM, Adler DG, Conway JD, et al. Overtube use in gastrointestinal endoscopy. *Gastrointest Endosc.* 2009;70(5):828-834.

13. Wilmer A, Rutgeerts P. Push enteroscopy. Technique, depth, and yield of insertion. *Gastrointest Endosc Clin N Am.* 1996;6(4):759-776.

14. Voron T, Rahmi G, Bonnet S, et al. Intraoperative enteroscopy: is there still a role? *Gastrointest Endosc Clin N Am.* 2017;27(1):153-170.

15. Chauhan SS, Manfredi MA, Abu Dayyeh BK, et al. Enteroscopy. *Gastrointest Endosc.* 2015;82(6):975-990.

16. Monsanto P, Almeida N, Lerias C, Figueiredo P, Gouveia H, Sofia C. Is there still a role for intraoperative enteroscopy in patients with obscure gastrointestinal bleeding?. *Rev Esp Enferm Dig.* 2012;104(4):190-196.

17. Iddan G, Meron G, Glukhovsky A, Swain P. Wireless capsule endoscopy. *Nature.* 2000;405(6785):417.

18. Yamamoto H, Sekine Y, Sato Y, et al. Total enteroscopy with a nonsurgical steerable double-balloon method. *Gastrointest Endosc.* 2001;53(2):216-220.

19. Yamamoto H, Kita H. Double-balloon endoscopy: from concept to reality. *Gastrointest Endosc Clin N Am.* 2006;16(2):347-361.

20. Matsumoto T, Moriyama T, Esaki M, Nakamura S, Iida M. Performance of antegrade double-balloon enteroscopy: comparison with push enteroscopy. *Gastrointest Endosc.* 2005;62(3):392-398.

21. Lo SK, Fujii-Lau LL, Enestvedt BK, et al. The use of carbon dioxide in gastrointestinal endoscopy. *Gastrointest Endosc.* 2016;83(5):857-865.

22. Early DS, Lightdale JR, Vargo JJ II, et al. Guidelines for sedation and anesthesia in GI endoscopy. *Gastrointest Endosc.* 2018;87(2):327-337.

23. Acosta RD, Abraham NS, Chandrasekhara V, et al. The management of antithrombotic agents for patients undergoing GI endoscopy. *Gastrointest Endosc.* 2016;83(1):3-16.

24. Khashab MA, Chithadi KV, Acosta RD, et al. Antibiotic prophylaxis for GI endoscopy. *Gastrointest Endosc.* 2015;81(1):81-89.

25. Lin S, Branch MS, Shetzline M. The importance of indication in the diagnostic value of push enteroscopy. *Endoscopy.* 2003;35(4):315-321.

26. Chavalitdhamrong D, Adler DG, Draganov PV. Complications of enteroscopy: how to avoid them and manage them when they arise. *Gastrointest Endosc Clin N Am.* 2015;25(1):83-95.

27. Ben-Menachem T, Decker GA, Early DS, et al. Adverse events of upper GI endoscopy. *Gastrointest Endosc.* 2012;76(4):707-718.

28. Levy I, Gralnek IM. Complications of diagnostic colonoscopy, upper endoscopy, and enteroscopy. *Best Pract Res Clin Gastroenterol.* 2016;30(5):705-718.

29. Yang R, Laine L. Mucosal stripping: a complication of push enteroscopy. *Gastrointest Endosc.* 1995;41(2):156-158.

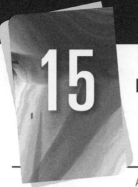

Deep Enteroscopy

Andrew J. Read, MD
Ryan Law, DO
Michael D. Rice, MD

Evaluation of the small bowel is difficult to endoscopically examine due to its length, distensibility, and tortuosity. Early methods for endoscopic evaluation of the small bowel were limited by efficacy. Push enteroscopy, as previously discussed, is suitable for evaluation of the proximal small bowel and distal ileum but is insufficient in visualizing the majority of the jejunum and more proximal ileum. To address this concern, Yamamoto el al. began to develop techniques for device-assisted enteroscopy which permitted evaluation of the entire small bowel and allowed for therapeutic intervention, if necessary. Currently, systems for single-balloon enteroscopy (SBE), double-balloon enteroscopy (DBE), and spiral enteroscopy exist. Use of these techniques is cumbersome, time-consuming, and require special training to perform. Furthermore, each platform includes dedicated equipment, both capital and disposable. This chapter will discuss single-balloon, double-balloon, and spiral enteroscopy including indications, contraindications, and the technical aspects of performing the procedure.

INDICATIONS

1. Diagnosis and/or therapy for suspected proximal small bowel bleeding
2. Overt gastrointestinal bleeding with a negative upper endoscopy and colonoscopy
3. Occult gastrointestinal bleeding or iron-deficiency anemia with a negative upper endoscopy and colonoscopy
4. Radiographic abnormalities found in the middle to distal small bowel
5. Evaluation of patients with polyposis syndrome
6. Placement of a percutaneous jejunostomy tube
7. Retrieval of foreign bodies

8. Access to altered anatomy (e.g., Whipple, Roux-en-Y gastric bypass, etc.)
9. Diagnosis and/or therapy for video capsule endoscopy findings in the middle to distal small bowel

CONTRAINDICATIONS (SIMILAR TO THOSE OF UPPER ENDOSCOPY)
Absolute
1. Bowel perforation, known or suspected
2. Bowel obstruction, known or suspected
3. Severe respiratory distress (unless the patient is on mechanical ventilation)
4. Atlantoaxial subluxation
5. Hemodynamic instability
6. Inability to provide adequate sedation

Relative
1. Uncooperative patient
2. Acute myocardial infarction
3. Small bowel ileus
4. Latex allergy. The balloons contain latex and thus DBE is contraindicated in severely latex allergic patients. Alternative procedures such as SBE, which are latex free, or premedication should be considered in consultation with anesthesia and/or allergy
5. Coagulopathy
   a. Elevated international normalized ratio (INR) >1.5
   b. Partial thromboplastin time (PTT) 20 seconds over control
   c. Bleeding time >10 minutes
   d. Platelet count <50,000/mL

EQUIPMENT
1. A dedicated SBE endoscope, 200 cm length with 2.8 mm working channel, and a corresponding overtube (13.2 mm outer diameter) **OR** DBE enteroscope, 180 to 230 cm length with a working channel ranging from 2.2 mm (pediatric) to 3.2 mm (therapeutic), and a corresponding overtube (range 12.2 to 13.2 mm outer diameter) **OR** spiral overtube, 118 cm length (22 cm spiral segment and 92 cm working length) with 48F (16 mm) outer diameter, including the locking coupler, green rotational handgrip, and spiral element. The 22 cm spiral segment is 70 cm distal to the green rotation handle. The spiral overtube does not contain latex. (The spiral overtube is intended to be used with 200 cm long enteroscopes with outer diameters between 9.1 and 9.5 mm.)

2. Light source and video system.
3. Balloon control unit.
4. Water supply and carbon dioxide insufflation. Carbon dioxide is highly recommended over room air for improved patient comfort and recovery, given extended duration of deep enteroscopy procedures.
5. Surgical lubricating jelly, gloves, eye protection, gown, shoe covers, and washcloth or gauze.
6. 60-mL syringe for flushes, biopsy forceps, electrocautery equipment (argon plasma coagulation (APC), where available, if bleeding is an indication), hemostatic clips, epinephrine injection, and glucagon.
7. Continuous electrocardiogram, pulse oximetry monitoring, and consideration of continuous waveform capnography monitoring.

PREPARATION

1. For an antegrade deep enteroscopy, we typically use 2L polyethylene glycol (PEG) electrolyte solution, taken the evening before the procedure. For a retrograde approach, an excellent colonic bowel preparation is required to maximize technical success of this procedure, and we typically use a 2-day bowel preparation with 6-8L of PEG solution.
2. Patients should fast a minimum of 2 hours from clear liquid ingestion and 6 hours from a light meal.
3. Therapeutic procedures are considered increased risk from a bleeding standpoint, and thus it is important to discontinue anticoagulation or dual antiplatelet therapy per periprocedural anticoagulation guidelines and in consultation with a patient's cardiologist or hematologist, where applicable.
4. Informed consent should be performed in writing prior to initiation of the procedure.
5. Place an intravenous line for administration of sedation.
6. Antibiotic indications are the same as for standard upper endoscopy or colonoscopy.
7. Sedation: Individual anesthesia plan is developed in conjunction with the anesthesia team based on the procedure and the patient's comorbidities. For antegrade procedures, we typically perform the procedure under general anesthesia with endotracheal intubation, but monitored anesthesia care could be considered. For retrograde procedures, we typically utilize monitored anesthesia care.
8. Position the patient in the left lateral decubitus position, as in standard upper endoscopy. Place a bite guard to protect the scope and patient's teeth for antegrade procedures.

9. The appropriate overtube should be back-loaded on the endoscope prior to insertion. The balloon should be installed and tested prior to insertion.

10. A trained assistant familiar with the deep enteroscopy technique is necessary.

11. Appropriate consent, protective radiation gowns, and shields should be available if fluoroscopy is used. Fluoroscopy for deep enteroscopy is rarely necessary.

SINGLE-BALLOON ENTEROSCOPY PROCEDURE

1. Antegrade SBE insertion: Gently flex the patient's head anteriorly prior to insertion of the enteroscope. The enteroscope is passed over the patient's tongue and across the epiglottis to the cricopharyngeus muscle. The upper esophageal sphincter is traversed, and the esophagus and stomach are closely examined.

2. After excluding esophageal varices, the overtube is advanced. If there is concern that the overtube cannot safely be advanced, either due to varices or mechanical stenosis, then the scope can be withdrawn, the overtube removed, and the scope reinserted without an overtube to address the source of obstruction.

3. A careful diagnostic examination of the esophagus and stomach, including a retroflexed view of the cardia and fundus, should be performed prior to advancing the enteroscope into the small bowel. Assess for the presence of varices, Cameron erosions/ulcers, and gastric antral vascular ectasia (GAVE). These can be overlooked but may explain iron-deficiency anemia or melena. "Scope trauma," or superficial mucosal injury, occurs frequently with device-assisted enteroscopy technique than with standard upper endoscopy or push enteroscopy.

4. The enteroscope should be shortened or straightened prior to entering the small bowel. This occurs by suctioning air from the stomach while gently withdrawing the enteroscope.

5. Small bowel insertion: The endoscope and overtube are advanced in a technique similar to push enteroscopy (see separate chapter) into the proximal jejunum. Prior to inflation of the balloon, it is important to ensure that the ampulla has been traversed to minimize potential balloon trauma in this region, thus mitigating the risk of pancreatitis.

6. Balloon basics: As there is only one balloon in SBE (present on the overtube), knowledge of balloon status (inflated/deflated) is simplified, and the mechanics are less complicated compared to DBE. However, the absence of a second balloon may lead to difficulty with enteroscope advancement and reduction.

7. Insertion technique: Once in the small intestine, the enteroscope is advanced to the point of maximal insertion. Anchoring is achieved by deflection of the endoscope tip toward the wall (in a hooking technique) and/or with use of continuous suction, as the overtube is advanced. Once both are maximally inserted, the overtube balloon is inflated, and the overtube and enteroscope are withdrawn together, while keeping the endoscope tip deflected in angled fashion to maintain positioning. This withdrawal aims to pleat the small bowel over the overtube. The scope is then advanced with the overtube balloon inflated, and the process is repeated as a cycle until the point of maximal insertion is reached.

8. Inspection of the mucosa should be done during intubation as well as during withdrawal of the endoscope. Frequent small bowel contractions may make visualization difficult. Intravenous (IV) glucagon (0.5 to 1 mg) may be given to reduce small bowel motility and improve mucosal examination. Care should be taken to look behind folds for small bowel pathology.

9. A working channel is present for diagnostic biopsies and therapeutic hemostasis. Cautery should be performed at lower energy settings because of the thinner wall of the small intestine. APC can be used for noncontact thermal treatment of small bowel angioectasias.

10. Retrograde SBE insertion: Insertion technique is similar to colonoscopy. The balloon can be utilized within the colon to aide in the colonoscopy. The most challenging part of the retrograde SBE procedure is terminal ileal intubation, which must be performed with the endoscope (as in ileocolonoscopy) and the overtube. To maximize the chance of success, reducing the enteroscope on insertion can help minimize looping. Once both the enteroscope and overtube are within the small intestine, the procedure progresses using the same technique as outlined above for antegrade SBE.

DOUBLE-BALLOON ENTEROSCOPY PROCEDURE

1. The initial steps of DBE parallel those of SBE above.

2. Balloon basics: Knowledge of balloon status (inflated/deflated) is essential at all times and can be readily assessed by the on-screen display. It is also critically important to pay attention to the position of the enteroscope relative to the overtube: a solid white line indicates the position on the enteroscope which cannot be withdrawn further (in relation to the overtube) and at which the overtube should not be inserted further—moving beyond this line risks shearing the balloons. With insertion, you should never advance either

component (endoscope or overtube) with the corresponding balloon inflated. Similarly, after the proximal small intestine, it is important to always have at least one balloon inflated at all times, as deflating both balloons risks significant loss of scope position.

3. Push-pull technique of insertion: Once in the small intestine distal to the ligament of Treitz, the two balloons can be used, in a series of maneuvers to allow for deeper insertion within the small bowel. The overtube balloon can be inflated ("overtube up"), providing relative stability within the small intestine, and then the enteroscope (with the balloon deflated) can be advanced through the overtube. Once advanced to the maximal position, the enteroscope balloon is inflated ("scope up") and the overtube balloon is deflated ("overtube down"). The assistant then advances the overtube, stopping at the solid white line. Next, the overtube balloon is inflated ("overtube up"), with both balloons inflated simultaneously. In this position, the endoscopist can now grasp the overtube and enteroscope together and gently withdraw them, reducing the formed loops by pleating the small bowel over the overtube or functionally shortening the small bowel. This process should be stopped when the endoscopist begins to encounter resistance or if the balloon pressure alarm sounds (Note: this alarm occurs frequently with deeper insertion and should be acknowledged on the control panel and then can proceed with the procedure). The length (distance in centimeters) of this reduction can be recorded by a second assistant and summed to estimate depth of insertion, although these do not represent exact distances, due to frequent slippage with reductions. Next, the enteroscope balloon can be deflated ("scope down") and insertion can proceed. This process is then repeated until the desired end point is reached (e.g., known pathology from a capsule study or CT scan), the cecum, or the point at which additional reductions do not yield additional advancement (due to increased looping, slippage, etc.). The point of maximal insertion can be marked with a submucosal tattoo if subsequent retrograde DBE is being considered.

4. Withdrawal technique: The withdrawal technique is essentially a reverse of the insertion technique. First, with the overtube balloon inflated ("overtube up") and the enteroscope balloon deflated ("scope down"), the enteroscope is withdrawn to the maximal point of withdrawal in relation to the overtube (as marked by the solid white line). In this position, the enteroscope balloon is inflated ("scope up") and the overtube balloon is deflated ("balloon down"), followed by the assistant's slow withdrawal of the overtube (with counter

pressure provided by the endoscopist). Next, the overtube balloon is again inflated ("overtube up") and the enteroscope balloon is deflated ("scope down"), and the withdrawal process resumes once again. As the endoscope/overtube near the proximal small intestine, both balloons should be deflated and the combined enteroscope/overtube withdrawn, as in push enteroscopy technique, to minimize potential balloon trauma in the region of the ampulla.

5. Inspection of the mucosa should be done during intubation as well as during withdrawal of the enteroscope, as mentioned above.

6. Working channels are present for diagnostic biopsies and therapeutic hemostasis, as mentioned above. A stiffening wire is available which can aid in insertion but should be used cautiously in the setting of prior surgeries or adhesions, given increased stiffness of the enteroscope. In addition, as there is only one working channel, the stiffening wire must be withdrawn prior to insertion of a therapeutic tool.

7. Retrograde DBE insertion: Insertion technique is similar to colonoscopy. The balloons can be utilized within the colon (using the standard antegrade DBE insertion technique) to aid in the colonoscopy. Similar to retrograde SBE, the most difficult aspect of retrograde DBE procedure is terminal ileal intubation, which must also be performed with the enteroscope and the overtube. The same techniques from SBE can be applied to DBE. With the overtube balloon inflated in the ascending colon ("balloon up") and the endoscope balloon deflated ("balloon down"), the tip of the endoscope can be advanced in the direction of the ileocecal (IC) valve. As in standard ileocolonoscopy, intubation of the IC valve can be aided by positioning the IC valve in approximately the 6 o'clock position. Once the enteroscope is advanced into the terminal ileum at the maximal position, the enteroscope balloon should be inflated ("scope up") to help anchor the enteroscope within the small bowel. Next, the overtube balloon can be deflated ("balloon down"), and the overtube can be advanced (using the same antegrade DBE technique as above). Once in the small bowel, the overtube balloon can again be inflated ("overtube up"). Depending on the scope/balloon positions at this stage, an additional insertion maneuver with the enteroscope balloon down ("scope down") may be needed to prevent slippage out of the small bowel on reduction. Once both the enteroscope and overtube balloons are relatively stable within the small intestine, the entire process can proceed following the same DBE push and pull technique as described in the antegrade DBE insertion technique.

SPIRAL ENTEROSCOPY

Special Preparation

1. Please see preparation above for DBE for basic preparation.
2. Prior to attaching the spiral overtube onto the enteroscope, liberally apply at least 1 oz of the recommended lubricant (or K-Y Jelly) inside the overtube. Lubrication can be reapplied through the injection port during the procedure as needed. Cover both ends of the overtube and shake back and forth to distribute the lubricant within the tube's entire length. Then lubricate the outside of the enteroscope prior to inserting it into the overtube. While advancing the enteroscope into the overtube, slowly rotate the overtube while covering its distal end to retain the lubricant. Once the enteroscope is inserted into the overtube, slide it back and forth to confirm sufficient lubrication.
3. Position the spiral overtube over the enteroscope so that its proximal end is at the 140 cm gradation mark on the scope (which subsequently aligns the tip of the spiral component approximately 22 cm from the tip of the scope).
4. Lock the spiral overtube onto the enteroscope by turning the coupler on the proximal end of the overtube clockwise. This will couple the enteroscope to the overtube. It is recommended to take note of the centimeter mark on the enteroscope just proximal to the coupler for reference when uncoupling from and recoupling with the overtube during the procedure.

PROCEDURE—INSERTION

1. Liberally apply lubrication to the entire length of the overtube prior to insertion.
2. Antegrade spiral enteroscopy insertion: With the patient in the left lateral decubitus position, slightly extend the neck to facilitate a straight initial passage of the enteroscope–spiral overtube apparatus.
3. If the patient is receiving general anesthesia, it is recommended to deflate the endotracheal tube (ET) balloon during both initial insertion and removal of the spiral overtube to facilitate passage and minimize esophageal mucosal trauma.
4. Under direct endoscopic visualization, pass the enteroscope along the patient's tongue and across the epiglottis to the cricopharyngeus muscle. With gentle pressure and slow clockwise rotation, advance the spiral overtube through the esophagus. If the ET was deflated during overtube insertion, reinsufflate the ET tube after passage through the esophagus.

5. Careful examination of the esophagus and stomach should be performed prior to advancing the enteroscope into the duodenum. While following the lesser curvature of the stomach, continue slow clockwise rotation of the overtube to advance through the stomach.

6. In order to facilitate initial spiral engagement in the small bowel, it is recommended to minimize insufflation of the stomach. Decompress the stomach prior to advancement into the duodenum. Application of abdominal counter pressure to the greater curvature of the stomach can assist in engagement of the spiral segment in the small bowel.

7. Advance the coupled overtube and enteroscope with a slow gentle rotational pressure into the duodenum (or until rotation becomes difficult).

8. Gently pull back the overtube while rotating clockwise (Cantero maneuver) to reduce any looping in the stomach, and create a straight position of the enteroscope overtube.

9. After engaging the spirals in the duodenum, spiral enteroscopy can begin.

PROCEDURE—SPIRAL ENTEROSCOPY TECHNIQUE

1. To rotationally advance the spiral apparatus deeper into the small bowel, rotate the overtube at a modest rate to pleat the small bowel over the overtube.

2. Perform examination of the small bowel during advancement of the spiral enteroscope.

3. While minimizing air insufflation, use gentle traction to facilitate spiral advancement. Irrigate with water to improve small bowel visualization.

4. Keep the scope short and straight to limit enteroscope looping.

5. Should advancement begin to slow down, a loop may have formed. Attempt to reduce the loop with a counterclockwise rotation while applying gentle traction to facilitate paradoxical advancement.

6. Never force rotation of the overtube. Should significant resistance be met, discontinue the maneuver.

7. Do not advance the locked overtube if the small bowel lumen cannot be clearly visualized.

8. Once rotational advancement becomes ineffective, a "hook and suction" maneuver can be performed to attempt to maximize depth of insertion. This is performed by unlocking the spiral overtube, pushing the enteroscope through the overtube (additional lubrication may be necessary), "hooking" the enteroscope while applying suction, and then pulling back

slowly with a clockwise rotation until the 140 cm mark on the enteroscope is reached. This step can be repeated until no longer effective.

9. The maximal point of insertion is reached when further rotational advancement becomes challenging due to resistance, and other techniques are no longer effective.

PROCEDURE—WITHDRAWAL

1. Examination of the small bowel can be performed during careful withdrawal of the enteroscope.
2. Uncouple the overtube and gradually pull the enteroscope through the overtube back to the 140 cm mark while evaluating the small bowel mucosa.
3. Recouple the overtube back onto the enteroscope at the 140 cm gradation mark.
4. Spiral withdrawal can begin by rotating the overtube counterclockwise very slowly.
5. It is important to never pull back the overtube without also rotating counterclockwise.
6. Initially apply gentle forward pressure during this counterclockwise rotation in order to facilitate smooth slow release of the small bowel. This gentle forward pressure helps to maintain the position of the spirals in the small bowel to avoid falling back into the stomach too quickly.
7. Pause after each full rotation for a few seconds to permit the small bowel to gradually unpleat and release over the enteroscope.
8. Once this maneuver is no longer effective in releasing the small bowel over the overtube, relax forward pressure to allow the spiral overtube to slowly retreat during counterclockwise rotation.
9. Continue this process until the 55 cm mark on the enteroscope reaches the mouth (the most proximal spiral on the overtube should now be approaching GE junction).
10. Uncouple the enteroscope from the overtube. Slowly pull the enteroscope and carefully examine the proximal jejunum back to the duodenum until the 130m mark on the enteroscope is reached.
11. Recouple the overtube to the enteroscope and begin slow counterclockwise rotational withdrawal through the esophagus.
12. If the patient is intubated, ask the anesthetist to deflate the ET balloon to permit safe passage of the spiral overtube through the proximal esophagus. Reinsufflate the balloon after the overtube is removed through the mouth.

RETROGRADE (PERRECTAL) SPIRAL ENTEROSCOPY

1. A retrograde spiral overtube (100 cm in length, 13.1 mm inner diameter, 18.5 mm outer diameter, and 30.6 mm outer diameter with the spiral element) is used. This can be preloaded and locked onto a pediatric colonoscope or an enteroscope.
2. Introduce the endoscope in the usual fashion through the anus and advance to the descending colon.
3. Unlock the overtube and rotationally advance over the endoscope in a clockwise rotation. The endoscope will typically further advance to the ascending colon with this maneuver.
4. Do not advance the overtube if the lumen cannot be clearly visualized. Minimize insufflation and use water irrigation to improve visualization. If the lumen cannot be satisfactorily visualized, gently pull back the scope and consider rotating the overtube counterclockwise until the lumen is again seen.
5. Once maximal insertion of the overtube was achieved in the colon (typically the ascending colon), the "Cantero maneuver" can be performed by uncoupling the overtube and applying suction, while concomitantly rotating the overtube clockwise and simultaneously pulling back on the endoscope.
6. Uncouple the overtube from the enteroscope and push the endoscope through the overtube to reach the cecum.
7. Intubation of the IC valve may require retroflexion of the endoscope in the cecum. The endoscope can then be advanced to evaluate the ileum.

NOVEL MOTORIZED SPIRAL ENDOSCOPE

A novel motorized spiral endoscopy is being clinically evaluated. This novel system integrates a motor in the handle of the endoscope which is coupled to and rotates a short disposable spiral overtube attached to the insertion tube. The endoscopist has control of the direction and speed of rotation with a foot pedal. This motorized spiral enteroscope similarly pleats the small bowel over the spiral threads analogous to manual spiral enteroscopy. Efficacy and safety studies are currently being conducted and show promise that this device may soon be in the endoscopist's tool box to evaluate the small bowel.

ADVERSE EVENTS

1. Discomfort
2. Bleeding (<1%)
3. Perforation (<1%)
4. Aspiration
5. Medication reactions
6. Mucosal damage

7. Oversedation
8. Hypotension
9. Tachycardia
10. Procedure intolerance
11. Hypoxia
12. Drug reaction
13. Major adverse events, which include perforation, bleeding, infection, and significant cardiovascular collapse such as arrhythmias and shock, may occur in 0.64% to 1% of procedures
14. Other adverse events reported in the literature, such as mucosal stripping, acute pancreatitis, and pharyngeal tears, are very rare and have been related to the use of the stiffening overtube

CPT CODES (15)

44360—Small intestinal endoscopy, enteroscopy beyond second portion of duodenum, not including ileum; diagnostic, with or without collection of specimen(s) by brushing or washing (separate procedure)

44361—Small intestinal endoscopy, enteroscopy beyond second portion of duodenum, not including ileum; with biopsy, single or multiple

44363—Small intestinal endoscopy, enteroscopy beyond second portion of duodenum, not including ileum; with removal of foreign body

44364—Small intestinal endoscopy, enteroscopy beyond second portion of duodenum, not including ileum; with removal of tumor(s), polyp(s), or other lesion(s) by snare technique

44365—Small intestinal endoscopy, enteroscopy beyond second portion of duodenum, not including ileum; with removal of tumor(s), polyp(s), or other lesion(s) by hot biopsy forceps or bipolar cautery

44366—Small intestinal endoscopy, enteroscopy beyond second portion of duodenum, not including ileum; with control of bleeding, any method

44369—Small intestinal endoscopy, enteroscopy beyond second portion of duodenum, not including ileum; with ablation of tumor(s), polyp(s), or other lesion(s) not amenable to removal by hot biopsy forceps, bipolar cautery, or snare technique

44370—Small intestinal endoscopy, enteroscopy beyond second portion of duodenum, not including ileum; with transendoscopic stent placement (includes predilation)

44372—Small intestinal endoscopy, enteroscopy beyond second portion of duodenum, not including ileum; with placement of a percutaneous jejunostomy tube

44373—Small intestinal endoscopy, enteroscopy beyond second portion of duodenum, not including ileum; with conversion of the percutaneous gastrostomy tube to the percutaneous jejunostomy tube

44380—Ileoscopy, through stoma; diagnostic, with or without collection of specimen(s) by brushing or washing (separate procedure)

44382—Ileoscopy, through stoma; with biopsy, single or multiple

Bibliography

1. Yamamoto H, Sekine Y, Sato Y, et al. Total enteroscopy with nonsurgical steerable double balloon method. *Gastrointest Endosc.* 2001;53(2):216-220.
2. Wilmer A, Rutgeerts P. Push enteroscopy. Technique, depth, and yield of insertion. *Gastrointest Endosc Clin N Am.* 1996;6(4):759-776.
3. Lin S, Branch MS, Shetzline M. The importance of indication in the diagnostic value of push enteroscopy. *Endoscopy.* 2003;35(4):315-321.
4. Chavalitdhamrong D, Adler DG, Draganov PV. Complications of enteroscopy: how to avoid them and manage them when they arise. *Gastrointest Endosc Clin N Am.* 2015;25(1):83-95.
5. Ben-Menachem T, Decker GA, Early DS, et al. Adverse events of upper GI endoscopy. *Gastrointest Endosc.* 2012;76(4):707-718.
6. Levy I, Gralnek IM. Complications of diagnostic colonoscopy, upper endoscopy, and enteroscopy. *Best Pract Res Clin Gastroenterol.* 2016;30(5):705-718.
7. Yang R, Laine L. Mucosal stripping: a complication of push enteroscopy. *Gastrointest Endosc.* 1995;41(2):156-158.
8. Akerman PA, Agrawal D, Cantero D, Pangtay J. Spiral enteroscopy with the new DSB overtube: a novel technique for deep peroral small-bowel intubation. *Endoscopy.* 2008;40(12):974-978.
9. Schembre DB, Ross AS. Spiral enteroscopy: a new twist on overtube-assisted endoscopy. *Gastrointest Endosc.* 2009;69(2):333-336.
10. Akerman PA, Cantero D. Spiral enteroscopy and push enteroscopy. *Gastrointest Endosc Clin N Am.* 2009;19:357-369.
11. Ali R, Wild D, Shieh F, et al. Deep enteroscopy with a conventional colonoscope: initial multicenter study by using a through-the-scope balloon catheter system. *Gastrointest Endosc.* 2015;82(5):855-860.
12. Lara LF, Singh S, Sreenarasimhaiah J. Initial experience with retrograde overtube-assisted enteroscopy using a spiral tip overtube. *Proc (Bayl Univ Med Cent).* 2010;23(2):130-133.
13. Neuhaus H, Beyna T, Schneider M, Devière J. Novel motorized spiral enteroscopy: first clinical case. *VideoGIE.* 2016;1(2):32-33.
14. Beyna T, Schneider M, Pullmann D, Gerges C, Kandler J, Neuhaus H. Motorized spiral colonoscopy: a first single-center feasibility trial. *Endoscopy.* 2018;50(5):518-523.

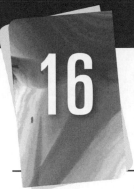

16

Placement of Enteral Self-Expandable Metal Stents

Aaron J. Small, MD
Shayan Irani, MD

Enteral self-expandable stents (SEMSs) have become an effective treatment option for malignant strictures of the esophagus, stomach, proximal small bowel, gastroenteric anastomoses, and the distal small bowel (terminal ileum) or the jejunum in select patients.[1,2] The goal is to achieve luminal patency, allowing food intake per os, and thereby obviating the need for more invasive operative alternatives. SEMSs although historically made of stainless steel now are almost exclusively made of nitinol (a shape-retaining alloy) and come in a variety of sizes and designs depending on the location of the stenosis. For the purposes of this chapter, we will focus on the application of metallic stenting within the lumen of the stomach and proximal small intestine, most commonly the duodenum. Endoscopic transmural stenting within the stomach and small intestine akin to the creation of an endoscopic anastomotic bypass is covered elsewhere in this handbook.

PATIENT SELECTION

Indications

Although enteral SEMSs have been used in both benign and malignant conditions, they have a limited role in benign diseases. Endoscopic stenting for palliation of a malignant gastroduodenal stricture from an intrinsic or extrinsic lesion has been shown to be safe and effective as therapy for restoring oral intake and improving patient quality of life.[3-7] Preoperative enteral stenting as a "bridge to surgery" is a less common scenario. Insertion of enteral stents for benign diseases is principally for temporary placement for postoperative complications such as strictures, leaks, and fistula, although there have been other indications listed below.[3]

Malignant

1. Gastric obstruction
   a. Primary or recurrent gastric cancer
   b. Gastrojejunal anastomosis—afferent and efferent limb obstruction
2. Duodenal obstruction
   a. Primary pancreatic cancer or metastatic disease to the pancreas
   b. Cholangiocarcinoma or gallbladder cancer
   c. Periampullary cancer
   d. Locally invasive tumors (e.g., colon)
3. Small bowel
   a. Metastatic disease involving the ligament of Treitz or jejunum
   b. Pelvic cancers affecting the distal terminal ileum

Benign

1. Gastric
   a. Postoperative fistula/leaks: sleeve gastrectomy, gastrojejunal anastomosis
   b. Gastric sleeve stricture
2. Duodenum
   a. Peptic ulcer disease stricture (short stricture more amenable)
   b. Fistula, e.g., pancreaticoduodenal or enterocutaneous fistula (low success rates)
   c. Perforation[8]
3. Small bowel
   a. Anastomotic-jejunal limb stenosis, leak, perforation

CONTRAINDICATIONS

There are very few absolute contraindications to enteral stent placement which are the same as those that preclude an upper endoscopy.[9] These include cardiopulmonary instability, recent myocardial infarction, or pulmonary embolus. Enteral stenting can be performed safely without cessation of antiplatelets or in anticoagulated patients. The presence of a transmural perforation which can sometimes be tumor-related, with or without associated peritonitis, may be too large of a defect for safe closure with a covered metal stent, and thus should be considered a relative contraindication.

Peritoneal carcinomatosis, while not an absolute contraindication, can portend a higher risk of primary stent failure since these patients will often have multifocal stenosis in more distal areas of the small intestine or have gastric or small bowel dysmotility from neural tumor invasion that is not alleviated by stent monotherapy.[10]

PATIENT PREPARATION
Preprocedural Planning and Equipment
Prerequisites

1. A basic prerequisite for placing enteral stents requires an endoscopy unit equipped with various endoscopes, stent types (discussed further below), high-quality fluoroscopy, and staff including endoscopic technicians/assistants, fluoroscopic operators, and anesthesia all of whom are comfortable with complex GI procedures.
2. In addition, knowledge of the patient's anatomy and any history of prior surgeries should be understood to determine the feasibility of endoluminal stenting.

Imaging

1. CT scan with oral contrast can elucidate the location, length, severity of the stricture, and the presence of a possible leak.
2. Upper GI series and/or small bowel follow through studies while more detailed than CT scans in defining gastroduodenal strictures may also aid in determining whether there are multiple other focal areas of stenosis in the more distal small bowel.

Procedural considerations

Precautions to minimize the higher risk of intraprocedural aspiration in these patients who may have complete gastric outlet obstruction should be undertaken. Some of the interventions that may reduce this aspiration risk are the following:

1. For gastric outlet obstruction, a nasogastric tube can be inserted for decompression of liquid and food contents in the stomach several hours prior to the procedure.
2. Either nil per os or clear liquid diet 24 hours prior to procedure.
3. Elective endotracheal intubation to protect the patient's airway during the procedure. In the rare circumstance that conscious sedation is the only option, the patient should be placed in left lateral position.
4. Use of large working channel endoscope for suctioning of semisolid food and excessive liquids on entry into the stomach.

Choice of endoscope

Routinely, an upper endoscope with a large-diameter working channel (≥3.8 mm) is most often used to place a through-the-scope (TTS) stent which commonly has a 10-French predeployment delivery system. Other endoscopes can be used depending on the location of the lesion and type of stent to be placed.

1. Therapeutic channel endoscope (working channel ≥3.8 mm).
2. Duodenoscope, particularly for patients that may require placement of a biliary stent during the same session.

3. Adult colonoscope can be used to reach proximal lesions beyond the third portion of the duodenum, the afferent limb in postsurgical anatomy, or for distal small bowel lesions (ileum) allowing for placement of TTS stents.
4. A double-balloon enteroscope with a large enough working channel diameter for TTS stent placement is on the horizon but not yet distributed in US centers.
5. Small caliber endoscope (outer diameter 5.4 mm) can be used in the rare case that to traversing the stricture in needed to advance a guidewire, then allow for backloading of a therapeutic upper endoscope for stent deployment.

Type of Stent

The indication, stricture characteristics (length and location), and stent availability within the endoscopy unit where the procedure will occur often determine the selection of the enteral stent used. To date, only uncovered metal stents are FDA approved and available in the United States for dedicated use in the enteral tract. These stents have the advantages of a low migration rate and TTS delivery for deployment across malignant strictures. Uncovered SEMSs should not be used ideally for benign enteric strictures given their, lack of removability.

While there are partially and fully covered SEMSs dedicated for enteral use, these are only available outside of the United States.[11] Thus, enteral stenting for benign disease is limited to the off-label use of available fully covered or partially covered esophageal SEMSs and less commonly biliary SEMSs which maximally expand to only 10 mm.

TECHNIQUES OF INSERTION

Enteral SEMSs can be placed with or without fluoroscopy when placing TTS stents or deployed under fluoroscopic guidance alone when using non-TTS techniques. Either approach requires advancement of a guidewire across the stenosis. Fluoroscopic views can better define the extent of the stricture including length, tortuosity, directionality, and presence of a leak. Advancing the endoscope beyond the obstructed region is not necessary, as is balloon dilation prior to stent placement in almost all cases. However, in the rare case where balloon dilation is required, it does significantly increase the risk of perforation. Basic steps for TTS stent placement are as follows:

Through-the-scope SEMS insertion

1. Passage of the endoscope to the site of the lesion (Fig. 16.1).
2. Water-soluble contrast injection through the working channel of the endoscope or through a biliary catheter to define the stricture characteristics and up- or downstream bowel.

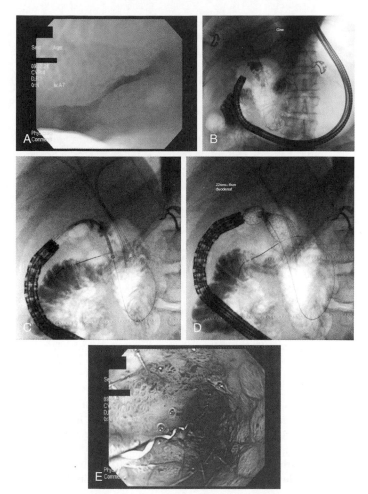

FIGURE 16.1 A, Endoscopic view of a high-grade duodenal stenosis from extrinsic compression in a patient with pancreatic cancer and concomitant biliary and gastric outlet obstruction. B, Guidewire advanced beyond the stenosis into the proximal duodenum. C, Placement of a constrained SEMS within the delivery sheath across the stenosis. D, Deployment of the uncovered SEMS with the distal end proximal to the ampulla and plastic biliary stents. E, Endoscopic view of the deployed SEMS traversing the duodenal stenosis.

3. Advancement of a guidewire of 0.025 or 0.035″ short 260 cm or long 450 cm biliary wire through the stricture.

4. Insertion of the constrained SEMS within the delivery sheath across the stricture. The position of the distal end is visualized under fluoroscopy as the assistant deploys the SEMS. The position of the proximal end of the SEMS

is confirmed under direct endoscopic visualization; the proximal stent end and its interstices can be seen through the catheter delivery system and watched as the assistant releases the stent.

There are a few tips and caveats to ensure successful TTS stent insertion:

1. The use of rotatable biliary catheters and occlusion stone extraction balloons can be helpful to define tortuous, high-grade strictures and facilitate advancement of a guidewire when the lumen cannot be seen. A small-diameter endoscope may also aid in this regard if able to be advanced beyond the stenosis.

2. The stricture length can be estimated by inflating the biliary extraction balloon against the most distal end of the stenosis, grasping the catheter at the biopsy port, then pulling back the deflated balloon until the tip of the catheter is visualized endoscopically. The stricture length will be the distance between the endoscopist's fingers and biopsy cap.

3. All braided enteral TTS stents foreshorten up to 40% after deployment. To account for this foreshortening, the endoscopist should watch the proximal end of the stent during deployment. The SEMS will appear to move away from the tip of the endoscope and will need to be gradually pulled back as the stent shortens and is pulled distally during expansion.

4. Most TTS enteral stents are able to be recaptured in the delivery sheath and repositioned if the stent is not in its desired place during deployment. There is a "point of no return" when the partially expanded SEMS is too far out of the constraining sheath and can no longer be recaptured, which generally is when less than a quarter of the stent remains in the delivery system.

5. After the stent is deployed, the delivery system is withdrawn. Caution should be taken to avoid dislodging the deployed SEMS while withdrawing the delivery catheter. This scenario can occur especially immediately post insertion while the stent is not yet maximally expanded within a tight stricture. To avoid this, the assistant can "recapture" the delivery sheath to its predeployment position toward the distal end of the stent, as the endoscopist gradually pushes the delivery catheter distally. The post-SEMS delivery system can then be carefully withdrawn toward the proximal end of the stent, no longer caught within the SEMS, and out of the endoscopic biopsy channel.

There are a few nuances for the ideally positioned stent. First, a well-placed SEMS should have a waist in the middle of the stent. As a general rule, a TTS stent of appropriate length should be 4 cm longer than the length of the stenosis with the lesion flared by 2 cm on both ends. In theory, this allows for: (1) stent foreshortening at both stent ends that can occur post procedure and (2) the maximal radial force that occurs in the middle of the stent to be applied within the targeted stenosis, making it less likely to spontaneously migrate post deployment.

Second, one must resist the urge to advance the endoscope through the stent immediately post deployment. This maneuver may dislodge the stent. If really needed, contrast injection through the endoscope working channel can confirm stent patency and adequacy of placement, with the guidewire left in place beyond the stricture/stent. Repositioning of the stent with a rat-tooth forceps or insertion of a second overlapping stent can be performed, if needed. Flow of contrast through the deployed stent should also verify that both the proximal and distal ends of the stent are not impinging the contralateral intestinal wall especially near fixed turns such as the ligament of Treitz.

Non–through-the-scope SEMS insertion

Placement of non-TTS enteral stents relies heavily on fluoroscopy for accurate stent deployment. As mentioned, there are no dedicated covered SEMSs for the enteral tract, so covered esophageal stents has been used for benign diseases of the stomach and small intestine. The esophageal-covered SEMSs manufactured in the United States have delivery systems that do not go through the endoscope. Consequently, being adept at non-TTS insertion of stents akin to interventional radiologists is a useful skill. Of note, two Korean manufacturers of covered esophageal SEMSs that have TTS delivery systems are now available in the United States. After the endoscope is advanced to the site of treatment, a guidewire is passed beyond the site of treatment and the endoscope is withdrawn leaving the guidewire in place. The non-TTS stent is loaded onto the guidewire and carefully advanced with an effort to avoid looping of the guidewire or the stent delivery system. Similar to placement of covered SEMS in the esophagus, external fluoroscopic markers or subcutaneous injections of contrast can be used to aid accurate stent placement.

Advancing a non-TTS SEMS delivery system to the small bowel can be challenging due to looping in an often dilated stomach even when working over a stiff spring-tip wire. In addition, covered esophageal stents available in the United States cannot be advanced far beyond the second portion of the duodenum limited by the length of the stent delivery system (assuming the patient has not had any prior surgeries). Some caveats to overcome the technical difficulties of non-TTS stent insertion are as follows:

1. Use of a super stiff guidewire, such as a Savary, Amplatz Super Stiff, or stiff Dreamwire. This can help to reduce looping in the stomach that may be grossly dilated.

2. Communication between the assistant and the endoscopist to maintain traction and counter-traction of the guidewire and stent delivery system as it is advanced.

3. Use of a transoral or transnasal small caliber endoscope alongside the non-TTS stent delivery system can allow for intraprocedural visualization of the proximal end of the stent during deployment.

4. In the small bowel, use of a single- or double-balloon enteroscope to allow use of the overtube for passage of the SEMS to places not traditionally reachable by the short delivery systems.[12]

POSTPROCEDURE

The postprocedural care of the patient after SEMS insertion depends on patient factors and the indication for stent placement. For patients with gastric outlet obstruction who have undergone enteral stent therapy, these patients do not necessarily need to stay in the hospital for stent-related care. However, the desired outcome to restore per oral intake and alleviate postprandial nausea/vomiting should be challenged while the patient is monitored. An upper GI series can be performed after a period of time (in our institution, the next morning) to allow the SEMS to reach its maximal diameter to confirm patency, positioning, and function, although this is not entirely necessary before allowing the patient to trial clears and advancing the patient's diet.

To date, there are no specific societal guidelines on dietary recommendations for patients with an indwelling enteral stent. Anecdotally, high-residue foods (vegetables, fruit, and peels of beans, etc.) can become entangled within the interstices of metallic stents and may result in stent occlusions especially as tissue ingrowth progressively narrows the stent over time,[3] although this phenomenon is not well substantiated in studies. At our institution, once the patient can tolerate food per os, we recommend that these patients try to adhere to a low-residue diet.

ADVERSE EVENTS

Both immediate and delayed adverse events can occur. Perforation and bleeding are the most serious adverse events, both of which can be immediate or delayed. Restenosis from stent occlusion either by tumor ingrowth/overgrowth or from benign tissue hyperplasia can also occur; however, it is often correctable by placement of an additional stent or less durably with argon plasma coagulationablation of the occluding tissue. Stent migration will occur more frequently when using covered stents (esophageal stents for benign strictures) and rarely with the uncovered metal stents placed for malignancy but in some series reported up to 10%. Fistula formation (from pressure necrosis at the end/s of the stent), biliary obstruction from the duodenal stent compromising an already partly obstructed bile duct, bleeding, and fevers are rare but can be significant.

Stent-induced perforation is the most dreaded complication and can occur either immediate or delayed. Two technical considerations can mitigate the perforation risk.

- Balloon dilation within the stent to aid in expansion immediate after deployment has been shown to increase the risk of stent-induced perforation and should be avoided.
- For strictures in the second portion of the duodenum, some advocate in final placement of the proximal end of the stent in the gastric antrum to avoid the edges of the stent ending in the duodenal bulb where there can be an increased perforation or bleeding risk from pressure necrosis.

SPECIAL CONSIDERATION

Concomitant Biliary and Duodenal Obstruction

In patients with gastric outlet obstruction and impending biliary obstruction, as is often the case with cancer involving the head of the pancreas, it is important, if possible, to be cognizant of not placing an enteral stent across the papilla making subsequent biliary access significantly more challenging.[13] Knowledge of the exact location of the papilla can be challenging though when the obstruction is proximal, but accurate stent placement is much easier when the obstruction is distal.

If the stenosis is proximal to the papilla, some advocate balloon dilation to advance the duodenoscope into the second portion to complete the endoscopic retrograde cholangiopancreatography. Insertion of the biliary SEMS first before placement of the duodenal stent is preferable and can be done in the same endoscopic session. If passage of the duodenoscope to the level of the papilla is not attainable despite balloon dilation, duodenal SEMS insertion with the distal end ending proximal to the papilla would be the next best option for later stenting of the bile duct after the SEMS expands over the ensuing 2 days. If biliary obstruction develops when there is already an indwelling gastroduodenal stent crossing the papilla or if the papilla is unrecognizable within the malignant stricture, endoscopic ultrasound or percutaneous access may be necessary, for antegrade or rendezvous retrograde biliary stent placement.

CPT CODES

43266—Esophagogastroduodenoscopy, flexible, transoral; with placement of endoscopic stent (includes pre- and post dilation and guidewire passage when performed)

44370—Small intestinal endoscopy, enteroscopy beyond the second portion of duodenum, not including ileum; with transendoscopic stent placement (includes predilation)

44384—Ileoscopy, through stoma; with placement of endoscopic stent (includes pre- and post dilation and guidewire passage, when performed)

76000—Fluoroscopy (separate procedure), up to 1 hour of physician time

References

1. Irani S, Kozarek RA. Gastrointestinal dilation and stenting. In: Podolsky DK, Camilleri M, Fitz JG, Kalloo AN, Shanahan F, Wang TC, eds. *Yamada Textbook of Gastroenterology.* 6th ed. Oxford: Wiley-Blackwell; 2015:2611-2626.
2. Kochar R, Shah N. Enteral stents: from esophagus to colon. *Gastrointest Endosc.* 2013;78:913-918.
3. Baron TH. Enteric stents: indications and placement techniques. In: Kozarek RA, Baron TH, Song H-Y, eds. *Self-Expandable Stents in the Gastrointestinal Tract.* 1st ed. New York: Springer; 2013:159-173.
4. Telford JJ, Carr-Locke DL, Baron TH, et al. Palliation of patients with malignant gastric outlet obstruction with the enteral wallstent: outcomes from a multicenter study. *Gastrointest Endosc.* 2004;60:916-920.
5. Adler DG, Baron TH. Endoscopic palliation of malignant gastric outlet obstruction using self-expanding metal stents: experience in 36 patients. *Am J Gastroenterol.* 2002;97:72-78.
6. Varadarajulu S, Banerjee S, Barth B, et al. Enteral stents. *ASGE Technology Committee Gastrointest Endosc.* 2011;74:455-464.
7. Kozarek RA, Ball TJ, Patterson DJ. Metallic self-expandable stent application in the upper gastrointestinal tract: caveats and concerns. *Gastrointest Endosc.* 1992;38:1-6.
8. Small AJ, Peterson BT, Baron TH. Closure of a duodenal stent-induced perforation by endoscopic stent removal and covered self-expandable metal stent placement (with video). *Gastrointest Endosc.* 2007;66:1063-1065.
9. Adler DG, Dua KS, Dimaio CJ, et al. Endoluminal stent placement core curriculum. ASGE Training Committee 2010-2011. *Gastrointest Endosc.* 2012;76:719-724.
10. Mendelsohn RB, Gerdes H, Markowitz AJ, et al. Carcinomatosis is not a contraindication to enteral stenting in selected patients with malignant gastric outlet obstruction. *Gastrointest Endosc.* 2011;73:1135-1140.
11. Chan GK, Choi IJ. Enteric prostheses. In: Kozarek RA, Baron TH, Song H-Y, eds. *Self-Expandable Stents in the Gastrointestinal Tract.* 1st ed. New York: Springer; 2013:103-120.
12. Ross AS, Semrad C, Waxman I, et al. Enteral stent placement by double balloon enteroscopy for palliation of malignant small bowel obstruction. *Gastrointest Endosc.* 2006;64:835-837.
13. Baron TH. Management of simultaneous biliary and duodenal obstruction: the endoscopic perspective. *Gut Liver.* 2010;4:S50-S56.

17 Endoscopic Mucosal Resection of Duodenal Lesions

Richard S. Kwon, MD, MS

This chapter will focus on duodenal adenomas which can present an endoscopic challenge. The prevalence of sporadic duodenal adenomas is roughly 5% of patients undergoing esophagogastroduodenoscopy (EGD)[1] and up to 90% in familial adenomatous polyposis (FAP) syndrome.[2] Sporadic ampullary adenomas are much rarer with a 0.12% prevalence.[3]

The treatment of choice for duodenal adenomas is endoscopic resection. The therapeutic goal is to resect these precancerous lesions before malignant degeneration, as well as, to avoid more invasive surgical resection. However, clinical decisions require consideration of the patient's comorbidities, age, preferences, and the relative risks of adverse events and malignancy.

NONAMPULLARY DUODENAL ADENOMAS
Preparation
1. NPO at least 6 hours prior
2. ASGE guidelines for antithrombotics, antiplatelets, and anticoagulation.[4] Discuss with appropriate healthcare providers
3. Preprocedure labs usually not necessary
4. Left lateral position
5. Sedation (anesthesia, monitored anesthesia, or conscious sedation) depending on comorbidities and availability of anesthesia services
6. Cardiopulmonary monitoring

Equipment
1. Gastroscope (diagnostic or therapeutic), duodenoscope, or pediatric colonoscope (preferably with high definition) as dictated by polyp location
2. Short transparent distal cap
3. Light source and image processor
4. Electrosurgical generator + pad

5. Endoscopic snare (hot or cold): size determined by target
6. Endoscopic biopsy forceps (hot or cold)
7. Argon plasma coagulation (APC) and appropriate processor
8. Sclerotherapy needle
9. Submucosal injectant (saline, hetastarch, colloid; low-viscosity emulsion (Eleview, Olympus America), viscous gel (ORISE, Boston Scientific); with or without epinephrine)
10. Dye—methylene blue, indigo carmine
11. Retrieval accessory: trap and/or retrieval net

Endoscopic Evaluation

1. Appropriate endoscope (may require multiple scopes, use of transparent distal cap)
2. White light or electronic chromoendoscopy or dye-based chromoendoscopy
3. Endoscopic considerations: evidence of submucosal invasion or malignancy, as well as, risks of incomplete/unsuccessful resection
   a. Size
   b. Percentage of lumen circumference (see Fig. 17.1)
   c. Length
   d. Relationship to the ampulla
   e. Location within the duodenal sweep
   f. Scar or fibrosis from prior resection attempts or nonlifting on submucosal injection
   g. Mucosal assessment for risk of dysplasia
      i. Paris classification[5]
      ii. Kudo pit pattern[6]
      iii. Spigelman criteria (for familial polyposis syndromes)[7]

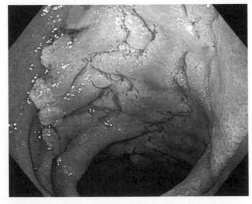

FIG. 17.1 Duodenal adenoma occupying ~75% of the circumference of the lumen and deemed endoscopically unresectable.

Methods of Duodenal Adenoma Resection

1. Conventional polypectomy
2. Endoscopic mucosal resection (with submucosal injection)[8] (see Fig. 17.2)
3. Underwater resection[3,9]
4. Band and slough[10]
5. Endoscopic submucosal dissection (should be reserved for expert endoscopists)[11]

Special Considerations

1. Polyps on duodenal sweep (anterior, medial wall) usually require a duodenoscope.
2. Duodenoscope challenges related to instrument manipulation through elevator.
3. Distal duodenal polyps may require a pediatric colonoscope to reach.
4. Identification of margins may be difficult due to villiform nature of both normal duodenal mucosa and adenomas— solution: dye or electronic chromoendoscopy.
5. Crevices/valleys may be challenging to lift and resect.
6. Limited room and maneuverability within the duodenal lumen may mean limitations to degree of lift and size of snares used for resection.

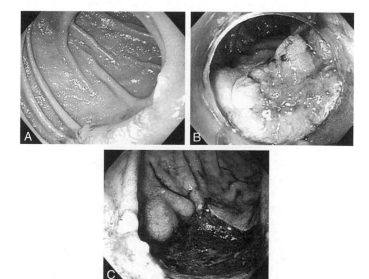

FIG. 17.2 A, Duodenal adenoma visualized with standard gastroscope. B, Margins of this duodenal adenoma better visualized using a standard gastroscope fitted with a clear cap. C, Resection site after lift with epinephrine and methylene blue and piece-meal resection with snare cautery.

Outcomes
1. Overall success rate = 70% to 100%[12,13]
   a. May require several procedures to achieve complete resection
2. Success rate based on lumen circumference[12]
   a. <25% = 95%
   b. 25% to 50% = 46%
   c. >50% = 0%

Possible Adverse Events
1. Perforation rate = 0% to 1.9%[12,13]
2. Bleeding rate = 0% to 14%[12,13]

Follow-up
1. Sporadic adenomas—usually every 3 to 6 months until eradication, then annually
2. Polyposis syndrome–related adenomas based on Spigelman criteria[14]

AMPULLARY ADENOMAS

Ampullary adenomas can be sporadic or associated with FAP. These are prone to malignant transformation. Endoscopic ampullectomy is considered the first-line treatment for benign adenomas with or without dysplasia. Ampullectomies are generally performed using a duodenoscope and should be reserved for interventional endoscopists or those comfortable performing ampullectomies with endoscopic retrograde cholangiopancreatography (ERCP). The goal of ampullectomy is complete excision, ideally en bloc. Piecemeal resections are required if the adenoma is large and extends along the duodenal wall.

Preparation: Same as for Duodenal Adenoma Resection Except
1. Prone position of patient
2. Consent should include risk of pancreatitis (see below)
3. Rectal indomethacin for prophylaxis[15]

Equipment: Same as for Duodenal Adenoma Resection Except
1. Duodenoscopes used exclusively
2. Fluoroscopy required for ERCP portion of the procedure
3. Catheter, guidewires, and stents typically used for ERCP

Assessment of Ampulla: Features of Benign Disease[16,17]
1. Size <4 cm
2. Localized or laterally spreading margins

3. Absence of any ulceration or spontaneous bleeding
4. Soft consistency
5. If concern about adequacy of candidacy, biopsy to look for malignancy. Sensitivity of biopsies is high but specificity is low (so risk of false negative)[18]

Role of endoscopic ultrasound (EUS): limited utility (malignancy or concern for intraductal extension)[19,20] (see Fig. 17.3)

1. Operator dependent
2. Meta-analysis shows moderate agreement between EUS and tumor staging by pathology.[21] Sensitivity 77% and specificity 78% in predicting T1 stage. Author reserves EUS for high risk of malignancy or very large lesion size

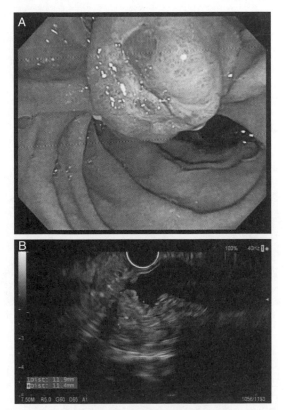

FIG. 17.3 A, Ampullary mass identified with a duodenoscope. The central ulceration is worrisome for malignancy. Biopsies confirmed adenocarcinoma. B, Linear endoscopic ultrasound (EUS) image of mass extending into the common bile duct. This patient subsequently underwent a Whipple procedure.

How the Author Performs (See Fig. 17.4)

1. Before resection, cannulate and inject contrast into one or both ducts for reference on fluoroscopy[20]
2. Small biliary sphincterotomy to help identify bile duct post ampullectomy
3. No submucosal injection
4. Snare (size dictated by adenoma size) cautery, endocut setting (ERBE, Tubingen, Germany)
5. Sample collection with Roth net immediately after resection so specimen is not lost
6. After ampullectomy, cannulate pancreatic duct for stent placement, usually 5 Fr, 5 or 7 cm stent with internal flanges. Consider placement of biliary stent if drainage is believed to be inadequate

Other Therapeutic Options

1. Wire cannulation of the pancreatic duct and perform ampullectomy using snare over wire[22]
2. Electrocautery settings: pure cut[23]
3. Submucosal injection of ampulla[16]
   a. May increase technical success and decrease adverse events
   b. Conversely may interfere with visualization and snare placement

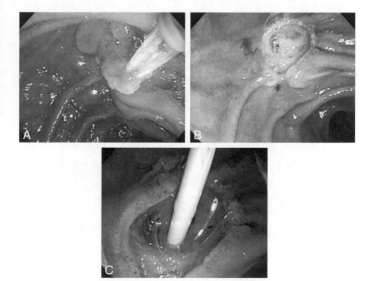

FIG. 17.4 A, Ampullary adenoma identified with a duodenoscope. B, Resection site with clean ulcer base. C, After placement of a pancreatic stent.

4. Methylene blue in preampullectomy pancreatic duct injection[24]
5. Tissue ablation using APC (requires 40-50W or higher for effective mucosal ablation), monopolar coagulation, ND:YAG laser, photodynamic therapy[25]
6. Sphincterotomy (biliary and/or pancreatic) post resection

Adverse Events—Overall Adverse Event Rate 15%, Mortality Extremely Rare[25,26]

1. Pancreatitis—up to 25%[26,27]
2. Bleeding—up to 25%[26,28]
3. Perforation (usually retroperitoneal)—<5%[27,29,30]
4. Cholangitis—2%[26]
5. Papillary stenosis—0% to 8%[26]

Outcomes

1. Success for endoscopic removal—45% to 90%[27,31]
2. Recurrence rate as high as 30%[32,33]
   a. Treatment options include snare polypectomy or ablation (hot avulsion with hot biopsy forceps, soft coagulation with a snare tip, APC, probe-based radiofrequency ablation)

Postprocedure

1. Monitor postprocedure per endoscopy unit
   a. Monitor post anesthesia
   b. Monitor abdominal pain (perforation or pancreatitis)
   c. Monitor bleeding
2. Resume antiplatelet, antithrombotic, and anticoagulation per endoscopist discretion
3. Repeat endoscopy in 1 to 3 months for initial check and PD stent pull. Repeat endoscopy yearly thereafter

References

1. Jepsen JM, Persson M, Jakobsen NO, et al. Prospective study of prevalence and endoscopic and histopathologic characteristics of duodenal polyps in patients submitted to upper endoscopy. *Scand J Gastroenterol*. 1994;29(6):483-487.
2. Bulow S, Björk J, Christensen IJ, et al. Duodenal adenomatosis in familial adenomatous polyposis. *Gut*. 2004;53(3):381-386.
3. Baker HL, Caldwell DW. Lesions of the ampulla of Vater. *Surgery*. 1947;21(4):523-531.
4. ASGE Standards of Practice Committee, Acosta RD, Abraham NS, Chandrasekhara V, et al. The management of antithrombotic agents for patients undergoing GI endoscopy. *Gastrointest Endosc*. 2016;83(1):3-16.
5. Endoscopic Classification Review Group. Update on the paris classification of superficial neoplastic lesions in the digestive tract. *Endoscopy*. 2005;37(6):570-578.
6. Kudo SE, Kashida H. Flat and depressed lesions of the colorectum. *Clin Gastroenterol Hepatol*. 2005;3(7 suppl 1):S33-S36.

7. Spigelman AD, Williams CB, Talbot IC, Domizio P, Phillips RK. Upper gastro-intestinal cancer in patients with familial adenomatous polyposis. *Lancet.* 1989;2(8666):783-785.

8. Alexander S, Talbot IC, Williams CB, Domizio P, Phillips RKS. EMR of large, sessile, sporadic nonampullary adenomas: technical aspects and long-term outcome (with videos). *Gastrointest Endosc.* 2009;69(1):66-73.

9. Binmoeller KF, Shah JN, Bhat YM, Kane SD. "Underwater" EMR of sporadic laterally spreading nonampullary duodenal adenomas (with video). *Gastrointest Endosc.* 2013;78(3):496-502.

10. Koritala T, Zolotarevsky E, Bartley AN, et al. Efficacy and safety of the band and slough technique for endoscopic therapy of nonampullary duodenal adenomas: a case series. *Gastrointest Endosc.* 2015;81(4):985-988.

11. Matsumoto S, Yoshida Y. Selection of appropriate endoscopic therapies for duodenal tumors: an open-label study, single-center experience. *World J Gastroenterol.* 2014;20(26):8624-8630.

12. Kedia P, Brensinger C, Ginsberg G. Endoscopic predictors of successful endoluminal eradication in sporadic duodenal adenomas and its acute complications. *Gastrointest Endosc.* 2010;72(6):1297-1301.

13. Navaneethan U, Lourdusamy D, Mehta D, et al. Endoscopic resection of large sporadic non-ampullary duodenal polyps: efficacy and long-term recurrence. *Surg Endosc.* 2014;28(9):2616-2622.

14. Syngal S, Brand RE, Church JM, et al. ACG clinical guideline: Genetic testing and management of hereditary gastrointestinal cancer syndromes. *Am J Gastroenterol.* 2015;110(2):223-262; quiz 263.

15. Elmunzer BJ, Scheiman JM, Lehman GA, et al. A randomized trial of rectal indomethacin to prevent post-ERCP pancreatitis. *N Engl J Med.* 2012;366(15):1414-1422.

16. Martin JA, Haber GB. Ampullary adenoma: clinical manifestations, diagnosis, and treatment. *Gastrointest Endosc Clin N Am.* 2003;13(4):649-669.

17. Cheng CL, Sherman S, Fogel EL, et al. Endoscopic snare papillectomy for tumors of the duodenal papillae. *Gastrointest Endosc.* 2004;60(5):757-764.

18. Yamaguchi K, Enjoji M, Kitamura K. Endoscopic biopsy has limited accuracy in diagnosis of ampullary tumors. *Gastrointest Endosc.* 1990;36(6):588-592.

19. Adler DG, Qureshi W, Davila R, et al. The role of endoscopy in ampullary and duodenal adenomas. *Gastrointest Endosc.* 2006;64(6):849-854.

20. ASGE Standards of Practice Committee, Chathadi KV, Khashab MA, Acosta RD, et al. The role of endoscopy in ampullary and duodenal adenomas. *Gastrointest Endosc.* 2015;82(5):773-781.

21. Trikudanathan G, Njei B, Attam R, Arain M, Shaukat A. Staging accuracy of ampullary tumors by endoscopic ultrasound: meta-analysis and systematic review. *Dig Endosc.* 2014;26(5):617-626.

22. Moon JH, Cha SW, Cho YD, et al. Wire-guided endoscopic snare papillectomy for tumors of the major duodenal papilla. *Gastrointest Endosc.* 2005;61(3):461-466.

23. Bohnacker S, Seitz U, Nguyen D, et al. Endoscopic resection of benign tumors of the duodenal papilla without and with intraductal growth. *Gastrointest Endosc.* 2005;62(4):551-560.

24. Poincloux L, Scanzi J, Goutte M, et al. Pancreatic intubation facilitated by methylene blue injection decreases the risk for postpapillectomy acute pancreatitis. *Eur J Gastroenterol Hepatol.* 2014;26(9):990-995.

25. Espinel J, Pinedo E, Ojeda V, Guerra Del Río M. Endoscopic ampullectomy: a technical review. *Rev Esp Enferm Dig.* 2016;108(5):271-278.

26. El H II, Cote GA. Endoscopic diagnosis and management of ampullary lesions. *Gastrointest Endosc Clin N Am.* 2013;23(1):95-109.

27. Napoleon B, Gincul R, Ponchon T, et al. Endoscopic papillectomy for early ampullary tumors: long-term results from a large multicenter prospective study. *Endoscopy.* 2014;46(2):127-134.

28. Moon JH, Choi HJ, Lee YN. Current status of endoscopic papillectomy for ampullary tumors. *Gut Liver.* 2014;8(6):598-604.

29. Tsuji S, Itoi T, Sofuni A, et al. Tips and tricks in endoscopic papillectomy of ampullary tumors: single-center experience with large case series (with videos). *J Hepatobiliary Pancreat Sci.* 2015;22(6):E22-E27.

30. Will U, Müller AK, Fueldner F, Wanzar I, Meyer F. Endoscopic papillectomy: data of a prospective observational study. *World J Gastroenterol.* 2013;19(27):4316-4324.

31. DePalma GD, Luglio G, Maione F, et al. Endoscopic snare papillectomy: a single institutional experience of a standardized technique. A retrospective cohort study. *Int J Surg.* 2015;13:180-183.

32. Irani S, Arai A, Ayub K, et al. Papillectomy for ampullary neoplasm: results of a single referral center over a 10-year period. *Gastrointest Endosc.* 2009;70(5):923-932.

33. Ceppa EP, Burbridge RA, Rialon KL, et al. Endoscopic versus surgical ampullectomy: an algorithm to treat disease of the ampulla of Vater. *Ann Surg.* 2013;257(2):315-322.

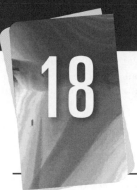

18 | Capsule Endoscopy

Salmaan A. Jawaid, MD
David R. Cave, MD

Video endoscopic capsules (PillCam, Medtronic, MN, USA; EC-10, Olympus America, PA; Mirocam, South Korea; and CapsoCam, Capsovision, CA) can be swallowed and images obtained from the entire small bowel without the need for sedation.[1] Individual digital images are transmitted out of the body by radio frequency to a recording device worn about the patient's waist (PillCam and EC-10 use human body conduction and CapsoCam capsule is recovered from the fecal stream). The images are processed and viewed as a video on a computer workstation after completion of the study.

INDICATIONS

Capsule endoscopy is indicated as a procedure for evaluation of suspected disease of the small intestine including the following:

1. Small intestinal bleeding (aka obscure gastrointestinal bleeding)[2]: These are patients with GI bleeding in whom no diagnosis has been made after upper endoscopy and colonoscopy. Capsule endoscopy has been shown to be superior to both push enteroscopy and radiographic imaging of the small bowel in the evaluation of these patients.[3] If a source of bleeding is detected by capsule endoscopy, a targeted deep enteroscopy (either through an anterograde or retrograde approach) has been shown to increase the diagnostic and therapeutic benefit in these patients.[4,5]

2. Known or suspected Crohn disease: In one study capsule endoscopy detected all the lesions seen on small bowel series and computed tomography scanning and detected additional lesions in 47% of cases.[6] In addition, capsule endoscopy findings can alter treatment strategies in a number of patients.[7]

3. Other suspected small bowel diseases. A growing body of literature supports the superiority of capsule endoscopy over other imaging modalities of the small bowel to detect and further characterize polyposis syndromes, celiac disease, and other malabsorption disorders.[8]

CONTRAINDICATIONS

1. Swallowing disorders (though the capsule can be placed endoscopically)
2. Implanted pacemakers and defibrillators. This is an FDA recommendation that has been questioned by multiple studies
3. Small bowel obstruction
4. Small intestinal strictures (degree of stricturing can be assessed with the patency capsule)

PREPARATION

The typical timing of a capsule exam is to begin the study at 8 AM. with completion of the study at 4 PM. This allows 8 hours of image acquisition during one working day. However, most manufactures now have capsules with a battery life of more than 12 hours, so the capsule recorder may be returned the following day.

1. Instruct the patient to present on the morning of the exam after a 12-hour fast. Some facilities use a 2 L polyethylene glycol preparation the night before.
2. Discontinue oral iron supplementation 3 days prior to the exam.
3. Advise them not to take medications, antacids, or sucralfate, since they can coat the intestinal lining, limiting visualization. Narcotics and antispasmodics can delay both gastric and intestinal emptying, making it difficult to visualize the entire small bowel during the 8-hour acquisition time.
4. Instruct patients to bring their medications with them to take during the day, if necessary. If a patient is diabetic, insulin doses may need to be adjusted.
5. Anticoagulants do not need to be stopped prior to the exam.
6. Instruct the patient to wear loose clothing on the day of the exam. Dresses should be avoided. A buttoned shirt and loose-fitting pants work best.
7. Charge the recorder's battery the evening prior to the study.
8. Bowel preparation may improve the quality of small bowel visualization but has minimal to no effect on transit times or visualization of the cecum, thus is not recommended.[9]

EQUIPMENT

1. **Small bowel capsules** are approximately 11 × 26 mm. They contain light-emitting diodes as a strobe type light source, a lens, a color camera chip, two silver oxide batteries, a radio frequency transmitter, and an antenna. The PillCam is a complementary metal oxide semiconductor chip while the EC-10 uses a CCD chip. The capsules obtain 2 to 3 images per second and transmit data via radio frequency or human body conduction to the recording device worn about the patient's waist. The capsules are disposable and do not need to be retrieved by the patient. They are passed naturally with a bowel movement. However, the CapsoCam, which has four cameras, needs to be recovered from the fecal stream with a simple collection kit. The video may be retrieved from the capsule and processed locally or mailed to a central reading facility.

2. **Recording devices:** These are mini-computers worn on a belt with up to 5 GB of memory, allowing for storage of the raw data obtained during a typical 8- to 12-hour examination. Once the study is completed, the recorded data are downloaded to a computer workstation with software that processes the images into a video for reading.

3. **The real-time viewer:** Recording devices with this capability can allow real-time viewing of the intestinal tract without having to wait for images to be downloaded. This allows for the quick detection of active bleeding or determining whether the capsule has left the stomach, without having to wait at least 8 hours before determining location of bleeding. CapsoCam does not have this facility.

4. **The workstation:** This contains software that interprets several aspects of the data obtained. In addition to the video images, the EC-10 system is designed to identify the capsule's location within the small bowel in 3-D.[10] A digital plot of the small bowel passage is produced that provides a location for each of the images obtained during the 8 hours. This localization is an estimate, since not only does the capsule move within the intestine, but the small bowel also moves within the abdominal cavity. For example, the small bowel can sag to the pelvis while a patient is standing. If the transit diagram produced is combined with the knowledge of the small bowel transit time, an approximation of the position of a lesion can be made.

In addition to localization software, the system also contains an image recognition algorithm that identifies red pixels in the data. This identifies possible areas of bleeding or the possible presence of vascular lesions.[11] False positives with this app are frequent. Each manufacturer provides software which has a variety of reading modes, speeds for viewing, and algorithms to remove repetitive images. The latter helps speed up viewing time.

PROCEDURE

This general set of instructions does not apply to the CapsoCam which is identified, activated, and swallowed.

1. Enter the patient's personal data into the computer workstation.
2. Initialize the recording device to the patient. This ensures that once completed, the recording device data cannot be confused with that of any other patient.
3. Apply the sensor array or sensor belt to the patient's abdomen. This will capture the signals from the capsule and transfer them to the recording device. The sensor array leads are attached by adhesive to the patient's abdomen. Some patients may need to be shaved prior to sensor attachment.
4. Place the empty recorder holster around the patient's waist or over the shoulder.
5. Place the recording device and battery pack into the holster and attach the sensor leads to the recording device.
6. Remove the capsule from its container. Removing the capsule from the magnet in the pack turns the capsule on, and it begins to flash and transmit its images twice per second. The recorder's light flashes in synchrony with the capsule, attesting to successful transmission of each image.
7. Instruct the patient to swallow the capsule, followed by a full glass of water.
8. Advise the patient that he or she may then leave the facility and carry on a normal day. The patient should (1) refrain from exercising and heavy lifting during the exam, (2) avoid large transmitters and magnetic resonance imaging (MRI) machines, (3) not stand directly next to another patient undergoing capsule endoscopy, (4) not touch the recorder or the antenna array leads, (5) not remove the leads, and (6) not take the belt or the shoulder straps off, if possible until the study is complete; in addition, the patient should be very careful when pulling up underwear over the sensors to avoid disconnection. The patient may (1) walk, sit, and lie down; (2) drive a car; (3) return to work; (4) use a computer, radio, stereo, or cell phone; (5) loosen the Velcro on the belt to facilitate going to the bathroom; (6) may drink clear liquids after 2 hours and eat 4 hours after swallowing the capsule; and (7) take his or her medications at that time.

POSTPROCEDURE

1. When the patient returns after 8 to 12 hours, remove the belt and the sensor arrays.
2. Instruct the patient to avoid having an MRI until the capsule passes. Should passage not be seen, an abdominal flat plate can be obtained after 2 weeks. The capsule read will confirm passage though the ileocecal valve.
3. Discharge the patient.
4. Attach the recorder to the workstation. Generally, downloads take less than 1 hour.
5. Once the download is complete, disconnect the recorder from the workstation, so that it can be recharged and initialized for a new patient.
6. Review the images on the workstation and create a report

INTERPRETATION

Before reading a capsule study, physicians should be familiar with the patient's medical history, not only including the indication for the study but also any surgical history. Prior knowledge of a surgical small bowel anastomosis can aid or simplify the interpretation of the study. In addition, physicians must have experience in interpreting endoscopic images. The reader should be able to make a diagnosis based on the images. This will allow the dismissal of normal variants and nonpathologic lesions, and the identification of specific pathologies require intervention. The images obtained at capsule endoscopy are slightly different from traditional endoscopy, since there is no air distention of the intestine. This is so-called "physiologic endoscopy." The bowel is not altered by the process of the examination. There is no sedation used, and thus there are no hemodynamic effects. There is no trauma caused by the capsule. There is no air insufflation to affect the microvasculature.

There are very specific steps that can be taken to ease the process of reading a capsule exam. A pattern of practice should be developed by the physician. The following is recommended:

1. Examine the very last image to assure that the colon has been entered. The presence of stool will confirm this finding.
2. After returning to the very first image, activate blood detection software (if the exam was performed in the setting of obscure gastrointestinal bleeding). To scan the entire study including the stomach, the first image is falsely identified as the first duodenal image on a thumbnail edit. This turns on the Suspected Blood Indicator (SBI) software. Any positive findings can be quickly examined, and thumbnails created. Once completed, the first image thumbnail is deleted.

3. Identify and thumbnail the first gastric image, and the first image of the duodenum and cecum. These are needed to determine both the gastric and small bowel emptying times. Increase the image rate to 25 frames/s, and play the images forward in an automatic mode—one- to four-frame viewing modes are available. The author's preference is to use the four-frame mode. The time that each image is on the screen is longer than in single-frame mode.

The esophagogastric junction is quickly seen, and the first gastric image is duly noted on a thumbnail edit. Using the time and color bar, quickly advance the images forward and backward until the first image of the duodenum is identified. This too is noted on a thumbnail edit. It should be remembered that the capsule can move backward and forward through the pylorus several times prior to its final passage and further advancement into the small bowel. Again, use the time/color bar to identify the ileocecal valve. This landmark proves to be quite difficult for many physicians. The presence of formed stool is a definite indicator of the colon, as is the disappearance of villi. It can take some time for the beginning reader to reliably identify this landmark, and then note it on a thumbnail edit.

4. Calculate transit times. The average gastric time is approximately 40 minutes, the average time in the small bowel is 240 minutes, and the average passage time to the colon is 300 minutes.[12] An 8-hour acquisition time assures that 80% to 85% of capsules will reach the colon, allowing for complete inspection of the small bowel. The new longer-battery-life capsules will nearly eliminate the problem of incomplete transit.

5. Once the landmarks have been thumbnailed, view the images. The gastric portion of the exam should be examined, but it can be viewed at a rapid rate since a recent upper endoscopy should have been performed. In the small bowel, starting at the first image of the duodenum, use the multiviewer function to scan two images or four images at a rate of 20 to 25 frames/s. A mouse with a scroll wheel is an essential tool. If reading is performed on a laptop computer, a mouse should be attached, since this greatly eases the reading process. When an area moves by too quickly or if a possible abnormality is seen, movement of the scroll wheel will stop the progress of the images and allow review of the passed images. The capsule moves extremely quickly in the proximal small bowel as compared to the distal sections. In the duodenum, the frame-to-finding ratio is quite high, and thus the duodenum often requires using the scroll wheel to examine each individual image. The frame-to-finding ratio in the ileum is quite low,

and the use of the scroll wheel diminishes distally. When an abnormality is identified, a thumbnail is created. Routinely creating thumbnails for every 30 minutes of images viewed is recommended. This allows the reader to stop, to read, and to find where the reading stopped and also prevents having to start over should the reader lose his or her place.

6. Review localization data. This allows the physician to know if an identified abnormality is within reach of a push entero-scope or requires deep enteroscopy. The information can also guide subsequent surgery. Generally, the localization image will identify the duodenum and ligament of Treitz. The physician derives location of an abnormality within the jejunum or ileum from a compilation of data. This includes the quadrant location provided by the localization image, the time of passage from the pylorus to the lesion, the amount of bowel visually traversed by the capsule en route to the lesions, and the amount of bowel traversed from the lesion to the ileocecal valve. This information is difficult to quantify, since a distance traveled algorithm is not yet available, but qualitative judgments by an experienced physician can be quite accurate in providing a location. Thus a differentiation between those patients treated with enteroscopic therapy (anterograde versus retrograde) and those requiring surgical intervention can be made. Lesions found within 30 minutes of passage from the pylorus and those located in the left abdomen are generally within reach of a 2.5-m-long push enteroscope or pediatric colonoscope. This statement is based on a typical small bowel passage time of 4 hours and a normal progression of the capsule within the proximal small bowel. Occasionally, a capsule may remain for a prolonged time in the duodenal bulb, altering the above generalizations. Lesions more than 1 hour beyond the pylorus may be reached by other forms of anterograde deep enteroscopy (double, single balloon or Spirus enteroscopes), but those beyond the 2- to 3-hour mark generally require surgical intervention for management. If a lesion is suspected in the distal small bowel, then a retrograde deep enteroscopy can be performed with the aforementioned instruments.

ADVERSE EVENTS

1. Capsule retention: A large study reveals that true retention for more than 2 weeks occurs in approximately 1% of examinations. The capsule is typically retained at a site of pathology that is likely to require surgery, such as strictures caused by non-steroidal antiinflammatory drugs or Crohn's strictures

or a partially obstructing tumor. It rarely becomes lodged in a diverticulum or in the appendiceal orifice. Retention only very rarely causes symptoms of obstruction. Use of a patency capsule, CT, or MR enterography is recommended in preference to a barium small bowel series for detection of small bowel stenosis.

OTHER USES FOR THIS TECHNIQUE

1. Initial diagnostic tool in nonhematemesis gastrointestinal bleeding[13]
2. Crohn disease; long-term management
3. Celiac disease; if patient refuses EGD or in the setting of refractory disease to assess activity
4. Chronic abdominal pain (very low yield)
5. Colorectal cancer screening—for patients who undergo incomplete screening colonoscopies

CPT CODES

91110—Gastrointestinal tract imaging, intraluminal (e.g., capsule endoscopy), esophagus through ileum, with physician interpretation and report

The diagnosis codes associated with capsule endoscopy are dependent on the indication and findings. The most common codes are those for GI bleeding, once colonoscopy and upper endoscopy are nondiagnostic.

References

1. Meron G. The development of the swallowable video capsule (M2A). *Gastrointest Endosc*. 2000;6:817-819.
2. Lewis B, Goldfarb N. The advent of capsule endoscopy — a not-so-futuristic approach to obscure gastrointestinal bleeding. *Aliment Pharmacol Ther*. 2003;17:1085-1096.
3. Costamagna G, Shah S, Riccioni M, et al. A prospective trial comparing small bowel radiographs and video capsule endoscopy for suspected small bowel disease. *Gastroenterology*. 2002;123:999-1005.
4. Fry LC, Neumann H, Jovanovic I, et al. Capsule endoscopy increases the diagnostic yield of double balloon enteroscopy in patients being investigated for obscure gastrointestinal bleeding. *Arch Gastroenterohepatol*. 2012;29:9-14.
5. Gay G, Delvaux M, Fassler I. Outcome of capsule endoscopy in determining indication and route for push-and-pull enteroscopy. *Endoscopy*. 2006;38:49-58.
6. Eliakim R, Fischer D, Suissa A, et al. Wireless capsule video endoscopy is a superior diagnostic tool in comparison to barium follow-through and computerized tomography in patients with suspected Crohn's disease. *Eur J Gastroenterol Hepatol*. 2003;15:363-367.
7. Kopylov U, Nemeth A, Koulaouzidis A, et al. Small bowel capsule endoscopy in the management of established Crohn's disease: clinical impact, safety, and correlation with inflammatory biomarkers. *Inflamm Bowel Dis*. 2015;21:93-100.

8. Scapa E, Jacob H, Lewkowicz S, et al. Initial experience of wireless-capsule endoscopy for evaluating occult gastrointestinal bleeding and suspected small bowel pathology. *Am J Gastro.* 2002;97:2776-2779.
9. Niv Y. Efficiency of bowel preparation for capsule endoscopy examination: a meta-analysis. *World J Gastroenterol.* 2008;14(9):1313-1317. doi:10.3748/wjg.14.1313.
10. Fischer D, Shreiber R, Meron G, et al. Localization of a wireless capsule endoscope in the GI tract. *Gastrointest Endosc.* 2001;53:AB126.
11. Liangpunsakul S, Mays L, Rex D. Performance of given suspected blood indicator. *Am J Gastroenterol.* 2003;98:2676-2678.
12. Appleyard M, Glukhovsky A, Jacob H, et al. Transit times for the capsule endoscope. *Gastrointest Endosc.* 2001;53:AB122.
13. Marya N, Jawaid S, Foley A, et al. A randomized controlled trial comparing efficacy of early video capsule endoscopy with standard of care in the approach to non-hematemesis. *Gastrointest Endosc.* 2019;89(1):33-43.e4.

PART FOUR

Colonoscopy Procedures

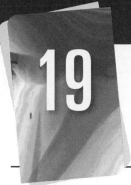

19

Basic Colonoscopy

Mishita Goel, MBBS
Rajesh Keswani, MD, MS

Colonoscopy permits the visual examination of the mucosal surface from the anal canal to the terminal ileum using a flexible digital instrument. A coordinated series of maneuvers are required for safe intubation of colon and associated diagnostic and therapeutic manuevers, such as polypectomy. The acquisition of these skills requires dedicated training, often obtained during a standardized training program such as a gastroenterology fellowship. Besides providing the ability to visualize suspected colon abnormalities (e.g., inflammation), it also permits biopsy and therapy (e.g., polypectomy) at any site; the ability to acquire tissue for histopathologic analysis allows for a confirmatory diagnosis to be made (e.g., inflammatory bowel disease). In contrast, other noninvasive imaging tests are unable to obtain biopsies or perform therapy and thus have a purely diagnostic role.

INDICATIONS[1]

The indications of colonoscopy are myriad including both diagnostic and therapeutic. Screening and surveillance are the most frequent indications for colonoscopy.

Diagnostic, Including

1. Screening for colorectal cancer[2-4]
   a. average-risk persons generally beginning at age 50 years, every 10 years
   b. if one first-degree relative diagnosed with colorectal cancer (or adenoma) at
      i. age >60 years: beginning at 40 years, with subsequent examination intervals based on initial colonoscopy findings

    ii. age <60 years: beginning at 40 years or 10 years before age of diagnosis of youngest relative, then every 5 years (also applies if two first-degree relatives diagnosed with colorectal cancer or adenomas)

  c. Lynch syndrome: beginning at age 20 to 25 years, every 1 to 2 years, until age 40 years, then annually

  d. Patients with familial adenomatous polyposis and identified colon polyps in whom surgery is being delayed: every 6 to 12 months

  e. Women with endometrial or ovarian cancer diagnosed at age <50 years: beginning at time of diagnosis, then every 5 years

2. Evaluation of gastrointestinal bleeding:

  a. Hematochezia (bright red blood per rectum) in absence of any definite anorectal source

  b. Melena (black, tarry stools) after an upper source has been excluded

  c. Iron-deficiency anemia

3. Positive fecal immunochemical test (FIT) (when FIT is used for colorectal cancer screening)

4. Evaluation of an abnormality on barium enema, flexible sigmoidoscopy, or CT colonography (virtual colonoscopy)

5. Surveillance:

  a. after removal of adenomas or serrated polyps

    i. US guidelines call for a 3-year interval examination in patients with three or more adenomas or when adenomas are >1 cm, contain high-grade dysplasia, or villous elements

    ii. US guidelines recommend a 5-year interval examination in patients with one to two adenomas

    iii. Guidelines vary when serrated polyps are removed during colonoscopy

  b. When colonoscopy is accompanied by an inadequate preparation, a repeat colonoscopy is recommended within a year regardless of findings

  c. after resection of colorectal cancer

6. In patients with ulcerative pancolitis or Crohn colitis of ≥8 years duration or left-sided colitis ≥15 years duration

7. Clinically significant diarrhea of unexplained origin

8. Evaluation for synchronous or metachronous malignancy in patients with colon cancer

9. Intraoperative lesion localization (e.g., polypectomy site, location of a bleeding site, or small mass)

Therapeutic, Including

1. Excision of precancerous colorectal lesions (i.e., polypectomy)

2. Hemostasis of bleeding lesions

3. Balloon dilation of strictures
4. Foreign body removal
5. Decompression of colonic pseudo-obstruction (Ogilvie syndrome) or volvulus
6. Endoscopic placement of a stent for a colorectal cancer causing large bowel obstruction
7. Percutaneous endoscopic cecostomy tube placement

CONTRAINDICATIONS
Absolute
1. Toxic megacolon
2. Fulminant colitis—Acute severe colitis characterized by toxic symptoms such as fever, anorexia, abdominal pain, diarrhea with shock or hypotension, ileus, or megacolon[5,6]
3. Known/suspected colonic perforation (however, if a colon perforation is caused during colonoscopy, colonoscopy may be continued to close the perforation)

Relative
1. Acute diverticulitis[7,8]
2. History of recent myocardial infarction or pulmonary embolus
3. Cardiopulmonary instability
4. Suspected poor bowel preparation

Although not a contraindication to colonoscopy, patients with coagulopathies (either due to intrinsic disease or medications) require a personalized approach to colonoscopy to determine appropriateness of procedure and whether the coagulopathy needs to be corrected.

Colonoscopy can safely be performed in pregnancy, but the potential risks and benefits should be carefully considered.

PREPARATION[9]
1. *Patient instructions*—Informed consent must be obtained after explaining the procedure, its benefits, risks, alternatives, and limitations in an understandable format. It is recommended that written instructions be provided at least a week prior to the procedure so that the patient can read them all and follow the medication and dietary changes required.
2. *Diet and medications*:
   a. Patients are recommended a low-residue diet for 2 to 3 days prior to colonoscopy
   b. On the prior to the colonoscopy, either a clear liquid–only diet *or* a strict low-residue diet is appropriate
   c. Most medications may be continued up until the time of colonoscopy

   d. Diabetic medications require an individualized approach in coordination with the prescribing provider as blood sugars fluctuate with the altered diet

   e. Iron must be stopped at least 5 days before colonoscopy since iron makes the residual feces black and difficult to purge

   f. Whether anticoagulant medicines are continued or stopped is an individualized decision based on the indication for the medicines and the intervention planned. Aspirin can always be continued for colonoscopy. NSAIDs should be discontinued if possible as they may result in colon erosions/ulcers

   g. Antibiotic prophylaxis is not required during colonoscopy

3. *Labs*—Routine preprocedure lab testing, chest imaging, or EKG is not required but may be used selectively based on patient's medical history and physical examination.

4. *Bowel preparation*—An excellent bowel preparation is required for effective colonoscopy. The ideal bowel preparation is safe, efficacious, palatable, and affordable. Multiple FDA-approved bowel preparations exist[10,11] like polyethylene glycol-electrolyte solutions (PEG-ELS),[12] low-volume PEG-ELS, sulfate-free PEG-ELS, sodium phosphate[13] etc., details of which are mentioned in Chapter 3.

5. *Anesthesia*—There are three approaches to anesthesia for colonoscopy: no sedation, moderate sedation[14] (also known as "conscious sedation"), and deep sedation. See Chapter 2 for details. Although not popular in the United States, colonoscopy is often performed without sedation in other countries. It has the particular advantage of a reduced cost and the ability for the patient to take themselves home without requiring an adult to accompany them.

EQUIPMENT

1. Colonoscope—The choice between an adult and pediatric colonoscope generally depends on the endoscopist's preference. Adult colonoscopes have a diameter of approximately 13 mm, whereas pediatric colonoscopes are approximately 11 mm. Pediatric colonoscopes are more flexible and can more easily navigate tighter colon turns such as in the sigmoid; however, they have a smaller accessory channel which may impair the ability to suction stool and does not accommodate some large devices (e.g., most colon stents). Occasionally, the colonoscopist might utilize an upper endoscope (gastroscope) to navigate a particularly difficult colon

2. Image processor

3. One or more screens projecting the colonoscope image

4. Hemodynamic monitoring equipment (pulse, blood pressure monitoring with/without continuous EKG); capnography is occasionally utilized but the data supporting its use are conflicting

5. Endoscopic devices such as biopsy forceps, polypectomy snares, retrieval nets, injection needles, hemostatic clips, and argon plasma coagulation probes

6. Universal precautions with gloves, gowns, and masks

Components of Colonoscope[15]

- a control section (two control knobs are present—a large knob for vertical adjustment and a smaller knob for lateral tip movement)
- an instrument channel (which allows the insertion of endoscopic accessories as described above)
- a shaft (portion of the instrument that gets inserted into the patient)
- the tip (distal end of the shaft; controlled from the control section)
- a connection section
- a connection line
- a lever to vary stiffness

PROCEDURE

Positioning

Colonoscopy is generally performed begun with the examinee in the left lateral decubitus position, but the patient position may be changed during the examination to facilitate cecal intubation. The position of the endoscopist varies between endoscopists but should take into account ergonomic principles.

Techniques[15]

1. Tip deflection: Vertical (up/down) and lateral (left/right) tip deflection; performed by using control knob.

2. Insufflation and suction: Although air was previously used for insufflation, carbon dioxide is preferred for patient comfort and safety; insufflation is performed using the air/water infusion valve and the suction valve buttons.

3. Torque: This is a critical maneuver in colonoscopy that is performed by turning the shaft clockwise or counter-clockwise; this results in changing the angle at which the colonoscope approaches the next turn and does not rely on using the wheels. This is best performed when there are no loops in the colonoscope. This is especially helpful when navigating colon turns or to place polyps in an optimal position for removal.

4. Advancing and reducing the colonoscope: Although advancing the colonoscope is intuitive, loops may form in the colon where the midportion of the colonoscope is stretching out a segment of colon. This results in patient discomfort and also makes colonoscope advancement challenging. At this point, reducing (or pulling back) the colonoscope is an essential maneuver to resolve colon loops and to keep the scope straight. In general, this is done by advancing beyond the colonoscope beyond a turn, applying torque to the colonoscope, and withdrawing the colonoscope. This results in removal of the loops and paradoxically can advance the colonoscope as the loop is resolved.

5. Water may be used instead of carbon dioxide to help navigate a challenging turn. In this case, water distends the lumen and often straightens a particularly angulated turn.

6. A transparent cap can be placed at the tip of the colonoscope to facilitate navigation through the turns of the colon by preventing what is known as "red out"—when the tip of the colonoscope is directly abutting the colon wall and the direction of the turn is not clearly seen.

7. Slide-by technique: This should infrequently be used and never by a novice. This involves slowly pushing the tip of the colonoscope forward in the anticipated direction of the lumen. As the colonoscope is being pushed against the wall, this may result in trauma and thus this should be performed carefully. It is suggested that the slide-by technique is safer with the use of a transparent cap, but this has not been clearly shown.

8. Abdominal pressure: To prevent formation of loops with colonoscope advancement, the endoscopist may ask the assisting technician or nurse to put pressure on the abdominal wall. This should be done in a targeted fashion. For example, if loop formation is suspected in the sigmoid colon, first the created loop should be reduced; second, abdominal wall pressure should be placed in the region of the sigmoid colon by the assistant; and third, the endoscopist should attempt to advance the colonoscope. If this does not work, the process should be restarted with adjustment of the abdominal wall pressure.

Examination[15]

1. Perform a perianal examination and digital rectal examination. This also lubricates the anal canal and relaxes the sphincters to facilitate colonoscope insertion.

2. Insert the scope into the rectum keeping the right hand on the shaft and using the left hand to control the up/down angulation knob for steering along with the right/left torque of the shaft to provide directional changes and prevent loop formation.

3. The rectum should be insufflated immediately upon colonoscope insertion. Advancement of the colonoscope through the rectum is performed without difficulty.

4. The advancement of the colonoscope into the sigmoid may be more challenging due to acute bends that might result in loop formation. Thus, the use of torque and, in some cases water to distend and straighten the colon, is helpful. As noted above, a transparent cap may also help identify the direction of the lumen.

5. Loops generally form in the sigmoid colon with colonoscope advancement. An attempt to reduce these loops should be made after reaching the descending colon utilizing torque and colonoscope withdrawal.

6. Advancing the colonoscope through the descending, transverse, and ascending colon requires careful attention to optimal technique with reduction of the colonoscope when loops are suspected after each turn, use of abdominal pressure to prevent loop formation, and occasionally changing patient position—generally to the supine position—if looping persists.

7. During advancement of the colonoscope, two major landmarks can often be identified to help determine progress—first the impression of the spleen can be seen at the junction of the descending colon/transverse colon, known as the splenic flexure; following this, the impression of the liver can be seen at the junction of the ascending colon/transverse colon, known as the hepatic flexure.

8. Advancement of the colonoscope into the cecum from the ascending colon is sometimes challenging due to looping. If the cecum cannot be reached despite external abdominal pressure, changing patient position to the supine or even right lateral decubitus position should be consider. The cecum is recognized by visualization of both the appendiceal orifice and ileocecal valve (ICV).

9. To intubate the terminal ileum, the ICV is generally placed at the 12 o'clock position. The colonoscope is then deflected in the direction of the ICV and the colonoscope withdrawn until the terminal ileum is intubated.

10. The scope can be retroflexed (U-turn) in two areas; the cecum, to evaluate the colon mucosa behind the thick ascending colon folds *and* the rectum, to evaluate the distal rectum and anal verge.

THERAPEUTIC COLONOSCOPY[16,17]

1. Tissue sampling and/or polyp removal for all visible lesions seen during colonoscopy is generally performed during withdrawal of the colonoscope. If required, a permanent marker can also be placed at a desired location by injecting carbon particles solution into the submucosa for future localization (either at future colonoscopy or surgery).

2. The most commonly performed therapeutic intervention is polypectomy. It can be done using various techniques depending on polyp size and characteristics. Cold forceps polypectomy for nonpedunculated polyps can be performed for polyps up to 2 mm but should be avoided for larger polyps. Cold snare polypectomy can be performed for polyps up to approximately 8 mm in size. Cautery (hot) polypectomy should not be routinely performed for polyps <8 mm but may be appropriate for the larger polyps.

3. When polyps are larger than 8 to 10 mm, a submucosal injection (sometimes with a contrast dye) is often performed beneath the polyp to lift away from the muscularis propria to facilitate safer removal. This is known as endoscopic mucosal resection.

4. Hemostasis can be achieved using endoscopic clipping (through-the-scope or over-the-scope) or cautery. Cautery techniques include monopolar forceps, bipolar probe, and argon plasma coagulation.

5. Benign colon strictures, often seen after surgery, can be treated with through-the-scope balloon dilators.

6. Malignant colonic obstruction can be treated via placement of self-expanding metal stents across the malignant obstruction. This can be done for either preoperative decompression or palliation of advanced cancer.

7. Decompression of the colon can also be performed via placement of a decompression tube, sometimes required for colonic pseudo-obstruction.

POST PROCEDURE

A detailed report following all colonoscopies should include the following:

- Patient's name, age, gender, and informed consent
- Date and time of colonoscopy
- Indication(s) for the procedure
- Type of instrument used
- Details of the sedation
- Bowel preparation quality

- Difficulties encountered during procedure and any special maneuver, if performed
- Description of colonoscopy findings
- Follow-up plan including timing of subsequent colonoscopies

ADVERSE EVENTS[9,18]

1. Cardiopulmonary—occur mostly due to procedural sedation; can range from transient hypoxemia to significant arrhythmias, respiratory arrest, myocardial infarction, and shock.

2. Bleeding—most often associated with polypectomy; may be immediate (treated immediately with colonoscopic hemostatic methods) or delayed that present up to 2 weeks after colonoscopy as hematochezia or melena depending on the location of the bleed. Delayed bleeding can be managed with colonoscopy and rarely requires angiographic embolization and surgery.

3. Postpolypectomy syndrome—occurs due to electrocoagulation injury that causes a transmural burn to the bowel wall leading to focal peritonitis without frank perforation. This often presents 1 to 5 days after procedure and is managed with IV hydration, parenteral antibiotics, and no oral intake until symptoms subside.

4. Perforation—generally occurs due to mechanical trauma and rarely (especially when carbon dioxide is used and in the absence of colitis), barotrauma. If a perforation is identified during colonoscopy, an attempt should be made to close the perforation with the colonoscope itself using endoscopic clips or (rarely) suturing. These patients can generally successfully be managed nonsurgically. In contrast, patients who present in a delayed manner with a perforation (i.e., unrecognized from time of colonoscopy) often require surgery.

5. Infection related to colonoscopy is very rare.

6. Gas explosion very rarely occurs and is due to use of electrosurgical energy (e.g., electrocautery or argon plasma coagulation) in the presence of combustible levels of hydrogen or methane gas in the colonic lumen; can occur due to use of incompletely absorbable carbohydrate preparations like mannitol, sorbitol, or lactulose.

CPT CODES[19,20]

45378—Colonoscopy, flexible; diagnostic, including collection of specimen(s) by brushing or washing, when performed (separate procedure)
45379—With removal of foreign body(s)

45380—With biopsy, single or multiple

45381—With directed submucosal injection(s), any substance

45382—With control of bleeding, any method

45384—With removal of tumor(s), polyp(s), or other lesion(s) by hot biopsy forceps

45385—With removal of tumor(s), polyp(s), or other lesion(s) by snare technique

45386—With transendoscopic balloon dilation

45388—With ablation of tumor(s), polyp(s), or other lesion(s) (includes pre- and post dilation and guidewire passage, when performed)

45389—With endoscopic stent placement (includes pre- and post dilation and guidewire passage, when performed)

45390—With endoscopic mucosal resection

45391—With endoscopic ultrasound examination limited to the rectum, sigmoid, descending, transverse, or ascending colon and cecum, and adjacent structures

45392—With transendoscopic ultrasound-guided intramural or transmural fine needle aspiration/biopsy(s), includes endoscopic ultrasound examination limited to the rectum, sigmoid, descending, transverse, or ascending colon and cecum, and adjacent structures

45393—With decompression (for pathologic distention) (e.g., volvulus, megacolon), including placement of decompression tube, when performed

45398—With band ligation(s) (e.g., hemorrhoids)

References

1. Bhagatwala J, Singhal A, Aldrugh S, Sherid M, Sifuentes H, Sridhar S. Colonoscopy – indications and contraindications. In: Ettarh R, ed. *Screening for Colorectal Cancer with Colonoscopy.* InTech; 2015.
2. Winawer S, Fletcher R, Rex D, et al. Colorectal cancer screening and surveillance: clinical guidelines and rationale – update based on new evidence. *Gastroenterology.* 2003;124(2):544-560.
3. Society AC. *American Cancer Society Recommendations for Colorectal Cancer Early Detection;* 2014.
4. ASGE|Press Release: Updates for Colon Cancer Screening Guidelines. Available at https://www.asge.org/home/about-asge/newsroom/news-list/2017/07/20/200803-press-release-updates-for-colon-cancer-screening-guidelines. Accessed June 1, 2018.
5. Lamont JT, Kelly CP, Bakken JS. *Clostridium difficile Infection in Adults: Clinical Manifestations and Diagnosis.* Waltham, MA: UpToDate; 2018. Available at https://www.uptodate.com/contents/clostridium-difficile-infection-in-adults-clinical-manifestations-and-diagnosis. Accessed May 1, 2018.
6. Peppercorn MA, Farrell RJ. *Management of Severe Ulcerative Colitis in Adults.* Waltham, MA: Wolters Kluwer; August 2014:13. Available at https://www.uptodate.com/contents/management-of-severe-ulcerative-colitis-in-adults. Accessed May 1, 2018.

7. Lahat A, Yanai H, Menachem Y, Avidan B, Bar-Meir S. The feasibility and risk of early colonoscopy in acute diverticulitis: a prospective controlled study. *Endoscopy.* 2007;39(6):521-524.
8. Gross M, Labenz J, Börsch G, et al. Colonoscopy in acute diverticulitis. *Visc Med.* 2015;31(2):124-129.
9. Lee L, Saltzman JR. *Overview of Colonoscopy in Adults.* UpToDate; 2013:1-56. Available at http://www.uptodate.com. Accessed May 1, 2018.
10. Standards of Practice Committee ASGE, Saltzman JR, Cash BD, et al. Bowel preparation before colonoscopy. *Gastrointest Endosc.* 2015;81(4):781-794.
11. Parekh PJ, Oldfield EC, Johnson DA. 9-Bowel preparation for colonoscopy. In: Chandrasekhara V, Elmunzer BJ, Khashab MA, Muthusamy VR, eds. *Clinical Gastrointestinal Endoscopy.* 3rd ed. Philadelphia: Content Repository Only!; 2019:102-109.e2.
12. Enestvedt BK, Tofani C, Laine LA, Tierney A, Fennerty MB. 4-Liter split-dose polyethylene glycol is superior to other bowel preparations, based on systematic review and meta-analysis. *Clin Gastroenterol Hepatol.* 2012;10(11):1225-1231.
13. UpToDate. Available at https://www.uptodate.com/contents/bowel-preparation-before-colonoscopy-in-adults. Accessed June 2, 2018.
14. Sonnenberg A. Sedation in colonoscopy. *Gastroenterol Hepatol.* 2016;12(5):327-329.
15. Lee S-H, Park Y-K, Lee D-J, Kim K-M. Colonoscopy procedural skills and training for new beginners. *World J Gastroenterol.* 2014;20(45):16984-16995.
16. Horiuchi A, Tanaka N. Improving quality measures in colonoscopy and its therapeutic intervention. *World J Gastroenterol.* 2014;20(36):13027-13034.
17. Forde KA. Therapeutic colonoscopy. *World J Surg.* 1992;16(6):1048-1053.
18. Standards of Practice Committee ASGE, Fisher DA, Maple JT, et al. Complications of colonoscopy. *Gastrointest Endosc.* 2011;74(4):745-752.
19. Colonoscopy – CPT Codes 45378-45398, G0105, G0121 – ASGE. Available at https://www.asge.org/docs/default-source/coding/colonoscopy_2018-coding-sheet.pdf?sfvrsn=4. Accessed May 1, 2018.
20. Colonoscopy Coding Guidelines|Screening Colonoscopy|ICD 10 & Modifier 33. Coding Intel; September 26, 2013. Available at http://www.codingintel.com/coding-for-screening-colonoscopy/. Accessed June 10, 2018.

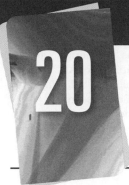

20

Anoscopy and Rigid Sigmoidoscopy

Ana DeRoo, MD
John C. Byrn, MD

The routine use of colonoscopy or flexible sigmoidoscopy to examine the rectum and distal colon has not alleviated the need for physicians to become proficient in the use of the anoscope and the rigid sigmoidoscope. The anoscope allows diagnosis and evaluation of conditions such as fistula in ano, perirectal abscess, anal fissure, anal cancer, or perianal Crohn disease and treatment of lesions in the anal canal and distal rectum.[1] Rigid sigmoidoscopy is useful for evaluation of and therapeutic maneuvers in the distal colon and rectum that cannot be performed with the flexible instrument, such as the topical application of formalin in radiation proctopathy and the removal of foreign bodies. In addition, rigid sigmoidoscopy can be performed anywhere there is an electrical outlet, with highly portable equipment that does not require expertise for cleaning or maintenance, as many components are disposable, and without the need for specially trained ancillary personnel. Therefore, rigid sigmoidoscopy is an expedient option in the intensive care unit, emergency department, or other situations requiring rapid use. This section will cover the techniques of anoscopy and rigid sigmoidoscopy.

INDICATIONS

1. Evaluation of symptoms referable to the colon, rectum, or anus: bleeding, discharge, protrusions or swellings, abdominal or anorectal pain, diarrhea, constipation or a change in bowel habits, severe itching
2. Surveillance of colorectal disease including anal and rectal neoplasms
3. Collection of specimen for histologic study (e.g., biopsies for anal intraepithelial neoplasia (AIN)) or stool and/or exudate for bacteriologic or parasitologic study

4. Removal of foreign bodies
5. Application of topical therapy such as formalin in cases of radiation proctopathy or trichloroacetic acid for AIN[2,3]
6. Injection of medications such as botulinum toxin injection into the anal sphincter for treatment of anal fissures
7. Basic rectal cancer screening examination in areas where flexible sigmoidoscopy or colonoscopy are not available

CONTRAINDICATIONS
Absolute
1. Lack of patient consent
2. Absent anus due to congenital condition or postoperative state
3. Severe pain during examination

Relative
1. Anal strictures
2. Recent anal surgery
3. Uncooperative patient
4. General medical condition
   - Acute peritonitis
   - Fulminant colitis/toxic megacolon
   - Acute, severe diverticulitis
   - Major anorectal trauma
   - Coagulopathy
   - Unstable cardiac disease

PREPARATION
1. Obtain informed consent.
2. Have chaperone in room.
3. Antibiotic prophylaxis is no longer recommended for patients undergoing GI endoscopy, unless a high-risk patient (e.g., prosthetic valve, previous infective endocarditis) has an established GI tract infection, at which point prophylactic antibiotics may be considered.[4]
4. Most patients can be examined with no prior bowel preparation.
5. If stool precludes an adequate examination, a bisacodyl suppository, tap water enema, or Fleet (or other proprietary small volume hypertonic phosphate) enema can be given and the examination carried out following evacuation. Outpatients may take the enema at home 1 to 2 hours prior to procedure.
6. Very rarely, an oral preparation with polyethylene glycol electrolyte solution or phospho-soda will be required the day prior to the procedure.

7. Premedication (sedation) is rarely necessary, although intravenous fentanyl and/or midazolam can be useful in unusual circumstances. Institutional sedation guidelines must be followed in such cases. Severely painful conditions may require scheduling examination with sedation or under anesthesia.

EQUIPMENT
Minimal Equipment

1. Anoscope and rigid sigmoidoscope: A variety of sizes are available if the institution uses reusable anoscopes. The disposable plastic anoscope allows for 360° visualization of the anal canal through the transparent plastic. Metal endoscopes frequently have angled tips, providing preferential viewing in one direction as well as end viewing of the anal canal on withdrawal of the instrument.[5] An adult rigid sigmoidoscope is adequate for all sizes of patient but the infant.
2. Light source: Anoscopes are available with and without an integrated light source.
3. Cotton swab sticks
4. Examination table or bed
5. Sheet to cover the patient
6. Gloves, 4 × 4-in. gauze pads, lubricant (2% topical lidocaine may be useful as a lubricant in painful anorectal disease)

Useful Equipment

1. Sigmoidoscopy table or routine examination table with availability of pillows/blankets to position the patient in knee-chest position if necessary
2. Suction
3. Air insufflator
4. Biopsy tools: either alligator-type (see "Procedure" section, "Rectal Biopsy with Alligator Forceps") or colonoscopic biopsy forceps
5. Medications to be used (epinephrine solution, silver nitrate sticks, botulinum toxin, 5% acetic acid and Lugol iodine solution for anal neoplasia surveillance)[6]
6. Colposcopes are an adjunct to a bivalve anoscope or angled anoscope, necessary for high-resolution anoscopy in anal neoplasia surveillance[6]

PROCEDURE

In order to successfully complete the procedure, the patient must be relaxed. Reassure the patient throughout and inform the patient what is to be done during the procedure. Advise the patient that a few deep breaths during the examination will often relax muscles and sphincters. A chaperone must be present during the procedure. Experienced chaperones are also helpful in the positioning of and providing reassurance to the patient.

Position

A variety of patient positions are adequate for anoscopy and rigid sigmoidoscopy: left lateral or Sims position, knee-chest position, and jackknife are the most common. Start by positioning the patient for the examination that best suits their comfort.[5,7]

Left Lateral (Sims) Position

This is best for bedridden or feeble patients. Be sure to get buttocks to the edge of the bed or table by placing the patient diagonally across the bed (Fig. 20.1A).

Knee-Chest Position

This is adequate for most examinations. It requires more patient stamina and cooperation (Fig. 20.1B).

Prone, Inverted (Jackknife) Position with Sigmoidoscopy Table

This is the most comfortable position for the patient and the examiner (Fig. 20.1C). Place the patient's knee rest high enough so that the "broken" table does not compress the abdomen. Angling the table allows the pelvic organs to "fall away" when the sigmoidoscope is advanced. Elbow rests are preferred so that the

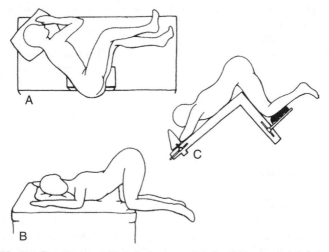

FIG. 20.1 Three major positions for anoscopy and sigmoidoscopy. A, Left lateral (Sims) position. B, Knee-chest position. C, Prone, inverted (jackknife) position.

patient does not slide off the end of the table. Care must be taken once the examination is complete, have the patient gradually resume an upright position, as some patients feel lightheaded or dizzy if they change position too quickly.

Digital Examination

1. Inspect the perianal area, and perform a digital examination.[5] Some practitioners wear two gloves on the examining hand, which can decrease in sensitivity of touch; however, time is saved because the soiled top glove can be removed, immediately proceeding with anoscopy or sigmoidoscopy.
2. Gently spread the buttocks apart and inspect the perineum and anal verge for cutaneous or anal pathology. This may be adequate to diagnose pathology (e.g., anal fissure or thrombosed hemorrhoid) and preclude need for anoscopy or sigmoidoscopy. If the examination is for hemorrhoids or prolapse, at this point the practitioner may ask the patient to perform a Valsalva maneuver.
3. Palpate the perianal and perineal tissues for abscesses or fistulae.
4. Perform the digital examination with a well-lubricated finger by inserting the finger slowly, directed toward the umbilicus of the patient. Advance the finger beyond the muscular sphincter, which measures approximately 3 to 5 cm in length. Sweep the finger circumferentially around the anal canal; a blind spot to sigmoidoscopy is directly posterior and proximal to the anal ring. Examine anteriorly for cul-de-sac lesions; do not mistake the cervix for tumor. Evaluate the prostate, if present. Ask the patient to bear down to evaluate sphincter tone, irregularity, or painful areas. Try to palpate any abnormalities to be visualized at anoscopy. Quality of stool from the examining finger should be noted and documented, and checked for occult blood if indicated.

Anoscopic Examination

The digital examination is part of a complete examination, but is also relaxes the anal sphincters and facilitates insertion of the scope. The anoscope is most useful to view fissures, fistula openings, internal hemorrhoids, papillitis and cryptitis, and neoplasms.

1. Insert a well-lubricated anoscope, stabilizing the obturator with the thumb.
2. Advance the anoscope, directed toward the umbilicus.
3. After inserting 3 to 4 cm, move the tip posteriorly.
4. If anal spasm is encountered, ask the patient to bear down or breathe through the mouth.

5. Visual examination of hemorrhoids with the anoscope is facilitated by having the patient strain (Valsalva) as you remove the anoscope. This is particularly important in the knee-chest position, where internal hemorrhoids may collapse.

6. To examine another quadrant of the anorectum, reinsert the obturator. Readvance and rotate the anoscope approximately 90°. Full evaluation generally requires a four-quadrant approach.

7. If there is access to a video-flexible sigmoidoscope, the end of the sigmoidoscope may be inserted into the anoscope with video evaluation (and magnification) on withdrawal of the instrument. This may increase diagnostic yield for small lesions.[8] Colposcopy may also be employed for high-resolution anoscopy of anal neoplasia.[6]

8. Document the findings of the examination, preferentially using left/right and anterior/posterior descriptors rather than the clockface due to variability of patient positioning.

Sigmoidoscopy Examination

If more proximal examination is required, proceed with rigid sigmoidoscopy.

1. Introduce the sigmoidoscope blindly only for the first 3 to 5 cm while stabilizing the obturator with the thumb. Direct the tip toward the umbilicus (Fig. 20.2A). Remove the obturator and, from this point on, advance the sigmoidoscope under direct vision.

2. Swing the tip of the sigmoidoscope posteriorly to follow the curve of the sacrum (Fig. 20.2B). Advance the scope as far as possible.

3. If the lumen is lost, the end of the sigmoidoscope is probably occluded by a valve or the rectal wall or is at the rectosigmoid junction (Fig. 20.2C). Do not push forward! Pull back 2 to 3 cm, rotate the scope until the lumen reappears, and then advance (Fig. 20.2D). Often, the tip of the advancing scope can "iron out" a fold or curve and aid in passage. Some examiners insufflate air if the lumen cannot be visualized; however, this may produce some discomfort. The rectosigmoid junction is encountered at 12 to 15 cm, and many sigmoidoscopies will end here. Often, this point can be negotiated by straightening the bend with the end of the scope or by insufflating air.

4. Withdraw the scope slowly, rotating the tip circumferentially to observe the entire rectal wall. Check the stool from this point for occult blood. Also test the mucosa for friability. Twirl a swab on the mucosa; remove it and look for capillary bleeding. Look behind the rectal valves of Houston.

5. Document the findings of the examination, preferentially using left/right and anterior/posterior descriptors rather than the clockface due to variability of patient position.

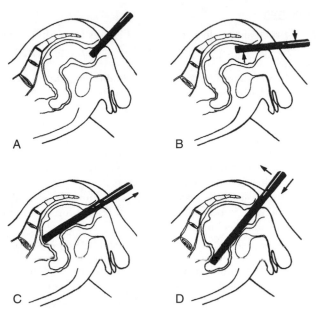

FIG. 20.2 Sequence of steps of the sigmoidoscopy. A, Sigmoidoscope, with obturator, is inserted, aimed toward the umbilicus. B, With the obturator removed, the tip of the scope is rotated posteriorly and advanced. C, If the lumen is lost, the sigmoidoscope is retracted until the lumen is found. D, The sigmoidoscope is then advanced.

Rectal Biopsy with Alligator Forceps

1. Unless a specific lesion is to be biopsied, a biopsy of the posterior rectal mucosa should be obtained below the peritoneal reflection (within 7 to 10 cm of the anal verge) to decrease the chance of free intraperitoneal perforation.
2. Bleeding can usually be stopped by applying pressure with dry cotton or with epinephrine-soaked swabs (1 mL of 1:1000 epinephrine diluted 1 to 10 with saline).
3. After the bleeding has stopped, the biopsy site may be cauterized with silver nitrate sticks.

POSTPROCEDURE

The patient may resume normal activity. Inform the patient that some "gas pains" may be experienced but to notify you if persistent pain or bleeding occurs. Inform the patient that fevers, severe abdominal pain, massive bleeding, or syncope are indications to seek immediate medical attention.

CPT CODES

45300—Proctosigmoidoscopy, rigid; diagnostic, with or without collection of specimen(s) by brushing or washing (separate procedure)

45303—Proctosigmoidoscopy, rigid; with dilation, any method

45305—Proctosigmoidoscopy, rigid; with biopsy, single or multiple

45307—Proctosigmoidoscopy, rigid; with removal of foreign body

45308—Proctosigmoidoscopy, rigid; with removal of single tumor, polyp, or other lesion by hot biopsy forceps or bipolar cautery

45309—Proctosigmoidoscopy, rigid; with removal of single tumor, polyp, or other lesion by snare technique

45315—Proctosigmoidoscopy, rigid; with removal of multiple tumors, polyps, or other lesions by hot biopsy forceps, bipolar cautery, or snare technique

45317—Proctosigmoidoscopy, rigid; with control of bleeding, any method

45320—Proctosigmoidoscopy, rigid; with ablation of tumor(s), polyp(s), or other lesion(s) not amenable to removal by hot biopsy forceps, bipolar cautery, or snare technique (e.g., laser)

45321—Proctosigmoidoscopy, rigid; with decompression of volvulus

45327—Proctosigmoidoscopy, rigid; with transendoscopic stent placement

46600—Anoscopy; diagnostic, with or without collection of specimen(s) by brushing or washing (separate procedure)

46604—Anoscopy; with dilation, any method

46606—Anoscopy; with biopsy, single or multiple

46608—Anoscopy; with removal of foreign body

46610—Anoscopy; with removal of single tumor, polyp, or other lesion by hot biopsy forceps or bipolar cautery

46611—Anoscopy; with removal of single tumor, polyp, or other lesion by snare technique

46612—Anoscopy; with removal of multiple tumors, polyps, or other lesions by hot biopsy forceps, bipolar cautery, or snare technique

46614—Anoscopy; with control of bleeding, any method

46615—Anoscopy; with ablation of tumor(s), polyp(s), or other lesion(s) not amenable to removal by hot biopsy forceps, bipolar cautery, or snare technique

References

1. Abcarian H, Alexander-Williams J, Christiansen J, et al. Benign anorectal disease: definition, characterization and analysis of treatment. *Am J Gastroenterol.* 1994;89:S182-S193.
2. Parikh S, Hughes C, Salvati E, et al. Treatment of hemorrhagic radiation proctitis with 4 percent formalin. *Dis Colon Rectum.* 2003;46:596-600.

3. Singh JC, Kuohung V, Palefsky JM. Efficacy of trichloroacetic acid in the treatment of anal intraepithelial neoplasia in HIV-positive and HIV-negative men who have sex with men. *J Acquir Immune Defic Syndr*. 1999;52(4):474-479.

4. Khashab MA, Chithadi KV, Acosta RD, et al. Antibiotic prophylaxis for GI endoscopy. *Gastrointest Endosc*. 2015;81(1):81-89.

5. MacKeigan J, Cataldo P. Disorders of the anorectum. In: DiMarino A, Benjamin S, eds. *Gastrointestinal Disease: An Endoscopic Approach*. Malden, MA: Blackwell Scientific; 1997.

6. Hillman RJ, Cuming T, Darragh T, et al. 2016 IANS international guidelines for practice standards in the detection of anal cancer precursors. *J Low Genit Tract Dis*. 2016;20(4):283-291.

7. Bateson M, Boucher I. *Clinical Investigations in Gastroenterology*. 2nd ed. Hingham, MA: Kluwer Academic Publishers; 1997.

8. Lazas D, Moses F, Wong R. Videoendoscopic anoscopy: a new technique for examining the anal canal. *Gastrointest Endosc*. 1995;42:351-354.

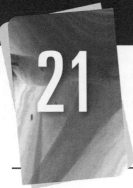

21

The Role of Endoscopy in the Management of Hemorrhoids

Shaffer R.S. Mok, MD, MBS
David L. Diehl, MD, FACP, FASGE

INCIDENCE

Approximately 2.2 million outpatient evaluations occur annually for hemorrhoidal adverse events.[1-3] Additionally, almost half of patients undergoing colonoscopy are found to have hemorrhoids. In the United States, 50% of adults age 50 years or older have reported gastrointestinal symptoms attributed to hemorrhoids.[4] As a result, it is vital for the endoscopist to be aware of the workup, staging, and indication for specific therapies aimed at hemorrhoids.

ANATOMY AND PATHOPHYSIOLOGY

Hemorrhoids are a normal part of the anatomy of the anal canal. They are described as clusters or "cushions" of vascular spaces, smooth muscle, and connective tissues within the anal canal. As hemorrhoidal vasculature has no muscular wall, hemorrhoids are strictly defined as sinusoids and thus are not anatomically categorized as veins or arteries.[5] Embryologically, the dentate line is a sharp division of the endoderm and ectoderm in the anal canal. This allows classifications of hemorrhoids into internal and external depending on whether they are above or below the dentate line. Somatic sensory neurons supply sensation to the perianal skin, therefore external hemorrhoids, when inflamed, can produce pain.

External hemorrhoids obtain vascular drainage via the inferior rectal vein, which drains via the pudendal vein into the internal iliac vein. In contrast, internal hemorrhoids receive their vascular drainage via the superior and middle rectal veins, which empty into the internal iliac vein directly.

Hemorrhoids are located in the anal canal in three major locations: left lateral, right anterior, and right posterior and can be internal, external, or both. For the purposes of this book, we will be discussing only internal hemorrhoids, as these are the target of endoscopic therapy.

GRADE

Hemorrhoids are usually graded based upon the Banov classification.[6] Grade I hemorrhoids are defined as nonprolapsing, grade II prolapse with defecation and spontaneously reduce, grade III prolapse with or without defecation and require manual reduction, and grade IV hemorrhoids are prolapsed permanently or are incarcerated. Grade I and II hemorrhoids can be treated conservatively (i.e., fiber, laxatives) or with endoscopic therapies. Grade III and IV hemorrhoids are typically managed surgically although there are some approved indications for endoscopic options.

INDICATIONS

Endoscopic therapy is indicated for symptomatic grade I, II, and III hemorrhoids and failure of conservative measures such as laxatives with fiber supplementation (Table 21.1).

CONTRAINDICATIONS

Absolute

1. Cardiopulmonary instability
2. Peritonitis or pelvic sepsis
3. Perforation
4. Fulminant colitis

Relative/Considerations

1. Immunosuppression
2. Portal hypertension
3. Active inflammation
4. Active inflammatory bowel disease
5. Torrential colonic bleeding

| TABLE 21.1 | Grade of Hemorrhoids Using the Banov Classification |

Therapy	Grade I	Grade II	Grade III	Grade IV
	Hemorrhoidal Grade			
Conservative Therapy (i.e., Laxatives, fiber)	X	X	X	X
Rubber Band Ligation	X	X	X[a]	
Sclerosant	X	X		
Infrared Coagulation	X	X	X[a]	
Bipolar Electrocautery	X	X		
Surgery		X	X	X

[a]Can be performed.[6]

6. Poor bowel preparation
7. Uncooperative patient
8. Active use of antiplatelet agents or anticoagulants

ADVERSE EVENTS

1. See Colonoscopy for general endoscopic adverse events
2. See below for unique potential adverse events

PREPARATION

The initial evaluation of the patient includes obtaining vital signs, history, and physical examination. An assessment by the physician of patient capacity to consent for an endoscopic procedure is a vital second step. The patient should undergo informed consent in an understandable language, and preprocedure discussion should include indications for the procedure, alternative therapy, possible adverse events, and the possibility of overlooking lesions.

Certain endoscopic hemorrhoidal therapies may require a bowel preparation. Please see below for which variations may require this. Procedures not requiring endoscopy can be performed safely in the office without the need of a bowel preparation or sedation. Endoscopic hemorrhoidal treatments may necessitate the use of IV sedation, again outlined in prior chapters.

THERAPIES

Rubber Band Ligation

Placement of the band over the hemorrhoid induces a pressure necrosis via ischemia, leading to subsequent ulceration and then fibrogenesis. This induces fixation of the hemorrhoid against the rectal wall.[7,8] Rubber band ligation (RBL) is the most commonly utilized endoscopic hemorrhoidal therapy. This treatment leads to an overall cure rate of as high as 93%.[1,9,10] Though some trials have demonstrated lower success rates, most patients in these trials were able to be retreated with repeat RBL. RBL also has demonstrated higher postprocedural pain and bleeding rates.[11-14] Globally, trial data have shown improved clinical response, lower adverse event rates, and need for fewer sessions using RBL.

At present the only device marketed for RBL is the Stiegmann-Goff Bandito Endoscopic Hemorrhoidal Ligator (ConMed Corp, Utica, NY). Similar banding devices have been developed for variceal banding which involves a wire or string that runs from the transparent cap through the working channel to a handle—SmartBand (Olympus, Tokyo, Japan), Speedband Superview Super 7 (Boston Scientific Corp, Malborough, MA), and SixShooter Universal Saeed, Multi-Band Ligator (Cook Medical

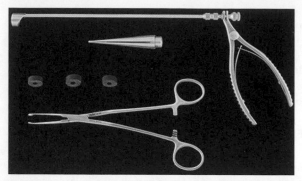

FIG. 21.1 The McGivney Hemorrhoidal Ligator (Miltex, York, PA) with bands and forceps. (Image used with permission from Integra York PA, Inc.)

Winston-Salem, NC). Several iterations of hemorrhoidal ligation using an anoscope alone have been created. The first is the McGivney Hemorrhoidal Ligator (Miltex, York, PA) (Fig. 21.1). This device is a stainless-steel 7-10-inch, gun-shaped ligation, holding four rubber ligation bands. This device is reusable, and the bands are latex-free. Another device that works via an anoscope is the ShortShot Saeed Hemorrhoidal Multi-Band Ligator (Cook Medical, Winston-Salem, NC) (Fig. 21.2).

Finally, two single-use devices, CRH O'Regan Disposable Hemorrhoid Banding System, CRH Medical Corp (Vancouver, BC, Canada) and SpaceBander (ConMed, Utica, NY), utilize direct suction to capture the hemorrhoid into the target area using a

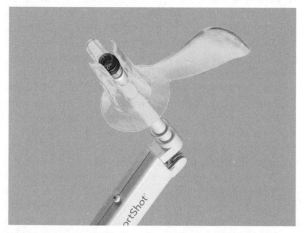

FIG. 21.2 Anoscope and ShortShot Saeed Hemorrhoidal Multi-Band Ligator. (Permission for use granted by Cook Medical, Bloomington, Indiana.)

FIG. 21.3 Single-use CRH O'Regan Disposable Hemorrhoid Banding System. (Image used with permission from CRH Medical Corp, Vancouver, BC, Canada.)

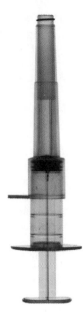

plunger at the end of the device (Fig. 21.3). The mechanism of hemorrhoidal therapy is the same for endoscopic and anoscopic RBL devices. Though studies performed have only evaluated older bipolar electrocautery technologies, RBL has also revealed higher success rates and symptom control as compared with this method.[8,15,16]

Equipment
1. Transparent plastic cap with preloaded bands OR preloaded device with preloaded bands
2. Suction
3. Hemorrhoidal grasping forceps
4. Adult upper endoscope or adult/pediatric colonoscope (for endoscope-based only)

Endoscopic Rubber Band Ligation Procedure
1. The patient is positioned in the left lateral decubitus position.
2. The transparent cap is affixed to the front of the adult endoscope.
3. After this device's transparent cap is affixed a long semistiff plastic introducer is placed through the working channel to the end of the scope.
4. A preloaded interlocking band/disk is clipped into the introducer.

5. The introducer is gently retracted into the transparent cap, by pulling on the introducer from the working channel.
6. Next, the target is suctioned into the endoscope.
7. Finally, the rubber bands are deployed by one of two means:
   a. The plastic introducer tugged retrograde, thus releasing the band.
   b. Tightening the trip wire via a rotating spool affixed to the working channel.[7,17-19]

Endoscope-Free Rubber Band Ligation

Reusable Stainless-Steel Device Procedure

1. This device operates through an anoscope and allows for hemorrhoidal targeting using hemorrhoidal grasping forceps.
2. Once the cushion is targeted, the hemorrhoid is grasped and retracted into the device.
3. The trigger is then pulled deploying the band over the hemorrhoid.

Handle-Shaped Single-Use Device Procedure

1. This single-use device is gun-shaped and includes a suction port at the base of the handle.
2. The hemorrhoidal cushion is centered.
3. Suction is then applied, capturing the hemorrhoid into the device.
4. Finally, the trigger is squeezed, deploying the band.

Conical-Shaped Single-Use Device Procedure

1. The device is introduced through the anus to the hemorrhoidal cushion target.
2. Counter-pulsing suction is the applied through a back-pull knob.
3. The bander is then moved gently forward deploying the band over the hemorrhoidal cushion.

Adverse Events[1,20-22]

1. Postprocedure pain
2. Bleeding (1% to 2.8%)
3. Thrombosed external hemorrhoids (1.5%)
4. Pelvic sepsis
5. Pelvic cellulitis
6. Bacteremia (0.09%)
7. Treatment failure (7% to 20%)

Sclerotherapy

The mechanism of action for sclerotherapy includes induction of an inflammatory response and thus fibrogenesis, with subsequent obliteration of the hemorrhoidal vascular spaces. The most commonly used agent is 5% phenol oil; however other used agents are polidocanol, 1% sodium tetradecyl sulfate, ethanolamine, quinine, aluminum potassium sulfate and tannic acid, and hypertonic saline. Though this method reveals a lower treatment success for grade III hemorrhoids, newer agents have demonstrated relatively high success for grade I hemorrhoids.[23-25] Not all of these agents are available in the United States (US).

Equipment
1. Adult upper endoscope or adult/pediatric colonoscope
2. Through-the-scope sclerosant needle
3. Sclerosant solution (5% phenol, polidocanol, 1% sodium tetradecyl sulfate, ethanolamine, aluminum potassium sulfate and tannic acid, or hypertonic saline)

Procedure
1. The endoscope is inserted through the anus to the hemorrhoidal cushion, which is centered into endoscopic view.
2. The needle is then placed through the working channel of an endoscope.
3. The sclerosant is attached to the proximal end of the sclerosant needle device.
4. 1 to 3 milliliters (mL) of a sclerosant are injected into the submucosa, typically above the hemorrhoid.

Adverse Events[26-31]
1. Postprocedure pain
2. Bleeding
3. Perforation
4. Fistula
5. Pelvic sepsis/abscess
6. Cellulitis/necrotizing fasciitis
7. Anal stricture
8. Treatment failure (12% to 80%)

Infrared Coagulation
Infrared coagulation is a therapeutic method for hemorrhoidal treatment that induces fibrogenesis by infrared-induced heat. These devices are FDA approved for grades I-III hemorrhoids. There are two types of infrared coagulation devices, one which works though the working channel of a colonoscope and the other with a slotted anoscope. The endoscopic device (Precision Endoscopic Technologies, Sturbridge, MA) works by insertion through the working channel via a 3.2 mm in diameter, 300 cm long fiberoptic probe. On the other hand, the handle-based infrared devices—IRC 2100 (Redfield Corp, Rochelle Park, NJ), Lumatec Infrared Coagulator (Lumatec, Munich, Germany, not

available in the United States)—involve a handle with quartz light tube and tungsten-halogen lamp for light delivery. The original trials evaluating this technology have proven high rates of therapeutic success for even grade III and IV hemorrhoids.[32]

Equipment

1. Through-the-scope infrared coagulation probe OR self-contained infrared coagulation device
2. Infrared coagulation power source
3. Adult upper endoscope or adult/pediatric colonoscope (for endoscope-based only)

Procedure Endoscopic Device

1. The endoscope is inserted through the anus and the hemorrhoidal cushion centered into endoscopic view.
2. The endoscope-driven device is inserted through the working channel via a 3.2 mm in diameter, 300 cm long fiberoptic probe.
3. The tip of the probe is deflected to the hemorrhoidal cushion targets at 3, 7, and 11 o'clock.
4. A foot pedal depressed delivering 1 to 5 seconds of infrared energy to the cushion.[1,33,34]

Procedure Handle-Base Device

1. The device is inserted through the patient's anus and the hemorrhoidal cushion centered within the device.
2. Actuation of the trigger via the devices handle, lead to delivery of infrared light through the lamp via the quartz tube to the cushion.

Adverse Events[1]

1. Postprocedure pain
2. Bleeding
3. Treatment failure (2% to 18%)

Bipolar or Direct Current Electrocautery

Using a similar mechanism of action to the above therapies, bipolar electrocautery–induced fibrogenesis of the hemorrhoidal cushion by delivering a high-frequency electrocautery energy, causing inflammation. This method was first introduced in 1987 and typically the device will deliver bipolar currents via two electrodes attached to either a grasper or anoscope device. The presently available anoscopic device (HET ConMed Corp, Utica, NY) involves a clear anoscope with built-in light source and utilizes two electrodes that attach to a power modulator and standard electrocautery system. Prior trial data suggested similar or slightly inferior results for bipolar electrocautery to

RBL.[8,15,34] However, newer device has been overall well tolerated and efficacious.[35-37]

Equipment

1. Adult upper endoscope or adult/pediatric colonoscope
2. Bipolar electrocautery device
3. Thermal regulation device
4. Electrosurgical generator
5. Hemorrhoidal grasping forceps

Procedure (Video 21.1)

1. The anoscope is introduced through the patient's anus, while lying in the left lateral decubitus position.
2. The device is then attached to the power modulator and into the electrocautery system set on bipolar mode at effect 1 and 8 W.
3. Next, the endoscope is placed through the anoscope to localize the target hemorrhoidal cushion.
4. Though suction and through-the-scope grasping forceps can be used, a true hemorrhoidal grasping forceps is best used to grab and retract the hemorrhoidal cushion.
5. After retraction, the hemorrhoidal cushion is then placed between the bipolar electrodes.
6. The pedal is then actuated, and bipolar energy delivered.
7. When the target temperature is reached, a green light will illuminate. Excessively high temperatures are indicated by a red light.
8. Once the target temperature is reached, the pedal is then released.
9. The device is then rotated, allowing targeting of the next area.

Adverse Events

1. Postprocedure pain
2. Bleeding
3. Treatment failure (0% to 38%)

Post Procedure

Certain hemorrhoidal therapies, as outlined above, do not require sedation and can safely be performed in an office setting. Alternatively, endoscopic hemorrhoidal therapies can require IV sedation and typically require 30 to 120 minutes of observation after the procedure in a monitored setting. Please see the colonoscopy section for a general summary of postendoscopic proceedings.

It is important otherwise to monitor patients for signs of worsening postprocedure pain, bleeding, and infection. Postprocedural pain may be treated with analgesic medication, Sitz baths, and topical rectal medications such as sucralafate or hydrocortisone. Postprocedure pain may be related to anal spasm induced by the treatment, but a high index of suspicion needs to be maintained to be aware of the dreaded adverse event of pelvic sepsis, which may present in a delayed fashion. This is thought to be due to full-thickness rectal wall necrosis, with a closed space infection spreading to the pelvis. Any signs of pelvic sepsis (e.g., fever, worsening pain, rigors, chills) require immediate antibiotic administration and emergent medical attention. Signs of clinical bleeding and sepsis may be immediate or delayed. Bleeding should be treated as would any other lower intestinal bleed with volume resuscitation, evaluation of hemodynamic parameters, blood product administration, and bleeding cessation. Clearly, proper pre- and postprocedural counseling is vital.

CONCLUSIONS

Endoscopic treatment of hemorrhoids involves an important understanding of anatomy, pathophysiology, and grade. Numerous modalities are available which are both endoscopy-driven and non–endoscopy-driven with varying levels of effectiveness, complexity, and procedure risks.

CPT Codes

46600—Diagnostic anoscopy

45300—Diagnostic proctoscopy

46221—Ligation of hemorrhoids by rubber band

45350—Sigmoidoscopy, flexible; with band ligation(s) (e.g., hemorrhoids)

45398—Colonoscopy, flexible; with band ligation(s) (e.g., hemorrhoids)

46500—Injection of sclerosing solution, hemorrhoids

45335—Sigmoidoscopy, flexible; with directed submucosal injection(s), any substance

44404—Colonoscopy, flexible; with directed submucosal injection(s), any substance

46930—Destruction of internal hemorrhoids by thermal energy (e.g., infrared coagulation, cautery, radiofrequency)

References

1. MacRae HM, McLeod RS. Comparison of hemorrhoidal treatments: a meta-analysis. *Can J Surg*. 1997;40(1):14-17. Available at http://www.ncbi.nlm.nih.gov/pubmed/9030078. Accessed June 27, 2018.

2. Wald A, Bharucha AE, Cosman BC, Whitehead WE. ACG clinical guideline: management of benign anorectal disorders. *Am J Gastroenterol.* 2014;109(8):1141-1157. doi:10.1038/ajg.2014.190.

3. Peery AF, Crockett SD, Barritt AS, et al. Burden of gastrointestinal, liver, and pancreatic diseases in the United States (Clinical—Alimentary Tract). *Gastroenterology.* 2015;149:1731-1741.e3. doi:10.1053/j.gastro.2015.08.045.

4. Johanson JF, Sonnenberg A. The prevalence of hemorrhoids and chronic constipation an epidemiologic study. *Gastroentrrology.* 1990;98:360-388. Available at https://www.gastrojournal.org/article/0016-5085(90)90828-O/pdf. Accessed June 26, 2018.

5. Shafik A. *Surgical anatomy of hemorrhoids.* In: *Surgical Treatment of Hemorrhoids.* London: Springer; 2009:7-13. doi:10.1007/978-1-84800-314-9_2.

6. Banov L, Knoepp LF, Erdman LH, Alia RT. Management of hemorrhoidal disease. *J S C Med Assoc.* 1985;81(7):398-401. Available at http://www.ncbi.nlm.nih.gov/pubmed/3861909. Accessed July 22, 2018.

7. Liu J, Petersen BT, Tierney WM, et al. Endoscopic banding devices. *Gastrointest Endosc.* 2008;68(2):217-221. doi:10.1016/J.GIE.2008.03.1121.

8. Jutabha R, Jensen DM, Chavalitdhamrong D. Randomized prospective study of endoscopic rubber band ligation compared with bipolar coagulation for chronically bleeding internal hemorrhoids. *Am J Gastroenterol.* 2009;104(8):2057-2064. doi:10.1038/ajg.2009.292.

9. El Nakeeb AM, Fikry AA, Omar WH, et al. Rubber band ligation for 750 cases of symptomatic hemorrhoids out of 2200 cases. *World J Gastroenterol.* 2008;14(42):6525-6530. doi:10.3748/wjg.14.6525.

10. Brown S, Tiernan J, Biggs K, et al. The HubBle trial: haemorrhoidal artery ligation (HAL) versus rubber band ligation (RBL) for symptomatic second- and third-degree haemorrhoids: A multicentre randomized controlled trial and health-economic evaluation. *Health Technol Assess (Rockv).* 2016;20(88):1-150. doi:10.3310/hta20880.

11. Ambrose NS, Hares MM, Alexander-Williams J, Keighley MR. Prospective randomised comparison of photocoagulation and rubber band ligation in treatment of haemorrhoids. *Br Med J (Clin Res Ed).* 1983;286(6375):1389-1391. doi:10.1136/BMJ.286.6375.1389.

12. Templeton JL, Spence RA, Kennedy TL, Parks TG, Mackenzie G, Hanna WA. Comparison of infrared coagulation and rubber band ligation for first and second degree haemorrhoids: a randomised prospective clinical trial. *Br Med J (Clin Res Ed).* 1983;286(6375):1387-1389. doi:10.1136/BMJ.286.6375.1387.

13. Poen AO, Felt-Bersma RJF, Knol W, Cuesta MA, Meuwissen SGM. A randomized controlled trial of rubber band ligation versus infrared coagulation in the treatment of hemorrhoids. *Eur J Gastroenterol Hepatol.* 2000;12(5):535-539. doi:10.1097/00042737-199812000-00108.

14. Marques CFS, Nahas SC, Nahas CSR, Sobrado CW, Habr-Gama A, Kiss DR. Early results of the treatment of internal hemorrhoid disease by infrared coagulation and elastic banding: a prospective randomized cross-over trial. *Tech Coloproctol.* 2006;10(4):312-317. doi:10.1007/s10151-006-0299-5.

15. Jensen DM, Jutabha R, Machicado GA, et al. Prospective randomized comparative study of bipolar electrocoagulation versus heater probe for treatment of chronically bleeding internal hemorrhoids. *Gastrointest Endosc.* 1997;46(5):435-443. doi:10.1016/S0016-5107(97)70037-3.

16. Randall GM, Jensen DM, Machicado GA, et al. Prospective randomized comparative study of bipolar versus direct current electrocoagulation for treatment of bleeding internal hemorrhoids. *Gastrointest Endosc.* 1994;40(4):403-410.

17. Cazemier M, Felt-Bersma RJF, Cuesta MA, Mulder CJJ. Elastic band ligation of hemorrhoids: flexible gastroscope or rigid proctoscope? *World J Gastroenterol.* 2007;13(4):585-587. doi:10.3748/wjg.v13.i4.585.

18. Trowers EA, Ganga U, Rizk R, Ojo E, Hodges D. Endoscopic hemorrhoidal ligation: preliminary clinical experience. *Gastrointest Endosc.* 1998;48(1):49-52. doi:10.1016/S0016-5107(98)70128-2.

19. Su MY, Chiu CT, Wu CS, et al. Endoscopic hemorrhoidal ligation of symptomatic internal hemorrhoids. *Gastrointest Endosc.* 2003;58(6):871-874. doi:10.1016/S0016-5107(03)02308-3.

20. Nelson RS, Ewing BM, Ternent C, Shashidharan M, Blatchford GJ, Thorson AG. Risk of late bleeding following hemorrhoidal banding in patients on antithrombotic prophylaxis. *Am J Surg.* 2008;196(6):994-999. doi:10.1016/j.amjsurg.2008.07.036.

21. Armstrong DN. Multiple hemorrhoidal ligation: a prospective, randomized trial evaluating a new technique. *Dis Colon Rectum.* 2003;46(2):179-186. doi:10.1097/01.DCR.0000049224.86580.41.

22. Albuquerque A. Rubber band ligation of hemorrhoids: a guide for complications. *World J Gastrointest Surg.* 2016;8(9):614-620. doi:10.4240/wjgs.v8.i9.614.

23. Moser KH, Mosch C, Walgenbach M, et al. Efficacy and safety of sclerotherapy with polidocanol foam in comparison with fluid sclerosant in the treatment of first-grade haemorrhoidal disease: a randomised, controlled, single-blind, multicentre trial. *Int J Colorectal Dis.* 2013;28(10):1439-1447. doi:10.1007/s00384-013-1729-2.

24. Yano T, Nogaki T, Asano M, Tanaka S, Kawakami K, Matsuda Y. Outcomes of case-matched injection sclerotherapy with a new agent for hemorrhoids in patients treated with or without blood thinners. *Surg Today.* 2013;43(8):854-858. doi:10.1007/s00595-012-0365-8.

25. Miyamoto H, Asanoma M, Miyamoto H, Shimada M. ALTA injection sclerosing therapy: Non-excisional treatment of internal hemorrhoids. *Hepatogastroenterology.* 2012;59(113):77-80. doi:10.5754/hge11089.

26. Barwell J, Watkins RM, Lloyd-Davies E, Wilkins DC. Life-threatening retroperitoneal sepsis after hemorrhoid injection sclerotherapy: report of a case. *Dis Colon Rectum.* 1999;42(3):421-423. Available at http://www.ncbi.nlm.nih.gov/pubmed/10223767. Accessed July 23, 2018.

27. Kaman L, Aggarwal S, Kumar R, Behera A, Katariya RN. Necrotizing fasciitis after injection sclerotherapy for hemorrhoids: report of a case. *Dis Colon Rectum.* 1999;42(3):419-420. Available at http://www.ncbi.nlm.nih.gov/pubmed/10223766. Accessed July 23, 2018.

28. Guy RJ, Seow-Choen F. Septic complications after treatment of haemorrhoids. *Br J Surg.* 2003;90(2):147-156. doi:10.1002/bjs.4008.

29. Adami B, Eckardt VF, Suermann RB, Karbach U, Ewe K. Bacteremia after proctoscopy and hemorrhoidal injection sclerotherapy. *Dis Colon Rectum.* 1981;24(5):373-374. doi:10.1007/BF02603422.

30. Schulte T, Fändrich F, Kahlke V. Life-threatening rectal necrosis after injection sclerotherapy for haemorrhoids. *Int J Colorectal Dis.* 2008;23(7):725-726. doi:10.1007/s00384-007-0402-z.

31. Mccloud JM, Jameson JS, Scott AND. Life-threatening sepsis following treatment for haemorrhoids: a systematic review. *Color Dis.* 2006;8(9):748-755. doi:10.1111/j.1463-1318.2006.01028.x.

32. Linares Santiago E, Gómez Parra M, Mendoza Olivares FJ, Pellicer Bautista FJ, Herrerías Gutiérrez JM. Effectiveness of hemorrhoidal treatment by rubber band ligation and infrared photocoagulation. *Rev Esp Enferm Dig.* 2001;93(4):238-247.

33. McLemore EC, Rai R, Siddiqui J, Basu PP, Tabbaa M, Epstein MS. Novel endoscopic delivery modality of infrared coagulation therapy for internal hemorrhoids. *Surg Endosc Other Interv Tech.* 2012;26(11):3082-3087. doi:10.1007/s00464-012-2325-1.

34. Pfenninger JL, Surrell J. Nonsurgical treatment options for internal hemorrhoids. *Am Fam Physician*. 1995;52(3):821-834, 839-841. Available at http://www.ncbi.nlm.nih.gov/pubmed/7653423. Accessed June 27, 2018.

35. Mok SRS, Khara HS, Johal AS, Confer BD, Diehl DL. Endoscopic treatment of internal hemorrhoids by use of a bipolar system. *VideoGIE*. 2017;2(10):290-292. doi:10.1016/j.vgie.2017.07.004.

36. Kantsevoy S V., Bitner M. Nonsurgical treatment of actively bleeding internal hemorrhoids with a novel endoscopic device (with video). *Gastrointest Endosc*. 2013;78(4):649-653. doi:10.1016/j.gie.2013.05.014.

37. Crawshaw BP, Russ AJ, Ermlich BO, Delaney CP, Champagne BJ. Prospective case series of a novel minimally invasive bipolar coagulation system in the treatment of grade I and II internal hemorrhoids. *Surg Innov*. 2016;23(6):581-585. doi:10.1177/1553350616660628.

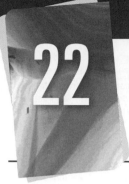

22

Polypectomy, Endoscopic Mucosal Resection, and Tattooing in the Colon

Sarah K. McGill, MD
Theodore W. James, MD
Ian S. Grimm, MD

Colonoscopy and removal of neoplasms prevents colorectal cancer. Techniques employed for resection include (1) cold snare polypectomy, (2) hot snare polypectomy, and (3) endoscopic mucosal resection. Recent research has provided a sound basis for choosing one method of polyp resection over another, based on polyp size and morphology. Endoscopic tattooing indelibly marks a lesion, facilitating localization for surgical resection or endoscopic surveillance.

POLYP EVALUATION

Carefully assess the size, shape, and probable histology of a polyp prior to resection. Estimate the polyp's size by comparing it to a device placed adjacent to the lesion, such as a standard snare catheter (2 mm), an open biopsy forceps (7 mm), or an opened snare of known diameter.

Polyp morphology can be described using the Paris classification: sessile polyps have a broad base (Paris 1s), pedunculated polyps have a narrow stalk consisting of normal tissue (Paris 1p), and nonpolypoid neoplasms are either slightly elevated but <2.5 mm in height (0-IIa), completely flat (0-IIb), or slightly depressed (0-IIc).

Study the color, surface pit pattern, and vascular pattern of a polyp to predict its most likely histology and the likelihood that it contains an invasive cancer. Advanced imaging techniques such as narrow band imaging (NBI) or i-Scan may help. The NBI International Colorectal Endoscopic (NICE) Classification is a simple and effective tool for visual prediction of polyp histology (Table 22.1).

	Type 1	Type 2	Type 3
Color	Same or lighter than background	Browner relative to background (verify that color arises from vessels)	Brown to dark brown relative to background; sometimes patchy whiter areas
Vessels	None, or isolated lacy vessels may be present coursing across the lesion	Brown vessels surrounding white structures	Has area(s) of disrupted or missing vessels
Surface pattern	Dark or white spots of uniform size, or homogeneous absence of pattern	Oval, tubular, or branched white structures surrounded by brown vessels	Amorphous or absent surface pattern
Most likely pathology	Hyperplastic or sessile serrated polyp	Adenoma	Deep submucosal invasive cancer

POLYPECTOMY INDICATIONS

1. Cold snare polypectomy: most polyps <10 mm in diameter.
2. Hot snare polypectomy: pedunculated polyps; sessile polyps 6 to 19 mm.
3. Endoscopic mucosal resection (EMR): *en bloc* resection of polyps 6 to 19 mm; piecemeal resection of lesions > 20 mm (see Video 22.1).

   a. Remove polyps encountered during screening colonoscopy at the time of their discovery, except for diminutive and small lesions with clear NICE 1 features that are located in the rectosigmoid colon. These hyperplastic polyps have no risk of progression to cancer.

   b. Polyps that have a high probability of deeply invasive cancer should NOT be removed endoscopically. Instead, the most concerning areas of the polyp (e.g., NICE 3 surface pattern, depressed areas, ulceration) should be biopsied. If invasive cancer is confirmed, refer the patient for surgical resection.

   c. Benign-appearing polyps too difficult to remove at the index colonoscopy should be photographed, with their location carefully documented, and in most cases, referred to an expert in advanced endoscopic mucosal resection. Partial colectomy for benign polyps is associated with greater risks and costs than endoscopic management, and is rarely necessary.

d. Nongranular laterally spreading tumor lesions with central depression that do NOT have NICE 3 features are considered ideal candidates for endoscopic submucosal dissection (ESD), an advanced technique performed at selected referral centers. Lesions with a high suspicion of superficial cancer invasion should be removed *en bloc*, either using EMR, ESD, or surgery.

POLYPECTOMY CONTRAINDICATIONS

1. The lesion has features suggestive of invasive carcinoma including ulceration, fixation, hard consistency, NICE 3 features. A nonlifting sign following submucosal injection is a relative contraindication; polyps that have been previously subjected to endoscopic therapy will often not lift well, but this should not be taken as a sign of invasive cancer.

2. Inability to complete the resection at the initial colonoscopy. Partial resection of a polyp should not be performed; the resulting submucosal fibrosis can complicate subsequent attempts at resection. Patients found to have large polyps during a screening examination may need to be rescheduled for a repeat procedure when adequate time and an experienced team are available to complete the resection in a single session.

3. Complete resection is not likely to be achieved. Polyps over 4 cm and those involving the ileocecal valve, appendiceal orifice, or anorectal junction are often very challenging, and may require referral to an expert in endoscopic resection techniques.

4. Unaddressed coagulation disorder.

5. Poor bowel preparation.

6. Poor general medical condition of the patient; excessive anesthetic risk.

7. Lack of the necessary staffing, training, and equipment needed to manage potential adverse events.

PREPARATION

Colonoscopic polypectomy is routinely performed on an outpatient basis following standard bowel preparation. Include polypectomy as part of the typical consent for colonoscopy. Consider asking patients to discontinue aspirin, nonsteroidal anti-inflammatory drugs (NSAIDs), and anticoagulants, especially when they are known in advance to have a large polyp requiring resection.

EQUIPMENT

Polypectomy

1. Colonoscope.
2. CO_2 insufflator.
3. Microprocessor-controlled electrosurgical generator (e.g., ERBE VIO, Tübingen, Germany).
4. Grounding pad, applied to the patient's flank. Avoid placing the pad over large bones such as the femur or pelvis.
5. Polypectomy snares in a range of sizes.
6. Retrieval apparatus (e.g., specimen container in circuit with suction line for small polyps that are aspirated through the accessory channel; grasping devices and nets for retrieval of larger lesions).
7. Hemostasis devices for postpolypectomy bleeding, such as clips and bipolar electrocautery probes.

Adjuncts for EMR

1. Standard sclerotherapy injection needle.
2. Submucosal injectate. Options include normal saline solution, hydroxyethyl starch, sodium hyaluronate, glycerol, or succi-nylated gelatin. Availability of these agents varies by region. Mix the fluid with methylene blue or indigo carmine to obtain a sky blue color. Commercial products specifically designed for submucosal injection are available in preloaded syringes (Orise, Boston Scientific; Eleview, Olympus). Dilute epineph-rine may be added to reduce intraprocedural bleeding, at a final concentration of 1:100,000 or 1:200,000.

Tattooing

1. Injection needle.
2. Tattooing agent: sterile carbon particle suspension (Spot, GI Supply, Camp Hill, PA).

PROCEDURE

Principles of Performing Effective Polypectomy, Regardless of the Modality Employed

1. Prior to beginning a resection, take the time to find a straight, relaxed scope position. Remove any loops using scope withdrawal and torque. This will greatly improve maneuverability.
2. Rotate the colonoscope until the polyp is located at the 5-o'clock position. Working on a polyp located in the upper half of the visual field is often inefficient or ineffective, because therapeutic devices exit the working channel of the scope at the bottom of the visual field.

3. Examine the full extent of the lesion. This will sometimes require retroflexion proximal to the lesion. For serrated polyps, electronic chromoendoscopy is often helpful in demarcating the edges of the lesion.
4. Stabilize the scope by anchoring it against the gurney with your hip, or by grasping the shaft of the scope between the fourth and fifth digits of your left hand.
5. Work close to the lesion. Place the snare accurately, to include a 1 to 2 mm margin of normal tissue beyond the edge of the polyp.
6. Following the polypectomy, carefully examine the base and perimeter of the resection defect for possible remnants.

Cold Snare Polypectomy

Cold snare polypectomy (CSP) is the preferred technique for resecting diminutive polyps (1 to 5 mm) and is also effective for removing small polyps (6 to 9 mm), most of which are also benign on histopathology. Cold snare polypectomy should be the dominant technique in screening examinations because thermal adverse events such as postpolypectomy bleeding and perforation are largely eliminated. Self-limited bleeding is commonly observed following cold snare polypectomy, but this is of no clinical consequence.

A key to successful cold snare polypectomy is to include a 2 to 3 mm margin of normal tissue surrounding the polyp, to avoid leaving any residual (Video 22.2). This requires use of a small, stiff snare, with a thin monofilament wire—ideally a device designed specifically for CSP. An *en bloc* cold polypectomy can be envisioned as a "fried egg"—the white portion representing normal tissue, and the yolk the polyp itself.

Removal of polyps with cold forceps is not recommended, except perhaps for tiny 1 to 3 mm lesions, because complete polyp resection is both more efficient and more effective with CSP than with forceps. Hot biopsy forceps removal is also not recommended, as this method entails risks of incomplete resection, cauterization of the resected specimen that can interfere with histopathological diagnosis, and serious adverse events resulting from thermal injury.

1. Carefully assess the margins of the lesion using electronic chromoendoscopy.
2. With the polyp positioned at 5 o'clock, open the snare completely to surround the polyp.
3. Maneuver the scope tip downward and verify that a rim of normal tissue surrounding the polyp remains encaptured within the snare as snare closure is initiated.

4. While maintaining firm downward pressure on the snare with tip deflection of the scope, ask the assistant to close the snare completely, transecting the polyp along with a rim of surrounding tissue.
5. Retrieve the specimen using suction and an in-line specimen trap.

Hot Snare Polypectomy

Use hot snare polypectomy (HSP) to resect pedunculated (stalked) lesions. HSP can also be used for sessile polyps in the 6 to 9 mm range; however, for lesions of this size, cold snare polypectomy has a superior safety profile and may be equally effective. Polyps that are 10 mm and larger can also be removed using the hot snare method, but EMR should be strongly considered for many of these polyps because (1) EMR can provide an *en bloc* specimen for lesions measuring up to 20 mm, (2) EMR may reduce the risk of deep thermal injury, and (3) EMR can result in higher rates of complete resection than HSP.

Techniques for Pedunculated Polyps

1. Optimize the localization of the polyp to the 5-o'clock position by repositioning the scope and/or the patient.
2. For very large pedunculated polyps, consider injecting the head of the polyp with 1:10,000 epinephrine in order to shrink it; this can facilitate snare placement, especially when the diameter of the polyp is greater than the largest available snare. Epinephrine injection into the stalk of a large polyp prior to resection may reduce immediate bleeding.
3. Polyps having a thick stalk can be prophylactically pretreated with clips or an endoloop, to reduce the risk of intraprocedural hemorrhage; however, placement of these mechanical devices onto a thick stalk can be challenging.
4. Select a snare that is larger than the diameter of the polyp head. Advance the closed snare and open the wire loop proximal to the lesion. By manipulating the endoscope controls and shaft, negotiate the snare loop over the polyp head and negotiate the snare down around the mid-section of the stalk, below the lower margin of the adenoma.
5. Gently push the base of the snare loop against the stalk. This will prevent the snare from riding up or down along the polyp stalk with snare closure.
6. Close the snare around the stalk until moderate resistance is encountered. While closing the snare, make sure that no portion of the head of the polyp or any surrounding tissue is unintentionally caught. Assess the mobility of the encaptured polyp by pushing and pulling on the closed snare, to

determine that the snare has not inadvertently entrapped adjacent mucosa. If surrounding tissue is caught within the snare, reopen it, and reposition it on the polyp. Once the stalk is confidently captured, apply electrosurgical energy using low-power pure coagulation or a blended cutting/coagulation current as the snare loop is very slowly tightened around the stalk. Pure cutting current should be avoided, because of an increased risk of intraprocedural bleeding. Look for visible whitening to indicate effective electrocautery. Large pedunculated polyps typically contain a central artery that should be thoroughly coagulated prior to completion of the stalk transection.

7. To avoid inadvertent mucosal burns at points of contact between the polyp head and the adjacent colonic wall, the snare may be moved back and forth as current is applied.

8. If excessive resistance is experienced, stop and reexamine for proper positioning of the snare. Do not pull through without coagulation. The rate of transection should be proportionate to the thickness of the polyp stalk.

9. Once transection is complete, retrieve the specimen with gentle snare capture or a retrieval device. Examine the stalk for bleeding or a visible artery.

10. If prompt bleeding is observed, and a portion of the stalk remains, this should be immediately re-snared and treated with prolonged strangulation, avoiding a second transection. Subsequent placement of a nylon loop (Polyloop, Olympus) over the remaining stalk or clip closure of the defect should be considered.

11. Over-the-scope (OTSC, Ovesco, Tübingen, Germany) clips can be applied to large stalks for postpolypectomy bleeding, or for prophylaxis against delayed bleeding in patients requiring anticoagulation.

Endoscopic Mucosal Resection

EMR is ideally suited for resection of polyps >2 cm, which need to be removed in multiple pieces (piecemeal). It demands more technical expertise than snare polypectomy and in some situations may require referring the patient to an expert center. There is no upper size limit for polyps that can be resected using piecemeal EMR. Sessile polyps <2 cm in diameter can often be resected *en bloc* (in a single piece) using EMR.

The injection of fluid into the submucosal space serves many purposes: it cushions the muscularis propria from thermal injury by electrocautery and makes flat lesions more polypoid, aiding in capture of the lesion with the snare. Dye in the injection fluid helps to delineate the lesion's borders, particularly helpful for sessile serrated polyps. Nonlifting of a lesion that has not previously been manipulated is suspicious for invasive cancer.

1. Depending on the lesion size, prepare one or more 10 mL syringes of sterile injectant.

2. If the polyp is in a dependent position, reposition the patient so that fluid and specimens cannot collect in the operative field. Maintaining a clean working field improves visualization and facilitates prompt treatment in the event of a complication.

3. Prime a standard injection needle with injectate and advance the needle tip. "Stab" the tip obliquely into the tissue at the edge of the lesion (insertion directly into the lesion is also allowed). The injected solution should promptly expand the submucosa and raise the lesion. If this does not happen, withdraw the needle slightly and reinject. Movement of the needle tip within the submucosal space during injection can help disperse the injection.

4. Select a stiff snare no more than 15 to 20 mm in diameter. Open the snare over the entire lesion (if it is under 20 mm), or over a section of the lesion, and deflect the scope tip firmly downward. Ideally the snare will be placed to capture a 1 to 2 mm margin of normal tissue at the lesion margin.

5. Gently tapping on the suction button will often encourage the polyp to jump up into the snare, at which point the assistant should gently enclose tissue within the snare.

6. Re-insufflate the lumen to flatten the muscularis propria.

7. Assess mobility of the lesion, to ensure that the muscularis propria is not entrapped in the snare.

8. "Tent" the ensnared polyp, by deflecting the tip of the scope toward the center of the lumen, to reduce thermal injury to the bowel wall.

9. Close the snare tightly and apply electrocautery to quickly transect the tissue using cutting current, such as Endocut Q, effect 3 (ERBE VIO, Tubingen, Germany). Avoiding the use of coagulating current may reduce thermal injury. If rapid transection does not occur, then reassess the snare capture, to verify that muscularis propria has not been entrapped within the snare.

10. Lesions <2 cm can be resected *en bloc* specimen, which is the best means to confidently confirm that all of lesion has been included within the resection margins. Following piecemeal resection, it is often difficult for pathologists to confirm that all of the lateral margins are free of pathology.

11. For large lesions resected piecemeal, perform contiguous resections, working from one end of the lesion to the other.

12. Repeat injections frequently as necessary, in order to retain a submucosal fluid cushion.

13. If any visible polyp cannot be snared, or does not lift due to submucosal fibrosis, then resect this tissue with forceps avulsion. Either hot or cold avulsion may be used. For hot avulsion, grab the tissue with hot biopsy forceps, and tent the tissue toward the lumen while applying cutting current to avulse the tissue. Cold avulsion using cold forceps is also effective and may preserve specimen quality. Avulsion is superior to argon plasma coagulation, which has fallen out of favor for this indication.

14. Following resection and ablation of all visible polyp, carefully examine the borders of the resection site and apply snare tip soft coagulation to destroy any microscopic dysplasia located at the perimeter of the resection and reduce polyp recurrence. The technician opens the snare a small amount, so that only 1 to 2 mm of snare tip protrudes past the end of the catheter; the electrocautery setting is switched to soft coagulation (ERBE Vio, Tubingen, Germany, soft coagulation settings of 80W, effect 4). Apply current circumferentially at the resection border until slight tissue whitening is visible. Hot biopsy forceps kept in the closed position are also effective for soft coagulation.

15. Retrieve all tissue for histopathology. Small specimens can be suctioned into a trap via the working channel of the scope. Options for retrieval of large specimens and *en bloc* resections include (1) use of a retrieval net, (2) grasping the specimen gently with a snare followed by scope withdrawal, or (3) suctioning the lesion into a cap, followed by scope withdrawal.

Endoscopic Tattooing

Tattoos aid surgeons to localize a lesion when viewing the colon from its peritoneal surface. In patients who will require surgery, multiple tattoos should be placed near the lesion. Inadvertent injection of the tattoo through the bowel wall can extensively stain peritoneal surfaces and obviate the intended benefits.

In general, for lesions that may require treatment with a subsequent endoscopic resection, avoid tattoos. Large polyps or those located near anatomical strictures such as the appendiceal orifice are easily located on follow-up colonoscopy without tattoos. Tattoo near a polyp is problematic as the carbon particles can lead to fibrosis and hinder subsequent attempts at resection. When a tattoo is necessary, a single injection > 3 cm distal to the lesion or on the opposite wall is least likely to interfere with a subsequent resection.

For postpolypectomy surveillance of resection sites that may be difficult to find at a later date, small tattoos placed on either side of the lesion are often helpful.

1. Obtain the tattooing agent (Spot, GI Supply, Camp Hill, PA), which comes in a prefilled syringe. Use of sterile India ink for tattoos is no longer recommended.
2. First perform a submucosal injection of ~1 mL of saline, forming a bleb. Then prime the injection catheter with Spot and inject ~1 mL into the bleb. This two-step method reduces the chances of an inadvertent transmural injection.
3. Inject at three or four locations surrounding the lesion if a surgical resection is required. For rectal lesions, some surgeons prefer tattoos to be placed a few centimeters distal to the lesion, to help ensure a safe margin of resection.
4. Document the site of tattoo injections in relation to the lesion, using both photography and accurate descriptions.

POSTPROCEDURE

1. Carefully assess the resection defect for completeness of resection, visible vessels, and signs of injury to the muscularis propria.
2. Postprocedure observation and recovery are the same as for any endoscopic procedure requiring sedation. Following colonic polypectomy and EMR, patients may resume a regular diet and can be discharged to home if asymptomatic. Significant pain that does not subside rapidly postprocedure requires evaluation for possible perforation, typically with abdominal radiographs.
3. Consider postprocedural hospitalization on an individual basis, such as for patients with coagulopathy or when adverse events are suspected.
4. Patients should be instructed to promptly report symptoms of pain, bleeding, or fever.
5. Antithrombotic medications are often held for a variable period of time following resection of large polyps, based on the perceived risk of delayed bleeding, medical indications for the medications, and recommendations of the prescribing physician.
6. Recurrence following piecemeal colonic EMR can occur in 10% to 30% of cases. These are usually small and unifocal and are easily treated on follow-up. Surveillance colonoscopy is often performed at 6 months following piecemeal EMR, especially for large lesions, and for lesions containing high-grade dysplasia.

INTERPRETATION

1. Postpolypectomy surveillance intervals are lesion- and pathology-dependent and are addressed in various guidelines, such as the 2012 US Multi-Society Task Force on Colorectal Cancer (Table 22.2).

2. Pathology reports indicating that a polyp contains intramucosal adenocarcinoma or carcinoma in situ are misleading, as these lesions are NOT malignant polyps and they are readily cured with a complete polypectomy.

TABLE 22.2	2012 Recommendations for Surveillance and Screening Intervals in Individuals With Baseline Average Risk	
Baseline Colonoscopy: Most Advanced finding(s)	**Recommended Surveillance Interval (y)**	**Quality of Evidence Supporting the Recommendation**
No polyps	10	Moderate
Small (<10 mm) hyperplastic polyps in rectum or sigmoid	10	Moderate
1-2 small (<10 mm) tabular adenomas	5-10	Moderate
3-10 tubular adenomas	3	Moderate
>10 adenomas	<3	Moderate
One or more tubular adenomas ≥10 mm	3	High
One or more villous adenomas	3	Moderate
Adenoma with HGD	3	Moderate
Serrated lesions		
Sessile serrated polyp(s) < 10 mm with no dysplasia	5	Low
Sessile serrated polyp(s) ≥ 10 mm OR Sessile serrated polyp with dysplasia OR Traditional serrated adenoma	3	Low
Serrated polyposis syndrome	1	Moderate

HGD, high-grade dysplasia.

3. Malignant polyps containing invasive cancer confined to the head of a pedunculated polyp are usually considered cured if favorable histological criteria are present: the carcinoma should be at least 2 mm from the resected margin, it cannot be poorly differentiated, and there can be no lymphovascular invasion.

4. Polyps that are resected *en bloc* and are found to have superficially invasive cancer with <1 mm of submucosal invasion are often considered cured, as the risk of metastasis is very low in such cases, but it is not zero. Consider consultation with pathologists and surgeons, especially for patients under age 60.

5. Endoscopically resected sessile polyps containing deeply invasive cancer have a significant risk of metastasis and partial colectomy is generally indicated.

ADVERSE EVENTS

1. **Intraprocedural bleeding** immediately following polyp transection occurs in about 10% of EMR procedures. This is often easily controlled with soft coagulation current (e.g., ERBE VIO, Tübingen, Germany: soft coagulation settings of 80W, effect 4) delivered via 1 to 2 mm of exposed snare tip applied directly to small bleeding sites. Larger bleeding sites and visible vessels can be effectively treated with soft coagulation current delivered via hot biopsy forceps or a coagulation grasper (Coagrasper, Olympus).

2. **Delayed bleeding** can occur as late as 2 weeks following polypectomy. Consider prophylactic clip closure for large right-sided lesions and polyps in patients who immediately resume antithrombotic medications. Bleeding stops spontaneously in many cases but may require endoscopic hemostasis following a rapid purge, especially if hemodynamic instability is noted.

3. **Perforation** occurs in 1% to 2% of colonic EMR procedures. If detected intraprocedurally, close small perforations with clips, either hemostatic clips or over-the-scope clips (OTSC, Ovesco, Tubingen, Germany), or with endoscopic suturing techniques. When using a contrast agent with submucosal fluid injection, a white round area of muscularis surrounded by a ring of blue-stained submucosa—known as a target sign—is a reliable indicator of muscularis injury, which should be repaired with clips.

Delayed recognition of a colonic perforation usually requires immediate surgical evaluation and exploratory laparotomy if peritoneal signs are present. Benign pneumoperitoneum in the absence of concerning clinical signs of perforation can usually be managed with observation alone.

4. **Transmural burn syndrome** (1%), also known as postpolypectomy syndrome, occurs when thermal energy during electrocoagulation extends into the muscularis propria and serosa, causing peritoneal inflammation. The patient typically reports abdominal pain and may have fever and leukocytosis, without free air on imaging studies. These symptoms usually resolve with conservative management after 1 to 2 days, with bowel rest, intravenous fluids, and antibiotics.

CPT CODES

45385—Colonoscopy, flexible, proximal to splenic flexure; with removal of tumor(s), polyp(s), or other lesion(s) by snare technique.
45381—With directed submucosal injection(s), any substance.
45390—With endoscopic mucosal resection.

Bibliography

1. Fertlisch M, Moss A, Hassan C, et al. Colorectal polypectomy and endoscopic mucosal resection (EMR): European Society of Gastrointestinal Endoscopy (ESGE) clinical guideline. *Endoscopy*. 2017;49:270-297.
2. Hayashi N, Tanaka S, Hewett D, et al. Endoscopic prediction of deep submucosal invasive carcinoma: validation of the narrow-band imaging international colorectal endoscopic (NICE) classification. *Gastrointest Endosc*. 2013;78:625-632.
3. Holmes I, Kim HG, Yang D, Friedland S. Avulsion is superior to argon plasma coagulation for treatment of visible residual neoplasia during EMR of colorectal polyps (with videos). *Gastrointest Endosc*. 2016;84:822-829.
4. Kim HG, Thosani N, Banerjee S, et al. Effect of prior biopsy sampling, tattoo placement, and snare sampling on endoscopic resection of large nonpedunculated colorectal lesions. *Gastrointest Endosc*. 2015;81:204-213.
5. Klein A, Bourke MJ. How to perform high-quality endoscopic mucosal resection during colonoscopy. *Gastroenterology*. 2017;152:46-471.
6. Klein A, Tate DJ, Jayasekeran V, et al. Thermal ablation of mucosal defect margins reduces adenoma recurrence after colonic endoscopic mucosal resection. *Gastroenterology*. 2019;156:604-613.
7. Kochhar G, Wallace MB. Virtual histology in everyday gastrointestinal endoscopy. *Clin Gastroenterol Hepatol*. 2018;16:1556-1561.
8. Lieberman DA, Rex DK, Winawer SJ, et al. Guidelines for colonoscopy surveillance after screening and polypectomy: a consensus update by the US Multi-society task force on colorectal cancer. *Gastroenterology*. 2012;143:844-857.
9. Rex DK, Hasan C, Bourke MJ. The colonoscopist's guide to the vocabulary of colorectal neoplasia: histology, morphology, and management. *Gastrointest Endosc*. 2017;86:253-263.
10. Strum WB. Colorectal adenomas. *N Engl J Med*. 2016;374:1065-1075.
11. Tate DJ, Bahin FF, Desomer L, et al. Cold-forceps avulsion with adjuvant snare-tip soft coagulation (CAST) is an effective and safe strategy for the management of non-lifting large laterally spreading colonic lesions. *Endoscopy*. 2018;50:52-62.

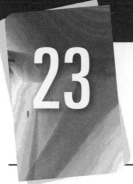

23 | Colonic Decompression

Karthik Gnanapandithan, MD, MS
Thiruvengadam Muniraj, MD, MRCP, PhD
Harry R. Aslanian, MD

Colonoscopy is a useful tool in the management of colonic obstruction and pseudo-obstruction. It can help determine the etiology of obstruction and play a role in treatment with decompression of retained gas and fluid from the colon.

INDICATIONS

Colonoscopy may be used to evaluate and potentially treat colonic obstruction of various etiologies that do not respond to conservative and medical treatment. Table 23.1 summarizes the indications of which, pseudo-obstruction, obstruction from colonic adenocarcinoma, and sigmoid volvulus are the most common.[1] Colonoscopy is contraindicated in the setting of perforation and peritonitis, while ischemia is a relative contraindication.[2]

APPROACH TO A PATIENT WITH COLONIC DILATION

The management of a patient with colonic obstruction or pseudo-obstruction is shown in Fig. 23.1. The first step is to rule out mechanical obstruction and treat any underlying medical conditions that may predispose to dysmotility. An abdominal radiograph will typically reveal dilated colon loops and allow for assessment of the degree of distention and aid in localizing the site of obstruction.[3] Fig. 23.2 shows distended colonic loops and increased stool burden in a patient with acute sigmoid volvulus. Abdominal computed tomography (CT) provides more detailed imaging that aids in evaluation of the etiology of obstruction. A conservative management approach is typically pursued in the absence of signs of peritonitis or impending perforation. This includes nothing by mouth, nasogastric tube placement, body positioning (knee-chest position or prone position with hip held high), intravenous hydration and correction of electrolyte

TABLE 23.1	Common Etiologies of Colonic Obstruction

1.	Benign obstruction	Volvulus
		Intussusception
		Hernia
		Strictures
		Extrinsic compression of colon
		Fecal impaction
2.	Malignant obstruction	Colonic adenocarcinoma
		Other primary colon malignancies
		Metastases to the colon
		Pelvic tumors with extrinsic compression
3.	Pseudo-obstruction	Risk factors:
		Abdominal surgeries
		Spinal trauma
		Other neurological disorders
		Dyselectrolytemias (hypokalemia, hypomagnesemia, hypophosphatemia)
		Medications (opioids, tricyclics, anticholinergics)
		Infections

abnormalities, enemas, and rectal tube placement. This is typically pursued for a period of 24 to 48 hours with close clinical monitoring. If these measures fail and obstruction is excluded radiologically, pharmacologic measures to treat pseudo-obstruction may be considered. Neostigmine is the most commonly used agent,[4] while metoclopramide, erythromycin, and cisapride (not available in the United States) are used less commonly. The risk of complications increase with increasing diameters of the colon[5] (more than 9 cm for the transverse colon and 12 cm for the cecum), although this also depends on the acuity and rate of progression of the increase in colon diameter.

COLONOSCOPIC DECOMPRESSION—PROCEDURE

Colonoscopic decompression can be accomplished by passing the scope proximal to the site of obstruction and suctioning retained air and fluid with or without the placement of a decompression tube (most commonly under fluoroscopic guidance). Patients are kept nothing by mouth. In the setting of colonic obstruction an oral bowel preparation is typically contraindicated. Tap water enemas may be pursued to aid in evacuation of rectal stool contents. Sedation with propofol or intravenous benzodiazepines alone is preferred, minimizing the use of opioid agents that may further impair colonic motility. Colonic insufflation should be minimized as insufflated gas in the proximal colon may acutely further increase distention and promote pain and perforation if not

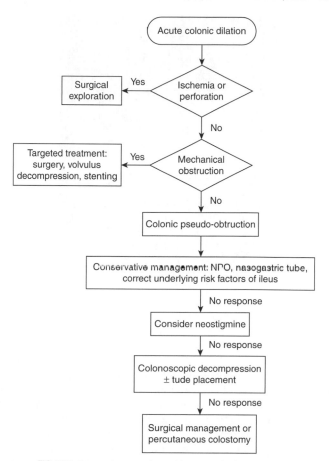

FIG. 23.1 Approach to a patient with acute colonic distension.

decompressed. Carbon dioxide insufflation should be utilized if available. The examination is primarily focused on relief of obstruction and a thorough examination of the mucosa is typically not possible given the limited bowel preparation and minimized insufflation. Cecal intubation is usually not needed as decompression at the hepatic flexure is therapeutic in most cases.[5] With gradual withdrawal of the scope, gas should be aspirated and the mucosa can be inspected for signs of ischemia or localization of a mass lesion.

COLONIC DECOMPRESSION TUBE PLACEMENT

When the colonoscope has reached the area of dilated bowel, it is typically readily apparent due to the increased diameter of the colon from distention with air and fluid. In some cases,

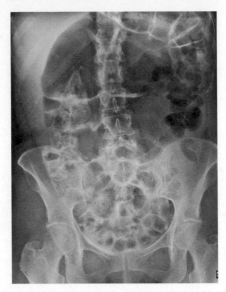

FIG. 23.2 Abdominal plain radiograph of a patient with sigmoid volvulus showing distended colonic loops and increased stool burden.

suctioning of air and fluid through the scope leads to a marked reduction in abdominal distention. If the colonoscope has not traversed the site of obstruction, fluoroscopic guidewire placement followed by passage of a decompression tube may be performed. Initial challenges in the placement of a decompression tube include traversing the colonic loops while preventing looping and maintaining tube position with removal of the scope and guidewire. Colonic stents are typically only utilized in the setting of obstruction due to known malignancy.

Decompression tube placement may be achieved with passage through the therapeutic channel of the scope over a guidewire or passage of the tube over the guidewire alone after the scope has been removed. If a distal site of obstruction is anticipated based on prior imaging, a therapeutic upper scope may be utilized to make guidewire exchange less cumbersome. Fluoroscopic guidance is typically utilized.

For passage over a guidewire, the guidewire is inserted into the instrument channel of the colonoscope and advanced into the dilated segment of the colon, with a stable loop of wire retained. The colonoscope is then gradually withdrawn with intermittent suction, carefully ensuring that the guidewire remains in position, with minimization of distal looping. The decompression tube (±guiding catheter) is flushed with water and is then advanced

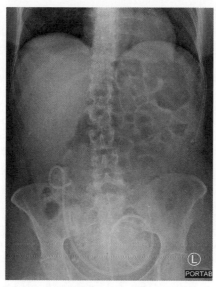

FIG. 23.3 Abdominal plain radiograph of the same patient after placement of colonoscopic decompression tube that shows improvement in the colonic dilation.

over the guidewire under fluoroscopic guidance. Once the tube is in position, the guidewire (±guiding catheter) is removed. The tube may be secured to the sacral crease with tape. Following placement, the patient's head is elevated to reduce aspiration risk and the tube is connected to gravity drainage, with regular flushing every 4 to 6 hours to prevent clogging. Postprocedure abdominal radiographs are useful in assessing tube placement and changes in colonic distension. Fig. 23.3 shows the abdominal radiograph of the patient with sigmoid volvulus (seen in Fig. 23.2) after the placement of a colonoscopic decompression tube.

ADVERSE EVENTS

Colon decompression tube efficacy may be limited by small luminal size leading to obstruction with stool contents and tube dislodgement. Recurrence of obstruction is common, with about 40% of patient having at least one recurrence after a decompression colonoscopy without tube placement.[6] There are no randomized controlled trials for comparison, but placement of a decompression tube has been shown to reduce recurrence rates in some studies.[1,7] Perforation is the most feared adverse event, described in 2% to 3% of patients undergoing decompression colonoscopy,[7] which is higher than in patients without colonic dilation. A mortality rate of 1% is reported.[6]

SURGICAL MANAGEMENT

Surgery is reserved for patients in whom medical and endoscopic measures fail or are not appropriate to treat the underlying cause of obstruction. In patients without signs of perforation or ischemia, cecostomy is typically the procedure of choice[8] for relief of acute colonic obstruction with consideration for the etiology and the overall health status of the patient. In those who are not surgical candidates, percutaneous endoscopic cecostomy is an option. When there are signs of ischemia or perforation, exploration and lavage is performed, usually with segmental resection of the affected bowel. This approach has a morbidity rate of 30% and mortality rate of 6%.

CONCLUSION

Patients with colonic distension should undergo diagnostic evaluation including imaging to exclude mechanical obstruction. Conservative management is the preferred initial approach while closely monitoring for potential complications of ischemia or perforation. In patients who fail conservative and medical therapy, colonic decompression has an important diagnostic and therapeutic role.

References

1. Saunders MD, Kimmey MB. Systematic review: acute colonic pseudo-obstruction. *Aliment Pharmacol Ther.* 2005;22(10):917-925. doi:10.1111/j.1365-2036.2005.02668.x.

2. ASGE Standards of Practice Committee ME, Harrison ME, Anderson MA, et al. The role of endoscopy in the management of patients with known and suspected colonic obstruction and pseudo-obstruction. *Gastrointest Endosc.* 2010;71(4):669-679. doi:10.1016/j.gie.2009.11.027.

3. Jaffe T, Thompson WM. Large-bowel obstruction in the adult: classic radiographic and CT findings, etiology, and mimics. *Radiology.* 2015;275(3):651-663. doi:10.1148/radiol.2015140916.

4. Valle RGL, Godoy FL. Neostigmine for acute colonic pseudo-obstruction: a meta-analysis. *Ann Med Surg.* 2014;3(3):60-64. doi:10.1016/j.amsu.2014.04.002.

5. Vanek VW, Al-Salti M. Acute pseudo-obstruction of the colon (Ogilvie's syndrome). An analysis of 400 cases. *Dis Colon Rectum.* 1986;29(3):203-210.

6. Kahi CJ, Rex DK. Bowel obstruction and pseudo-obstruction. *Gastroenterol Clin North Am.* 2003;32(4):1229-1247.

7. Geller A, Petersen BT, Gostout CJ. Endoscopic decompression for acute colonic pseudo-obstruction. *Gastrointest Endosc.* 1996;44(2):144-150.

8. Duh QY, Way LW. Diagnostic laparoscopy and laparoscopic cecostomy for colonic pseudo-obstruction. *Dis Colon Rectum.* 1993;36(1):65-70.

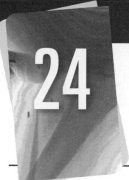

24

Placement of Colonic Self-Expandable Metal Stents

Amy Hosmer, MD

The placement of self-expandable metal stent (SEMS) in the colon is performed for the palliation of malignant disease within or adjacent to the colon and for preoperative decompression. Placement of colonic SEMS for the treatment of benign disease is rarely indicated. Several FDA-approved colonic SEMS with varying deployment mechanisms and proprietary features are currently available; however, their functionality is largely similar. All currently available colonic SEMS are uncovered. Based on meta-analysis data, the overall technical and clinical success is well over 90%.[1]

INDICATIONS[2]
1. Colorectal cancer:
   a. Palliation of advanced disease (partial obstruction or complete obstruction and no evidence of systemic toxicity)
   b. Preoperative decompression/bridge to surgery[3]
2. Extracolonic pelvic malignancies (i.e., ovarian cancer, sarcomas, etc.)

CONTRAINDICATIONS
1. Benign etiologies for colonic obstruction
2. Concurrent therapy with bevacizumab (Avastin)[4] or prior radiation therapy
3. Those associated with routine colonoscopy

PREPARATION
1. Consider imaging with rectal contrast (i.e., barium enema, CT scan w/ rectal contrast) prior to stent placement to provide an anatomical roadmap.

2. Cautious bowel preparation can be considered for patients with partial colonic obstruction, generally more proximally lesions.
   a. For patients with subtotal or total colon obstruction, oral bowel preparations should be avoided and replaced with enema preparations to clean the colon distal to the obstruction.
3. Obtain informed consent from the patient or patient representative that outlines the possible complications of the procedure as well as alternative methods of treatment.
4. Start an intravenous line for administration of systemic sedation.
5. Consider preprocedure antibiotics in patients with complete bowel obstruction as microperforations with bacterial translocation can occur with insufflation during the procedure.

EQUIPMENT

1. Therapeutic gastroscope or pediatric/adult colonoscope with an appropriate working channel to accommodate through-the-scope colonic stent catheter
2. Carbon dioxide (CO_2) insufflation, water irrigation, or air insufflation set to low if CO_2 is not available (to avoid over-insufflation of the colon lumen in setting of obstruction, as may already be dilation proximal to lesion)
3. Guidewire (450 cm in length)
4. Occlusion balloon catheter (this can be utilized to confirm positioning with the colon and to define the stricture length)
5. Fluoroscopy (Stents can be placed safely without fluoroscopy by experienced endoscopists, but only in setting of incomplete obstruction with the stricture can be traversed.)
6. Water-soluble contrast
7. A variety of self-expandable metal stent lengths (6 to 12 cm in length) should be available. Currently available colonic self-expandable metal stents are uncovered.
8. Radiopaque markers, either endoclips or contrast solution for injection through a sclerotherapy needle
9. Leaded aprons for radiation safety
10. Radiation dosage badges for personnel
11. Lubricant
12. Personal protective equipment

PROCEDURE

1. Assessment and marking of the lesion. Perform a diagnostic colonoscopy/sigmoidoscopy to assess lesion location and characteristics to determine the appropriate SEMS. If an obstructive lesion does not allow the passage of a standard

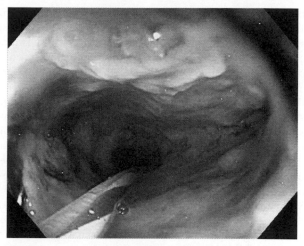

FIG. 24.1 Left-sided obstructive colon cancer. The occlusion balloon catheter pre-loaded with a long guidewire can be seen traversing the obstructive lesion.

adult colonoscope/gastroscope, a neonatal gastroscope can be used to traverse the stenosis. Alternatively, a guidewire and extraction balloon catheter can be passed across the lesion. The balloon can then be inflated and withdrawn until resistance is met, thereby defining the proximal extent of the stricture (Fig. 24.1). Alternatively, contrast injection via the extraction balloon catheter can define the characteristics of the stenosis (i.e., shape, length, luminal diameter). Balloon dilation of a colonic stenosis can be performed to allow endoscope passage; however, this may increase the risk of adverse events, particularly in malignant strictures. Since SEMS are placed under fluoroscopy, the distal and proximal extent (if possible) of the lesion should be marked with radiopaque markers. We recommend placement of taped paperclips on the patient's skin to identify these landmarks. Alternatively, if the C-arm is not moved, the clips can be placed on the fluoroscopy screen.

2. Choosing the correct SEMS. Ideally, the correct colonic SEMS should aim to allow for a minimum of 2 cm on both the proximal and distal extent of the straddled lesion after stent foreshortening (if applicable).[5] The endoscopist should be familiar with the concept of foreshortening, as discussed in Chapter 13: Placement of Esophageal Self-Expandable Metal Stents.

3. Placement of the stent delivery system. After marking the tumor, a long guidewire is passed across the stenosis and coiled proximally. The endoscopist should be aware that

placement of a colonic stent will require an endoscope with a 10 Fr working channel, most commonly a therapeutic gastroscope or adult colonoscope. The stent introducer is placed over the guidewire. Using the fluoroscopic markers for the proximal and distal ends of the stricture, position the stent to allow for at least 2 cm on each side of the stricture. Though there are individual differences based on the manufacturer, stent delivery systems usually entail a folded wire mesh stent that is compressed over a semirigid plastic catheter that can be introduced over a wire. The stent can be released from its compressed state by withdrawing a plastic sheath housing the stent through various proprietary deployment mechanisms.

4. Stent deployment. After catheter positioning, the stent is then deployed proximal to distal, with the endoscopist continually monitoring deployment under fluoroscopy and/or endoscopy. When using woven stents, vigilant monitoring of stent deployment and expansion is necessary. Woven stents exhibit foreshortening (as mentioned above) which requires constant back tension on the delivery catheter during deployment to ensure correct placement. For many currently available stents, adjustments can be made to the stent position until a specified portion of the stent is deployed (i.e., point of no return); however, at that point the stent can no longer be reconstrained by the stent delivery system.

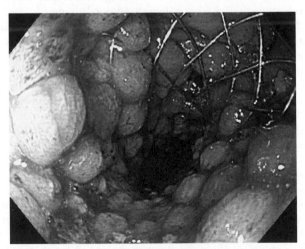

FIG. 24.2 Complete deployment of an uncovered self-expandable metal stent within the left colon for the management of an obstructive colon cancer.

5. Withdrawal of the stent delivery system. Once the stent is fully deployed, the delivery system and guidewire can be removed (Fig. 24.2). In cases with very tight strictures care must be taken during removal of the delivery catheter. Fluoroscopic and/or endoscopic monitoring of the stent while removing the delivery system will minimize the risk of stent displacement. Rarely, the catheter tip can catch at the stricture, thereby increasing the risk for stent dislodgement.

ADVERSE EVENTS

The most common adverse events of colonic stent placement are perforation, stent migration, bleeding, and abdominal pain.

1. Perforation[3,6]: The risk of perforation in experienced hands is likely less than 5%. Perforation can be immediate or delayed. It occurs more commonly in the distal colon where sharp angulation and tissue redundancy can make stent placement challenging. The risk of perforation is increased in patients receiving bevacizumab or those with prior radiation therapy in the region of stent placement.

2. Stent migration[3,7]: Stent migration occurs more frequently in patients receiving a shorter or smaller caliber stents. It occurs typically within 1 week of placement, and in patients with a nonobstructive stricture or extraluminal compression. Patients with prior stent placement who subsequently have a therapeutic response to oncologic therapy are also at higher risk for migration.

3. Bleeding: Intra- and postprocedural bleeding is usually minor and self-limited and relates to stent expansion.

4. Abdominal pain: Transient mild abdominal pain is quite common and typically occurs in the first few days after stent placement while the stent continues to expand.

POSTPROCEDURE

1. Dietary guidelines: Patients with left-sided lesions should adhere to a low-residue diet (i.e., Virginia Easy to Chew and Swallow Diet: https://med.virginia.edu/ginutrition/wp-content/uploads/sites/199/2014/04/Easy-To-Chew-and-Swallow-Diet-02.17-2.pdf) with regular laxative usage (suggest polyethylene glycol) to avoid fecal impaction. Foods which are high in fiber (i.e., raw fruits and vegetables) should be avoided. For lesions in the right colon, these recommendations can be softened as stool in this area of the colon is typically liquid.

2. **Failure to provide decompression:** In a small subset of patients, successful stent placement does not provide adequate decompression. This may occur due to a variety of technical and/or anatomical issues and may require placement of a percutaneous cecostomy to provide adequate decompression.

3. **Tumor/tissue ingrowth or overgrowth:** In patients with prior stent placement, they may develop tissue ingrowth, either from tumor or from reactive hyperplasia, within the stent interstices or overgrowth at the stent flanges. Subsequent stent placement may be necessary in such situations.

References

1. Watt AM, Faragher IG, Griffin TT, et al. Self-expanding metallic stents for relieving malignant colorectal obstruction: a systematic review. *Ann Surg.* 2007;246:24.

2. van Hooft JE, van Halsema EE, Vanbiervliet G, et al. Self-expandable metal stents for obstructing colonic and extracolonic cancer: European Society of Gastrointestinal Endoscopy (ESGE) Clinical Guideline. *Endoscopy.* 2014;46:990.

3. Matsuda A, Miyashita M, Matsumoto S, et al. Comparison of long-term outcomes of colonic stent as "bridge to surgery" and emergency surgery for malignant large-bowel obstruction: a meta-analysis. *Ann Surg Oncol.* 2015;22:497.

4. Imbulgoda A, MacLean A, Heine J, et al. Colonic perforation with intraluminal stents and bevacizumab in advanced colorectal cancer: retrospective case series and literature review. *Can J Surg.* 2015;58:167.

5. Chandrasekhara V, Elmunzer BJ, Khashab M, et al. *Clinical Gastrointestinal Endoscopy*; 2018.

6. Choi JH, Lee YJ, Kim ES, et al. Covered self-expandable metal stents are more associated with complications in the management of malignant colorectal obstruction. *Surg Endosc.* 2013;27:3220.

7. Khot UP, Lang AW, Murali K, Parker MC. Systematic review of the efficacy and safety of colorectal stents. *Br J Surg.* 2002;89:1096.

Endoscopic Retrograde Cholangiopan-creatography

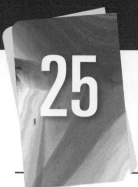

25 Basics of ERCP

Larissa Fujii-Lau, MD

Since endoscopic retrograde cholangiopancreatography (ERCP) was first introduced in 1968 and endoscopic sphincterotomy in 1974, it has become the standard of care in the therapeutic management of many pancreaticobiliary diseases.[1,2] ERCP remains one of the most technically challenging of all procedures performed by gastroenterologists and typically requires an additional year of training to become comfortable with its nuances. This chapter reviews the basics of ERCP through the periprocedural period but does not focus on the interventional aspect of this procedure as that is covered in later chapters.

PREPROCEDURAL CONSIDERATIONS

Indications

ERCP has evolved from a diagnostic procedure to a predominately therapeutic intervention. Cross-sectional imaging with abdominal ultrasound (US), computed tomography (CT) scan, and/or magnetic resonance cholangiopancreatography (MRCP) as well as endoscopic ultrasound (EUS) or intraoperative cholangiogram (IOC) is often used to decide which patient requires therapeutic ERCP. It is important to review all of these images prior to the case to assist in procedural planning. Table 25.1 lists the indications of ERCP.

Contraindications

- Risks of procedure are thought to outweigh benefits.
- Lack of consent.
- Suspected luminal perforation.
- Lack of necessary equipment/accessories needed to complete the procedure.
- If a sphincterotomy is being planned, then patients with coagulopathies and/or taking antithrombotic medications.[3]

TABLE 25.1	Indications for ERCP		
Biliary Indications	**Pancreatic Indications**	**Other**	
Choledocholithiasis	Pancreatic duct stones	Ampullectomy for adenoma	
Biliary stricture	Pancreatic duct stricture		
Bile leak	Pancreatic duct leak		
Obstructive jaundice	Pseudocyst drainage		
Cholangitis			
Biliary pancreatitis			
Papillary stenosis (type 1 SOD)			
Choledochocele (type III choledochal cyst) treatment			

SOD, sphincter of Oddi dysfunction.

- Aspirin and nonsteroidal anti-inflammatory drugs (NSAIDs) may be continued perioperatively.
- If a patient is coagulopathic and requires urgent ERCP, then alternatives such as balloon sphincteroplasty or stent placement without preceding sphincterotomy can be considered.

Periprocedural Administration of Antibiotics
- Routine use of periprocedural administration of antibiotics (typically a fluoroquinolone, beta-lactam, or third-generation cephalosporin) does not decrease the risk of infectious complications.[4,5]
- Judicious use of antibiotics in certain situations does have benefit in certain patients:
  - Complex strictures where there is a risk of retained contrast (i.e., hilar strictures, primary sclerosing cholangitis).
  - Immunosuppressed patients.
  - Contrast is injected during failed cannulation attempts.

Equipment
- Side-viewing duodenoscope (Fig. 25.1)
  - Up/down and left/right dials, elevator that allows for upward/downward movement
  - Typically 11.5 mm in diameter and has a large diameter working channel (typically 4.2 and 4.8 mm) allowing for 10 French (Fr) equipment
- Sphincterotome (Fig. 25.2)
  - Advantage of being capable of performing a sphincterotomy, has the capability to bow/flex, and studies have shown improved cannulation rates compared to standard cannulas.[6,7]
  - Teflon catheter that contains a continuous wire loop with 2 to 3 cm of exposed wire to allow for sphincterotomy.

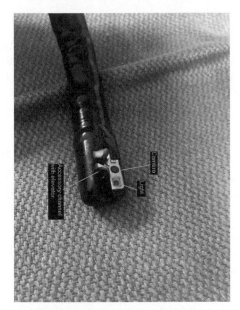

FIG. 25.1 Side-viewing duodenoscope. Notice how the camera is proximal to the tip of the duodenoscope. It is important to keep this in mind as pushing the duodenoscope under resistance can lead to perforation caused by the tip of the scope.

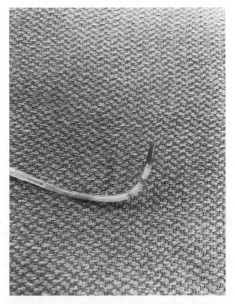

FIG. 25.2 Sphincterotome with a slight bow/flex of the wire.

- Electrocautery unit for sphincterotomy.
- Cannulas
  - Can be helpful in some situations such as the tapered tip cannula for dilation of tight strictures to allow for passage of larger accessories or the needle-tip catheter for cannulation of the minor papilla (Cramer cannula, Cook Medical, Bloomington, IN).
- Guidewires
  - Important for cannulation and maintaining access in the desired duct and facilitate placing and exchange of any accessory.
  - Vary in diameters (ranging from 0.018 to 0.035 inch), length (ranging from 260 to 480 cm), coating (i.e., Teflon), tip material (i.e., hydrophilic, platinum, tungsten), and tip shape (straight or angled).
  - Guidewires that are more hydrophilic, maneuverable, and flexible are used for cannulation and to pass through tight strictures.
  - Stiffer guidewires are useful to assist with advancement of any accessory.
- Locking device if the short-wire system is preferred.
  - Examples: Rapid Exchange Biliary System (Boston Scientific), Fusion system (Cook Medical), or V-system (Olympus)
- Fluoroscopy is required in majority of ERCPs.
  - Full strength contrast theoretically decreases the amount of contrast required to delineate the anatomy, particularly during cannulation to limit inadvertent pancreatic duct injection.
  - Diluted contrast to half strength decreases the risk of obscuring small stones during contrast injection.

INTRAPROCEDURAL CONSIDERATIONS
Sedation

Each institution differs in regard to preference for the type of sedation administered during an ERCP. Most institutions use an anesthesiologist or nurse anesthetist to provide sedation for ERCP cases, but some also provide nurse-administered sedation under the guidance of the endoscopist.

It is important to take into account the patient's inherent risk of sedation based on cardiopulmonary status, physical examination (including the body measurement index [BMI] and Mallampati score), and presence of cervical spine disease when determining the level of sedation. In addition, the anticipated length and complexity of the planned procedure should be considered when deciding how to sedate the patient. If the indication is for stent removal, a lower level of sedation may be required than for an ERCP planned in a patient with a hilar stricture. Furthermore, patient positioning may dictate the type of sedation given. In the prone position, airway patency and assessment of respirations are more difficult than in the left lateral or supine position. Therefore, general anesthesia is often preferred, but not required, if the patient is prone.

Patient Positioning

Typically patients are positioned either left lateral or prone during ERCP. Patient positioning is determined by endoscopist preference, anesthesiologist concerns (airway, respiratory stability), and patient factors (BMI, neck flexibility, abdominal wounds, abdominal distention). The prone position typically allows for better fluoroscopic imaging of the distal bile and pancreatic duct systems (easier to determine what duct is being cannulated) and the intrahepatic system. In addition, secretions tend to obscure duodenoscope visualization less in the prone position. Despite these theoretical advantages, studies have not shown a significant difference in technical success or adverse events between the two positions.[8-10]

Technique
Duodenoscope Insertion

Duodenoscope insertion is often the first step to learn during ERCP training. As compared to the standard gastroscope, the duodenoscope is side-viewing and has stiffer tip. With this side view, to gain passage through any opening (i.e., upper esophagus, lower esophagus, pylorus), the orifice needs to be positioned below the view of the scope. If the endoscopist can see the opening, the scope is not positioned correctly and will not advance through it. It is important not to push with significant force while advancing the duodenoscope to decrease the risk of perforation.

Tips to advance the duodenoscope to the papilla:

- When inserting into the mouth, slightly reflect the up/down knob downward toward you in a counterclockwise fashion (tip up) until you pass the tongue.
- Then reflect the up/down knob upward away from you in a clockwise fashion (tip down) to advance the scope to the back of the throat.
- Use your right hand to make small right/left motions of the scope while gently advancing the duodenoscope to pass the cricopharyngeus and enter into the esophagus.

- Passing through the esophagus should be relatively straight-forward, continuing with the small right/let torquing movements of the duodenoscope shaft using your right hand while advancing the duodenoscope.

- In the esophagus, be cautious in older patients or those with esophageal disorders who may have a tortuous esophagus.

- At the lower esophageal sphincter, make sure you do not see the opening of the gastroesophageal junction in direct view. If you see the gastroesophageal opening in view, then reflect the up/down knob downward toward you in the counterclockwise direction (tip up) to put the opening at the 6-o'clock position, then gently advance the duodenoscope into the stomach.

- In the stomach, similar to an upper endoscopy, torque the duodenoscope shaft to the right (clockwise) using your right hand while advancing the duodenoscope.

- When you reach the antrum, reflect the up/down knob downward toward you in the counterclockwise direction (tip up) until you reach the pylorus.

- Often when advancing the duodenoscope in the antrum, the pylorus can often be seen *en face*. Position the pylorus so it is lying in the 6-o'clock position below the duodenoscope and your view of the pyloric opening is lower and lower (similar to a "setting sun") by reflecting the up/down knob downward toward you (tip up).

- Once the duodenoscope enters the posterior duodenal bulb, rotate the duodenoscope shaft toward the right (clockwise), turn your body a little to the right, continue to hold the up/down knob a little downwards toward you (tip up) until you reach the descending duodenum

- Shorten the scope by keeping the right torque of the duodenoscope shaft (some endoscopists lock it in this position), right torque of your body, then pull the duodenoscope back to allow it to naturally advance to the second/third portion of the duodenum. Continue to pull back on the scope until you see the papilla.

- On fluoroscopy, the duodenoscope should look like a curved L in the *short position*, which is preferred in majority of cannulations (Fig. 25.3). Sometimes the *long position* is required for appropriate alignment of the papilla (Fig. 25.4). To move the scope into the long position, push the scope in with a right torque. Using fluoroscopy often helps to ensure that the scope is moving appropriately and it is important not to push against too much resistance as this is a technique that can rarely lead to a perforation.

Aligning the Papilla for Selective Cannulation

Selective cannulation into either the bile or pancreatic duct is the most important step in performing ERCP, but it remains one

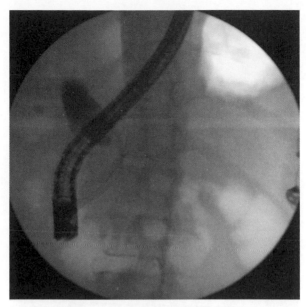

FIG. 25.3 Short position of the scope on fluoroscopic view.

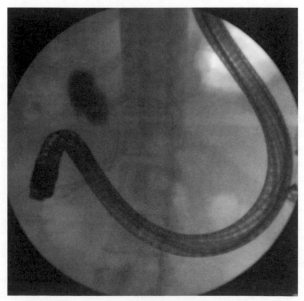

FIG. 25.4 Long position of the scope on fluoroscopic view.

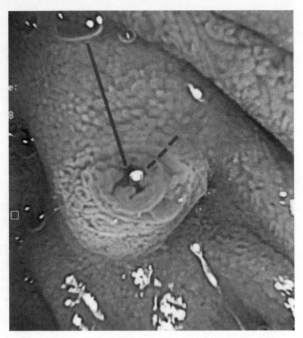

FIG. 25.5 Alignment of the papilla. The straight line delineates the bile duct orientation while the perforated line delineates the pancreatic duct orientation.

of the most challenging steps. Aligning the papilla in the correct position is critical to allow for selective cannulation. Prior to inserting your cannulation device, taking time to examine the papilla to determine the orientation of the ducts is important and should not be overlooked.

In a normal papilla, the bile duct orifice lies in the 11-o'clock position while the pancreatic duct orifice lies in the 1-o'clock to 5-o'clock position (Fig. 25.5). The bile duct axis continues upward in the 11-o'clock position, so it often requires an approach from below with the view of the papilla on the upper portion of your screen and an upward reflection of your cannulation accessory. In contrast, the pancreatic duct lies in a more straight axis and can be approached more *en face* without any or minimal reflection of the cannulation device tip.

Sphincterotomy
See Chapter 26 for tips on how to perform a sphincterotomy and Chapters 27 to 28 for techniques on therapies performed during ERCP.

Fluoroscopic Imaging

In addition to becoming comfortable with the side-viewing endo-scopic views, when learning ERCP one needs to become familiar with interpreting fluoroscopic images. Majority of ERCP cases are guided by the images provided by fluoroscopy.

Tips on obtaining and interpreting the fluoroscopy images:

- A scout film taken prior to scope insertion is helpful to deter-mine whether there are calcified stones, prior stent/drains in place, cholecystectomy clips, and other intervening structures (i.e., colonic air, retained contrast) that may obscure imaging.

- To calculate the size of any structure seen on fluoroscopy, com-pare it to the diameter of the duodenoscope (standard width is 11.5 mm). A normal bile duct diameter ranges from 3 to 9 mm, while a normal pancreatic duct diameter is up to 4 mm in the head, 3 mm in the body, and 2 mm in the tail.

- If choledocholithiasis is suspected, start injecting contrast with the catheter in the proximal duct and bring the catheter down slowly to decrease the risk of pushing the stones proximally into the intrahepatic ducts which makes it harder to remove.

- As air can obscure visualization of stones, adequate contrast injection to delineate the anatomy and presence of stones is preferred prior to performing a sphincterotomy (which will introduce air into the duct).

- If the duodenoscope is obscuring views of portions of the bile duct (typically if needing to visualize the suprapancreatic por-tion of the bile duct), change the position of the scope into the long position by pushing the scope in with a right torque.

- With the patient in the left lateral or prone position, the left intrahepatic ducts will preferentially opacify due to the force of gravity. Placing the patient in the right lateral or supine posi-tion or a balloon occlusion cholangiogram with the balloon inflated may help to opacify all intrahepatic ducts.

- A focal change in caliber of the duct of interest likely indicates pathology and should undergo further evaluation with ade-quate contrast injection starting from above the level of the narrowing.

- Distinguishing between air bubbles and stones may require tilting the head of the table up as gallstones will move distally down the duct while air will move proximally up the duct in this position.

- If stent insertion is planned, the extraction balloon catheter can be used as a measuring tool as the length of the balloon (distance between the two black markers) is 1 cm. The bal-loon should be deflated when using it as a measuring tool as resistance to the inflated balloon may tamper with the true measurements.

- Another simplified principle to assist in determining adequate stent length for distal bile duct strictures is if the entire stricture is below the lower aspect of the scope shaft as it crosses the bile duct while the scope is in the short position, a 5 cm long stent should be adequate. If it is proximal to the upper aspect of the scope shaft as it crosses the bile duct with the scope in the short position, a stent that is at least 7 cm in length should be used.

POSTPROCEDURAL CONSIDERATIONS

Adverse Events

The ASGE standards of practice committee provided an excellent review of the adverse events associated with ERCP.[11] As a comprehensive review of the adverse events of ERCP is too exhaustive for this chapter, only some general tips on the adverse events unique to this procedure will be provided.

Pancreatitis

Post-ERCP pancreatitis (PEP) is the most common serious adverse event of ERCP and occurs up to 10% in average-risk patients and 15% in high-risk patients.[12-14] Table 25.2 summarizes the risk factors for PEP.

Tips to decrease the risk of pancreatitis:

- Ensure appropriate patient selection by using other imaging modalities such as EUS and MRCP to determine which patient will require therapeutic intervention during ERCP.

TABLE 25.2	Risk Factors for Post-ERCP Pancreatitis[11,15]
Patient-Related Risk Factors	**Procedure-Related Risk Factors**
Female gender	Difficult cannulation (i.e., >10 min)
Younger age (<40 y old)	Repeated pancreatic duct wire
Previous post-ERCP pancreatitis or	cannulation
recurrent pancreatitis	Pancreatic duct injection
Suspected sphincter of Oddi	Pancreatic sphincterotomy
dysfunction	Late use of precut sphincterotomy
Normal serum bilirubin	Endoscopic papillary large-balloon
Absence of chronic pancreatitis	dilation without a preceding
Nondilated extrahepatic bile duct[a]	sphincterotomy
	Intraductal ultrasound[a]
	Endoscopist with low ERCP volume[a]

[a]Likely risk factors.
Data from Chandrasekhara V, Khashab MA, Muthusamy VR, et al. Adverse events associated with ERCP. *Gastrointest Endosc.* 2017;85(1):32-47 and Dumonceau JM, Andriulli A, Elmunzer BJ, et al. Prophylaxis of post-ERCP pancreatitis: European Society of Gastrointestinal Endoscopy (ESGE) guideline – updated June 2014. *Endoscopy.* 2014;46(9):799-815.

- Avoid ERCP in patients with suspected sphincter of Oddi dysfunction type 3 (patients with right upper quadrant pain without a dilated bile/pancreatic duct and normal liver/pancreatic enzymes).
- Guidewire cannulation is preferred over contrast injection–assisted cannulation as it has been shown to decrease the risk of PEP and increase rates of cannulation.[16]
- Minimize the number and volume of contrast injected into the pancreatic duct.
- If the pancreatic duct is repeatedly cannulated and/or if the dual guidewire technique is employed for biliary cannulation, place a prophylactic pancreatic duct stent. Preferably, a 5 Fr stent should be used over a 3 Fr stent.[17]
- Early precut sphincterotomy should be considered in cases of difficult biliary cannulation. Needle-knife fistulotomy in which the cut starts above the orifice is preferred in patients with dilated bile duct as it has the lowest risk of PEP.[15]
- If endoscopic papillary balloon dilation (EPBD) is utilized, maintain the duration of dilation to >1 minute.[18,19]
- Consider rectal indomethacin administration in high-risk patients.[20] Meta-analyses have shown that rectal indomethacin helps prevent PEP in high-risk, but not low-risk, patients and should preferably be administered before, rather than immediately after, the procedure.[21,22]
- Consider aggressive IV hydration with lactated Ringer's solution in patients without the risk of fluid overload (i.e., those with sepsis, cholangitis, acute or chronic pancreatitis, heart problems).[23,24]

Bleeding

Bleeding most commonly occurs after sphincterotomy. It has been reported in up to 2% of ERCP and can occur up to several weeks after sphincterotomy.[25,26]

Tips to decrease or treat the risk of bleeding:
- Hold antithrombotic medications for the recommended interval and correct any coagulopathy.[3]
- Use a blended cut is recommended over pure cut current.[27]
- In patients that are at high risk for bleeding, EPBD can be considered over sphincterotomy.[28]
- If post-sphincterotomy bleeding occurs, epinephrine injection at the apex and around the sphincterotomy site is often effective at stopping the bleeding.
- Other techniques such as thermal therapy (bipolar, argon plasma coagulation) and clip placement may also be used with caution of avoiding the pancreatic duct orifice.
- If all else fails, placement of a fully covered metal stent should be considered but requires an additional ERCP to remove the stent in 2 to 4 weeks.

TABLE 25.3	ERCP-Related Perforations[11,29-31]		
Stapfer Type (%)	Location	Cause	Management
I (17.8%)	Duodenal wall	Duodenoscope	Endoscopic clip/suture closure Surgery
II (58.4%)	Periampullary	Sphincterotomy	Placement of a fully covered metal stent
III (13.2%)	Bile duct, pancreatic duct	Guidewire injury, stone extraction, stent placement	Most likely to heal spontaneously Placement of a biliary or pancreatic stent
IV (10.6%)	Retroperitoneal	Excessive insufflation during endoscopy, sphincter manipulation	Observation with IV antibiotics only

Data from Chandrasekhara V, Khashab MA, Muthusamy VR, et al. Adverse events associated with ERCP. *Gastrointest Endosc.* 2017;85(1):32-47; Enns R, Eloubeidi MA, Mergener K, et al. ERCP-related perforations: risk factors and management. *Endoscopy.* 2002;34(4):293-298; Cirocchi R, Kelly MD, Griffiths EA, et al. A systematic review of the management and outcome of ERCP related duodenal perforations using a standardized classification system. *Surgeon.* 2017;15(6):379-387; Kumbhari V, Sinha A, Reddy A, et al. Algorithm for the management of ERCP-related perforations. *Gastrointest Endosc.* 2016;83(5):934-943.

Perforation

The incidence of perforations during ERCP is low at 0.35%.[29] Risk factors for perforation include surgical or altered anatomy, older age, suspected sphincter of Oddi dysfunction, sphincterotomy, longer procedure duration, biliary stricture dilation. There are different mechanisms of perforation that may occur during ERCP compared to general endoscopy. Table 25.3 addresses these different perforation types and their management. Early recognition and treatment is the key to management. If needed, CT scan with oral contrast administration should be performed.

CONCLUSION

ERCP is a technically challenging procedure that requires many unique periprocedural preparations. Understanding the indications, contraindications, and how to handle any adverse event that occurs is important while learning how to perform ERCP. Furthermore, ERCP calls for the endoscopist to not only need to interpret endoscopic images, but also fluoroscopic images. Therefore, ERCP should only be performed by physicians who have undergone the recommended training to learn the complexities of this procedure.

References

1. McCune WS, Shorb PE, Moscovitz H. Endoscopic cannulation of the ampulla of vater: a preliminary report. *Ann Surg.* 1968;167(5):752-756.
2. Kawai K, Akasaka Y, Murakami K, Tada M, Koli Y. Endoscopic sphincterotomy of the ampulla of Vater. *Gastrointest Endosc.* 1974;20(4):148-151.
3. Acosta RD, Abraham NS, Chandrasekhara V, et al. The management of antithrombotic agents for patients undergoing GI endoscopy. *Gastrointest Endosc.* 2016;83(1):3-16.
4. Harris A, Chan AC, Torres-Viera C, Hammett R, Carr-Locke D. Meta-analysis of antibiotic prophylaxis in endoscopic retrograde cholangiopancreatography (ERCP). *Endoscopy.* 1999;31(9):718-724.
5. Bai Y, Gao F, Gao J, Zou DW, Li ZS. Prophylactic antibiotics cannot prevent endoscopic retrograde cholangiopancreatography-induced cholangitis: a meta-analysis. *Pancreas.* 2009;38(2):126-130.
6. Cortas GA, Mehta SN, Abraham NS, Barkun AN. Selective cannulation of the common bile duct: a prospective randomized trial comparing standard catheters with sphincterotomes. *Gastrointest Endosc.* 1999;50(6):775-779.
7. Schwacha H, Allgaier HP, Deibert P, Olschewski M, Allgaier U, Blum HE. A sphincterotome-based technique for selective transpapillary common bile duct cannulation. *Gastrointest Endosc.* 2000;52(3):387-391.
8. Ferreira LE, Baron TH. Comparison of safety and efficacy of ERCP performed with the patient in supine and prone positions. *Gastrointest Endosc.* 2008;67(7):1037-1043.
9. Tringali A, Mutignani M, Milano A, Perri V, Costamagna G. No difference between supine and prone position for ERCP in conscious sedated patients: a prospective randomized study. *Endoscopy.* 2008;40(2):93-97.
10. Mashiana HS, Jayaraj M, Mohan BP, Ohning G, Adler DG. Comparison of outcomes for supine vs. prone position ERCP: a systematic review and meta-analysis. *Endosc Int Open.* 2018;6(11):E1296-E1301.
11. Chandrasekhara V, Khashab MA, Muthusamy VR, et al. Adverse events associated with ERCP. *Gastrointest Endosc.* 2017;85(1):32-47.
12. Masci E, Mariani A, Curioni S, Testoni PA. Risk factors for pancreatitis following endoscopic retrograde cholangiopancreatography: a meta-analysis. *Endoscopy.* 2003;35(10):830-834.
13. Andriulli A, Loperfido S, Napolitano G, et al. Incidence rates of post-ERCP complications: a systematic survey of prospective studies. *Am J Gastroenterol.* 2007;102(8):1781-1788.
14. Kochar B, Akshintala VS, Afghani E, et al. Incidence, severity, and mortality of post-ERCP pancreatitis: a systematic review by using randomized, controlled trials. *Gastrointest Endosc.* 2015;81(1):143-149.e9.
15. Dumonceau JM, Andriulli A, Elmunzer BJ, et al. Prophylaxis of post-ERCP pancreatitis: European Society of Gastrointestinal Endoscopy (ESGE) guideline – updated June 2014. *Endoscopy.* 2014;46(9):799-815.
16. Tse F, Yuan Y, Moayyedi P, Leontiadis GI. Guide wire-assisted cannulation for the prevention of post-ERCP pancreatitis: a systematic review and meta-analysis. *Endoscopy.* 2013;45(8):605-618.
17. Afghani E, Akshintala VS, Khashab MA, et al. 5-Fr vs. 3-Fr pancreatic stents for the prevention of post-ERCP pancreatitis in high-risk patients: a systematic review and network meta-analysis. *Endoscopy.* 2014;46(7):573-580.
18. Liao WC, Lee CT, Chang CY, et al. Randomized trial of 1-minute versus 5-minute endoscopic balloon dilation for extraction of bile duct stones. *Gastrointest Endosc.* 2010;72(6):1154-1162.
19. Liao WC, Tu YK, Wu MS, et al. Balloon dilation with adequate duration is safer than sphincterotomy for extracting bile duct stones: a systematic review and meta-analyses. *Clin Gastroenterol Hepatol.* 2012;10(10):1101-1109.

20. Elmunzer BJ, Scheiman JM, Lehman GA, et al. A randomized trial of rectal indomethacin to prevent post-ERCP pancreatitis. *N Engl J Med.* 2012;366(15):1414-1422.
21. Inamdar S, Han D, Passi M, Sejpal DV, Trindade AJ. Rectal indomethacin is protective against post-ERCP pancreatitis in high-risk patients but not average-risk patients: a systematic review and meta-analysis. *Gastrointest Endosc.* 2017;85(1):67-75.
22. Wan J, Ren Y, Zhu Z, Xia L, Lu N. How to select patients and timing for rectal indomethacin to prevent post-ERCP pancreatitis: a systematic review and meta-analysis. *BMC Gastroenterol.* 2017;17(1):43.
23. Buxbaum J, Yan A, Yeh K, Lane C, Nguyen N, Laine L. Aggressive hydration with lactated Ringer's solution reduces pancreatitis after endoscopic retrograde cholangiopancreatography. *Clin Gastroenterol Hepatol.* 2014;12(2):303-307.e1.
24. Shaygan-Nejad A, Masjedizadeh AR, Ghavidel A, Ghojazadeh M, Khoshbaten M. Aggressive hydration with Lactated Ringer's solution as the prophylactic intervention for postendoscopic retrograde cholangiopancreatography pancreatitis: a randomized controlled double-blind clinical trial. *J Res Med Sci.* 2015;20(9):838-843.
25. Freeman ML, Nelson DB, Sherman S, et al. Complications of endoscopic biliary sphincterotomy. *N Engl J Med.* 1996;335(13):909-918.
26. Cotton PB, Garrow DA, Gallagher J, Romagnuolo J. Risk factors for complications after ERCP: a multivariate analysis of 11,497 procedures over 12 years. *Gastrointest Endosc.* 2009;70(1):80-88.
27. Morris ML, Tucker RD, Baron TH, Song LM. Electrosurgery in gastrointestinal endoscopy: principles to practice. *Am J Gastroenterol.* 2009;104(6):1563-1574.
28. Park DH, Kim MH, Lee SK, et al. Endoscopic sphincterotomy vs. endoscopic papillary balloon dilation for choledocholithiasis in patients with liver cirrhosis and coagulopathy. *Gastrointest Endosc.* 2004;60(2):180-185.
29. Enns R, Eloubeidi MA, Mergener K, et al. ERCP-related perforations: risk factors and management. *Endoscopy.* 2002;34(4):293-298.
30. Cirocchi R, Kelly MD, Griffiths EA, et al. A systematic review of the management and outcome of ERCP related duodenal perforations using a standardized classification system. *Surgeon.* 2017;15(6):379-387.
31. Kumbhari V, Sinha A, Reddy A, et al. Algorithm for the management of ERCP-related perforations. *Gastrointest Endosc.* 2016;83(5):934-943.

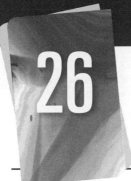

26

Endoscopic Sphincterotomy

Todd H. Baron, MD

Endoscopic sphincterotomy (ES) is often used as a primary therapeutic modality or a secondary tool to facilitate minimally invasive management of a variety of pancreaticobiliary disorders. When deep cannulation of the duct of interest fails, several different precut sphincterotomy techniques can be performed. In this chapter, the indications, techniques, and adverse events of endoscopic sphincterotomy will be discussed.

INDICATIONS AND CONTRAINDICATIONS

The indications and contraindications for ES are shown in Table 26.1 and can be subdivided into those that require selective biliary, pancreatic, or dual sphincterotomies, and/or to facilitate access in cases of difficult cannulation often referred to as "precut sphincterotomy." Dual sphincterotomy (biliary and pancreatic) is sometimes utilized pre- or postendoscopic ampullectomy (papillectomy) with the intention of decreasing postampullectomy adverse events such as pancreatitis, cholangitis, and papillary stenosis or for improved diagnostic accuracy in detecting intraductal involvement.

Precut sphincterotomy refers to techniques utilized to gain access to the bile and pancreatic ducts when efforts at prior deep selective cannulation have failed. These techniques utilize electrosurgical energy to cut papillary tissue and expose underlining ducts to facilitate deep cannulation of the duct of interest. In patients with Billroth II anatomy, a needle knife sphincterotomy can be performed over a biliary stent since standard sphincterotomes orient in the opposite direction of the intended cut.

Patient Preparation
1. Informed consent
2. NPO per guidelines[1]
3. Correction of coagulopathy

TABLE 26.1	Sphincterotomy Techniques	
Technique	**Indications**	**Contraindications**
Biliary sphincterotomy	■ Choledocholithiasis ■ Biliary leaks ■ Sphincter of Oddi dysfunction ■ Benign or malignant papillary stenosis ■ Choledochocele ■ Sump syndrome ■ Biliary parasites ■ Facilitate access for biliary interventions	■ Unstable or uncooperative patient ■ Uncorrected coagulopathy ■ Difficult anatomy precluding appropriate trajectory and visualization of the cut (e.g., intradiverticular papilla)
Pancreatic sphincterotomy/minor duct sphincterotomy	■ Sphincter of Oddi dysfunction (pancreatic type) ■ Papillary stenosis/stricture ■ Pancreatic divisum ■ Facilitate further pancreatic duct interventions such as transpapillary drainage of pseudocysts, pancreatic duct fistula, and pancreatic duct obstruction	■ Low ERCP volume (relative <200 per year) ■ Uncorrected coagulopathy ■ New surgical anastomosis ■ Difficult anatomy precluding appropriate trajectory and visualization of the cut
Precut sphincterotomy	■ Failure of standard cannulation ■ Impacted gallstones in the ampulla ■ Consider in Billroth II and altered anatomy ■ Consider for minor duct sphincterotomy	■ Low ERCP volume (relative) ■ Uncorrected coagulopathy ■ Difficult anatomy precluding appropriate trajectory and visualization of the cut

4. Withholding of antithrombotics per guidelines, drug package inserts, and after discussion with healthcare providers (primary provider of patient's antithrombotic agents)[2]
5. Management of cardiac pacemaker/defibrillator per guidelines[3]

Equipment Needed

1. Standard duodenoscope (native gastroduodenal anatomy)
2. Electrocautery pad
3. Electrosurgical generator (preferably controlled to allow precise control of the length of the cut and to eliminate "zipper cut")
4. Standard sphincterotome of choice (many available)
5. Needle knife (many available)

6. Standard ERCP guidewires and catheters
7. Pancreatic stents for prevention of post-ERCP pancreatitis[4]
8. Rectal indomethacin for prevention of post-ERCP pancreatitis[4]
9. Secretin (ChiRhoStim) for minor papilla cannulation
10. Fully covered metal biliary stents
11. Coagulation devices for management of bleeding (bipolar probes, hemostatic forceps, clips)

TECHNIQUES[5]

Biliary and Pancreatic Sphincterotomy

1. Administration of rectal indomethacin 100 mg for prevention of post-ERCP pancreatitis.
2. Select electrosurgical current. A commonly used electrocautery option is the "Endo Cut" mode of the ERBE generator to allow precise control of the length of the cut and eliminate "zipper cuts," while blending cut and coagulation currents. Pure cut can be considered for pancreatic sphincterotomy to reduce risk of stenosis but carries risk of uncontrolled cutting.
3. Deep cannulation of the duct of interest and passage of guidewire into the duct.
4. Withdraw sphincterotome toward the duodenum leaving the guidewire in place to allow about one-fourth to one-third of the cutting to be located inside the papilla.
5. Bow the tip of the sphincterotome to contact the roof of the papilla, making sure that no more that 5 mm of the cutting wire is inside the papilla (Fig. 26.1).
6. Orient the cutting wire between the 11-o'clock (biliary) and 1-o'clock (pancreatic) position to reduce bleeding and perforation adverse events. In the event the cutting wire is oriented outside these parameters toward the 3-o'clock direction, rotate the right/left ratchet to the left while simultaneously advancing the duodenoscope into the long position.
7. Step on the cutting pedal to allow cut to be initiated. Upward pressure is needed to continue the cut. This can be achieved by one or more of the following: closing the elevator, slightly withdrawing the endoscope, or rotating the shaft of the endoscope to the left.
8. Continue until the length of the sphincterotomy is deemed adequate. The length varies depending on the size of the intraduodenal portion of the bile duct and the indication for the sphincterotomy. It must not extend beyond the junction of the duodenal wall and the intraduodenal portion of the bile doctor pancreatic duct since additional cutting results in perforation (Fig. 26.2).

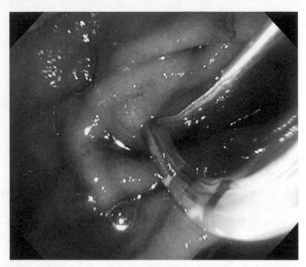

FIG. 26.1 Sphincterotome in position and bowed just prior to initiating biliary sphincterotomy.

9. In selected cases to facilitate removal of large biliary stones, a small endoscopic sphincterotomy combined with large-balloon (≥12 mm) dilation seems to be a safer alternative than a large sphincterotomy with balloon dilation.[6]

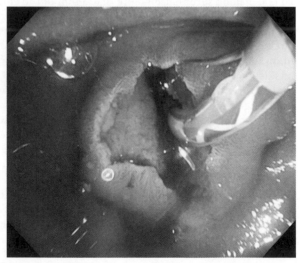

FIG. 26.2 Subtotal biliary sphincterotomy. There is a small remaining intraduodenal portion that could be cut.

10. Extension of a previous sphincterotomy might be warranted in certain settings such as recurrent bile duct stones or symptoms after initial sphincterotomy for SOD. The same techniques and instructions as defined above can be used.

11. For pancreatic sphincterotomy, a smaller cut is used and care must be taken not to extend the cut that would involve the pancreatic duct as this leads to stenosis. Pancreatic stents are placed to prevent post-ERCP pancreatitis.

12. In patients with periampullary duodenal diverticula, traditional landmarks may be obscured when the papilla is located at the edge of the diverticulum. In this case the sphincterotomy should be performed over a guidewire with only few millimeters of the cutting wire inside the papilla while strictly avoiding directing the cut toward the base of the diverticulum. Conversely, when the papilla is located in the middle of a diverticulum, the intraduodenal portion is outlined and the landmarks are more obvious than in normal anatomy.

13. In the setting of altered anatomy such as after Billroth II surgery where the papilla is rotated 180° as compared to native anatomy, options include use of a special push-type sphincterotome that cuts in the 5- to 6-o'clock direction. Alternatively, a plastic stent can be placed into the duct of interest and cut the roof of the papilla with a needle knife.

Precut Sphincterotomy

Precut sphincterotomy refers to techniques utilized to gain access to the bile or pancreatic ducts when efforts at deep selective cannulation have failed (pre = cut before cannulation). These techniques often utilize a needle knife where electrosurgical current is applied to a diathermy wire at its end to cut papillary tissue and expose underlining ducts to facilitate deep duct cannulation. The indications for precut sphincterotomy are shown in Table 26.1.

There are multiple techniques to perform precut sphincterotomy.[7] These include the free-hand needle knife sphincterotomy (NKS) technique, the needle -knife fistulotomy (NKF) technique, and the use of a traditional sphincterotome and a transpapillary pancreatic sphincterotomy (TPS), for biliary cannulation.

NKS Technique

1. Insert the needle knife just at or just into the papillary orifice.

2. Superficial incisions are made in an upward motion directed superiorly toward the 11-o'clock position (for biliary cannulation) and toward the 1-o'clock position (for pancreatic cannulation) using the elevator and/or the up-down wheel. The size of the cut is determined by the anatomy, size of the papilla,

and length of the intraduodenal segment. Repetitive cuts in the same direction are made in efforts to dissect down and expose the duct to be accessed with the retracted needle knife catheter and guidewire, or standard sphincterotome. The bile duct opening is sometimes not obvious and appears as a nipple representing the circular muscles of the sphincter choledochus. Gentle probing in the middle of the incision line or use of methylene blue after secretin stimulation (for pancreatic access) can be helpful to gain deep access.

3. Placement of a prophylactic pancreatic stent. The stent can be placed before or after NKS.

NKF Technique

1. The needle knife is used and the incision is begun a few millimeters above the papillary orifice. Cutting can proceed from a point close to the duodenal wall and progress in a downward direction or begin closer to the papilla and progress in an upward fashion until the underlying duct is exposed.

2. The decision to place a stent is based upon the length of time cannulation is attempted prior to undertaking precut and number of PD injections or guidewire passages.

TPS Technique[8]

1. After cannulation of the pancreatic duct over a guidewire that has been passed deeply, the tip of the sphincterotome is positioned in the pancreatic duct for few millimeters.

2. A small pancreatic sphincterotomy is performed directing the cut toward the bile duct and through the inter-ductal septum to open the common channel and separate the biliary and pancreatic orifices.

3. The sphincterotome and guidewire are withdrawn from into the duodenum, and the upper portion of the cut is gently probed to gain deep biliary access.

4. Placement of a prophylactic pancreatic duct stent after the cut while the guidewire remains in the PD and prior to cannulation of the bile duct.

Minor Papilla Sphincterotomy (and Precut Minor)

Sphincterotomy of the minor papilla is performed for treatment of acute recurrent pancreatitis in the setting of pancreas divisum (complete and incomplete) as well as to facilitate pancreatic ductal interventions such as stricture dilation and stone removal.

There are two methods to perform minor papilla sphincterotomy after deep cannulation is achieved: pull sphincterotomy and needle knife over a stent.

Standard Pull Sphincterotome

1. In most patients the landmarks are not as well-defined and the cut is made in the orientation that the sphincterotome and guidewire align and the cut length is usually 5 to 8 mm.
2. It is important not to have cutting wire in contact with the pancreatic duct as cautery-induced stenosis may occur.

Needle Knife Over Pancreatic Duct Stent

1. After deep cannulation and wire placement a pancreatic duct stent is placed (5 Fr, 2 to 4 cm in length).
2. A needle knife is used to perform a sphincterotomy over the stent using the stent as a guide. The tip of the needle knife can be placed at the orifice just inside the stent entry and incremental incisions are made to progressively expose more of the intraduodenal portion of the stent, which is reflective of incision of the minor papilla sphincter.

Minor Papilla Precut

Minor papilla precut is riskier than precut at the major papilla because of poorly defined landmarks, and if cannulation is not successful, then placement of a prophylactic pancreatic duct stent is not possible.

1. Administer secretin or equivalent agent to allow the papillary opening and intraduodenal segment of the minor papilla to be better defined.
2. A needle knife is used and the incision begun at, or just above, the opening in small increments. When clear, colorless output is seen, the opening is probed with a catheter and wire.
3. Dye spraying with methylene blue after the precut can help define the opening. Once the duct is cannulated, the sphincterotomy might be extended using the techniques described above for minor papilla sphincterotomy.
4. A stent is placed for prevention of PEP.

ADVERSE EVENTS

1. Pancreatitis
2. Bleeding
3. Cholangitis
4. Cholecystitis
5. Perforation

Treatment of Adverse Events

1. PEP is managed as for pancreatitis of any other etiology.
2. Bleeding can be intraprocedural or delayed up to 10 to 14 days. Intraprocedural bleeding, including oozing that continues beyond 5 minutes or at the end of all therapeutics should

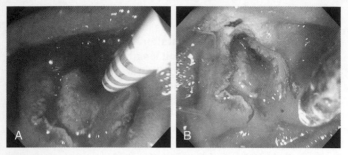

FIG. 26.3 Management of post-sphincterotomy bleeding. A, Active bleeding from the apex of the biliary sphincterotomy. A 7 Fr bipolar electrocautery probe is in position. B, After coagulation there is cavitation and complete hemostasis.

be treated. Options include epinephrine injection, thermal therapy (bipolar probes or coagulation grasping devices; Fig. 26.3), and mechanical methods (endoclips), alone or in combination. In difficult to control post-ERCP bleeding, the use of fully covered self-expandable metal stents (SEMS) can control bleeding by tamponade effect.[9]

3. Refractory post-sphincterotomy bleeding may require angiographic embolization

4. Most sphincterotomy-related perforations are retroperitoneal (type II or IV) and rarely require surgical intervention. The presence of intra- or retroperitoneal free air is not a determinant of operative management and generally correlates with the amount of air insufflation and manipulation during the procedure. Careful endoscopic examination of the sphincterotomy site with contrast injection should be performed in cases of suspected sphincterotomy perforation. Closure of a periampullary defect with endoclips and/or placement of a fully covered SEMS,[9] plastic stent, or placement of nasobiliary tube should be attempted in cases where a defect is identified endoscopically or by contrast extravasation demonstrated fluoroscopically.

5. If the defect cannot be repaired endoscopically or access to the bile duct fails, surgical intervention or placement of an internal-external drain by interventional radiology may be necessary.

References

1. SGE Standards of Practice Committee, Early DS, Lightdale JR, et al. Guidelines for sedation and anesthesia in GI endoscopy. *Gastrointest Endosc.* 2018;87(2):327-337.
2. ASGE Standards of Practice Committee, Acosta RD, Abraham NS, et al. The management of antithrombotic agents for patients undergoing GI endoscopy. *Gastrointest Endosc.* 2016;83(1):3-16.

3. Parekh PJ, Buerlein RC, Shams R, Herre J, Johnson DA. An update on the management of implanted cardiac devices during electrosurgical procedures. *Gastrointest Endosc.* 2013;78(6):836-841.
4. Rustagi T, Jamidar PA. Endoscopic retrograde cholangiopancreatography (ERCP)-related adverse events: post-ERCP pancreatitis. *Gastrointest Endosc Clin N Am.* 2015;25(1):107-121.
5. Testoni PA, Mariani A, Aabakken L, et al. Papillary cannulation and sphincterotomy techniques at ERCP: European Society of Gastrointestinal Endoscopy (ESGE) clinical guideline. *Endoscopy.* 2016;48(7):657-683.
6. Manes G, Paspatis G, Aabakken L, et al. Endoscopic management of common bile duct stones: European Society of Gastrointestinal Endoscopy (ESGE) guideline. *Endoscopy.* 2019;51(5):472-491.
7. Mammen A, Haber G. Difficult biliary access: advanced cannulation and sphincterotomy technique. *Gastrointest Endosc Clin N Am.* 2015;25(4):619-630.
8. Miao L, Li QP, Zhu MH, et al. Endoscopic transpancreatic septotomy as a precutting technique for difficult bile duct cannulation. *World J Gastroenterol.* 2015;21(13):3978-3982.
9. Akbar A, Irani S, Baron TH, et al. Use of covered self-expandable metal stents for endoscopic management of benign biliary disease not related to stricture (with video). *Gastrointest Endosc.* 2012;76(1):196-201.

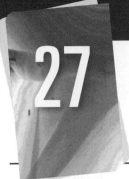

27

Management of Biliary Lithiasis

Sean Bhalla, MD
Ryan Law, DO

Over 20 million Americans are estimated to have gallbladder disease.[1] Choledocholithiasis has been estimated to be present in 10% to 20% of individuals with symptomatic gallstones.[2] Biliary lithiasis can be associated with acute cholangitis and/or acute biliary pancreatitis. Choledocholithiasis often requires prompt endoscopic treatment prior to surgical cholecystectomy in symptomatic biliary lithiasis or cholangitis, to aid in resolution of pancreatitis, or to minimize subsequent episodes of pancreatitis. Nearly all bile duct stones can be treated endoscopically using various methods. Small bile duct stones can easily be extracted via sphincterotomy in conjunction with balloon or basket extraction. Large bile duct stones, defined as a stone ≥1.5 cm in diameter, can be more challenging to extract. Multiple procedures and techniques may sometimes be required in the treatment of larger stones. The American Society for Gastrointestinal Endoscopy (ASGE) provides an up-to-date guideline of endoscopic management of choledocholithiasis, but does not provide explicit guidelines or technical interventions needed for stone extraction.[3] This chapter will outline and review available techniques for removal of bile duct stones.

INDICATION
1. Choledocholithiasis
2. Cholangitis
3. Gallstone pancreatitis
4. Mirizzi syndrome

ABSOLUTE CONTRAINDICATIONS
1. Refer to Chapter 5 on Basic Upper Endoscopy
2. Refer to Chapter 25 on Basic ERCP

RELATIVE CONTRAINDICATIONS

1. Coagulopathy, INR >1.5
2. Baseline platelet count <50,000/mm
3. Refer to Chapter 25 on Basic ERCP

EQUIPMENT

- Duodenoscope and accompanying tower/processor/monitor
- CO_2 insufflator with full canister or wall attachment
- Guidewire (minimum 270 cm length)
- Sphincterotome (Needle knife papillotome should be available for freehand precut.)
- Stone retrieval basket and/or extraction balloon
- Dilating balloons and inflation device (size range 8 mm up to 20 mm)
- Mechanical lithotriptor
- Digital, single-operator cholangioscopy with electrohydraulic lithotriptor and accessories (SpyGlass DS; Boston Scientific, Marlborough, MA)
- Fluoroscopy
- Water-soluble contrast
- Leaded aprons for radiation safety
- Radiation dosage badges for personnel

PREPROCEDURE

1. Patient should be NPO at least 6 hours to procedure.
2. Patients on anticoagulants and antiplatelet agents should stop or alter their medication after discussion with the prescribing physician (if unable to stop anticoagulation, consider balloon sphincteroplasty) (see Chapter 4 on Anticoagulant and Antiplatelet Agents).
3. Obtain standard preoperative consent by the endoscopist and anesthesiologist outlining possible risks, benefits, and alternative methods of treatment.
4. Position patient per endoscopist preference (i.e., prone, supine, or left lateral).
5. ERCP is generally performed under anesthesia assistance.
6. Consider a single dose of indomethacin 100 mg per rectum to reduce the risk of post-ERCP pancreatitis, if no contraindications are identified.
7. Consider preprocedure initiation of intravenous fluids (specifically lactated Ringer's solution) with continuation to the postprocedure setting to reduce the risk of pancreatitis.

PROCEDURE

Techniques for Stone Extraction

Balloon Sphincteroplasty + Balloon/Basket Extraction

Balloon sphincteroplasty (without sphincterotomy) was initially described for removal of small stones with goal of preserving the sphincter of Oddi.[4] This technique may be particularly useful in patients with surgically altered anatomy (e.g., Billroth II gastrojejunostomy[5]), periampullary diverticulum, coagulopathy, thrombocytopenia, and/or need for ongoing anticoagulation where sphincterotomy is less desirable. It is important to note that there have been reports increased adverse event rates such as post-ERCP pancreatitis with sphincteroplasty.

1. Cannulate the bile duct and pass a guidewire into the biliary tree (see Chapter 25 on Basic ERCP).
2. Dilating balloon (<12 mm diameter) is passed over the guidewire and placed across the ampullary orifice.
3. Inflate the balloon to the desired diameter and pressure using iodinated contrast.
4. Hold the balloon in place across the papilla for at least 30 seconds.
5. Adequate dilation has been achieved when the waist of the balloon is no longer visible.
6. Deflate the balloon.
7. Evaluate the dilation to ensure the stone can be extracted (dilation can be repeated).
8. If necessary, balloon or basket extraction can be used to remove stones.

Sphincterotomy + Balloon/Basket Extraction (Video 27.1)

Sphincterotomy is a commonly performed technique in ERCP. It is important as it improves the ability for biliary stone removal and may facilitate additional endotherapy (i.e., stent placement, dilation, etc.).

1. After guidewire cannulation is achieved (see Chapter 25 on Basic ERCP), insert the sphincterotome cannula into the ampulla over the guidewire.
2. Perform a cholangiogram by injecting iodinated contrast into the biliary tree to determine the location and size of bile duct stones.
3. A complete biliary sphincterotomy is performed using electrocautery to divide the sphincter of Oddi to the level of the first transverse duodenal fold. The luminal impression of the intraduodenal bile duct to provide directionality (usually between 11 and 1 o'clock) (see Chapter 25 on Basic ERCP).
4. Once the sphincterotomy has been completed proceed with balloon or wire basket extraction as described in the next section.

Balloon Extraction

1. The balloon catheter is passed over the guidewire into position above the bile duct stone.
2. The balloon is inflated to match the diameter of the bile duct, thereby allowing capture of the stone upon withdrawal. Extraction balloons can be inflated from 8.5 to 20 mm.
3. Using gentle tension, the inflated balloon is withdrawn. When the balloon and captured stone reach the ampulla, a quick clockwise torque often delivers the stone and balloon through the ampulla.
4. Multiple sweeps may be required to clear the biliary duct of additional stones. The endoscopist should take care to avoid attempted removal of more than one stone per sweep.

Basket Extraction

1. Introduce the basket over the guidewire that is in the common bile duct.
2. Place the basket proximal to the stone.
3. Open the basket to its full extent.
4. Gently pulling and pushing the basket to and fro will trap the stone within the basket.
5. Close the basket.
6. Withdraw the basket through the ampulla to remove the entrapped stone.
7. Extract one stone at a time to prevent stone impaction within the basket wires.

Mechanical Lithotripsy

Using this technique, large stones not easily extracted with balloons or baskets can be pulverized. Two commonly used tools available are made by different manufacturers. One can be used through the scope and requires assembly, while the other is guided over a wire after the scope is removed and a hand crank is used to crush the stone.

1. After guidewire cannulation is achieved (see Chapter 25 on Basic ERCP), insert the sphincterotome cannula into the ampulla over the guidewire.
2. Create sphincterotomy (see section on sphincterotomy in Chapter 26).
3. Advance mechanical lithotripsy basket over the guidewire into common bile duct.
4. Open the basket and gently rotate it in order to trap the stone.
5. Once captured, advance the metal sheath to the level of the stone to secure it.

6. Close the basket taking care to prevent slippage of the basket and/or loss of the stone.

7. Closing the basket will increase tension on the wires and pulverize the stone.

8. Pull the basket back into the duodenum to remove stone fragments.

9. If multiple stones are present, each stone should be crushed individually.

10. Balloon sweep may be required to clear the bile duct of all stone fragments.

Combined Endoscopic Sphincterotomy and Papillary Large Balloon Dilation

This technique uses a combination of sphincterotomy and papillary large balloon dilation to remove large bile duct stones, with the intent to avoid lithotripsy. Large balloon dilation is defined as ≥12 mm (Fig. 27.1A–C). If prior sphincterotomy has been performed, a repeat is not necessary. Since balloon dilation will be performed, a large sphincterotomy is not needed. The goal of sphincterotomy is to reduce the risk of post-ERCP pancreatitis, and to orient the dilation and possible resultant tear away from pancreatic orifice.

1. After guidewire cannulation is achieved (see Chapter 25 on Basic ERCP), insert the sphincterotome cannula into the ampulla over the guidewire.

2. Create sphincterotomy (see section on sphincterotomy in Chapter 26).

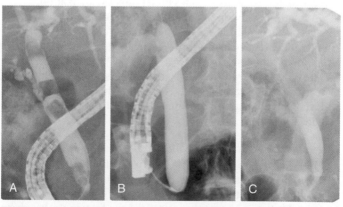

FIG. 27.1 A, Several large stones within the common hepatic and common bile duct. B, Endoscopic papillary large balloon dilation (EPLBD) with effacement of the waist at the ampulla. C, Final cholangiogram following duct clearance after EPLBD demonstrates no remaining bile duct stones.

3. Insert balloon over guidewire until it crosses the ampulla.
   a. Given that biliary dilation balloons are limited to 10 mm, nonbiliary dilating balloons (i.e., esophageal, pyloric or colonic balloons will be required).
   b. The size of the balloon should be matched to the distal bile duct.
4. Position the balloon so the waist is located at the site of sphincterotomy.
5. Inflate the balloon with iodinated contrast under fluoroscopic and endoscopic guidance.
6. Perform a gradual dilation to prevent excessive bleeding.
   a. If the balloon waist does not resolve at 75% of maximal pressure, further inflation should be avoided.
7. Hold the balloon in place for 30 to 60 seconds.
8. Deflate the balloon.
9. Extract the stone using the basket or balloon extraction technique (see section on balloons/baskets above).

Cholangioscopy with Intraductal Lithotripsy

Cholangioscopy can be performed using a direct peroral cholangioscope or a disposable digital single-operator cholangioscope which is passed into the bile duct via the working channel of the duodenoscope. The disposable single-operator, mother-daughter system is most common. Once biliary access has been achieved via the cholangioscope, electrohydrolic lithotripsy or laser therapy can be used for successful intraductal lithotripsy. It should be noted that a cholangioscopy-guided extraction basket has recently been made available to remove stones under direct visualization.

1. Sphincteroplasty or sphincterotomy is needed to aid in passage of the cholangioscope.
2. A guidewire is placed into the intrahepatic ducts via the duodenoscope.
3. The single-operator, mother-daughter system is advanced into the biliary tree just distal to the bile duct stone of interest.
4. Lithotripsy is then performed using either electrohydraulic energy or laser.

Electrohydraulic Lithotripsy (Video 27.2)

Electrohydraulic lithotripsy (EHL) uses high-voltage electric sparks delivered in short pulses that expand in surrounding aqueous medium to create shock wave oscillations and fragment stones.

1. Once cholangioscope is in position in the bile duct, straighten the cholangioscope.
2. Flush water through the working channel and simultaneously advance the EHL fiber.
3. Ensure the EHL fiber tip is visible outside the cholangioscope on endoscopy and fluoroscopy.

4. EHL fiber tip should be pushed close to but not touching the center of the stone.
5. Continuous saline irrigation into the bile duct is necessary to allow for magnification of the power of EHL.
6. Pulsed energy (i.e., power and shots) is delivered directly at the stone with care to touch the walls of the bile duct as this may cause injury.
7. Once stone fragmentation is complete, remove the EHL fiber and cholangioscope.
8. An extraction balloon can be used to remove the remaining stone fragments.

Laser Lithotripsy

1. Once cholangioscope is in position in the bile duct, straighten the cholangioscope.
2. Use standard laser safety precautions and appropriate eye protection.
3. Pass the laser catheter system into working channel of cholangioscope.
4. Ensure correct location of the laser system with fluoroscopy.
5. Irrigate saline into the common bile duct.
6. The laser beam should be perpendicular to the stone.
7. Fire the laser at the stone. The pulsed laser system generates high-energy shock waves by the creation and expansion of excited plasma that oscillates to fragment biliary stones.[6]
8. Once the stone has been fragmented, remove the laser system and the cholangioscope.
9. Using balloon sweep of the bile duct, stone fragments should be removed.

POSTPROCEDURE

1. Monitor for postprocedure adverse events which generally occur within the first 6 hours.
2. Continue intravenous fluids to mitigate risk for post-ERCP pancreatitis.
3. Patients should be referred for interval cholecystectomy, ideally within 2 weeks after stone extraction from the bile duct.

ADVERSE EVENTS

Across multiple studies, significant adverse events (i.e., pancreatitis, sepsis, bleeding, perforation) range from 5% to 12%, and mortality ranges from 0.1% to 1.4%.[7–12]

1. Post-ERCP pancreatitis
2. Bleeding
3. Infection/sepsis

4. Perforation
5. Cardiopulmonary adverse events (aspiration, hypoxemia, arrhythmia) related to procedural sedation
6. Rare instances of procedure-related death

CONCLUSION

More than 85% of biliary stones can be removed by sphincterotomy or balloon sphincteroplasty with assistance of basket or balloon extraction.[13] However, larger stones or altered gastrointestinal anatomy can make stone removal challenging and thus the alternative methods described above may need to be utilized. If complete stone extraction cannot be performed in a single session, it is recommended that biliary stent be placed to prevent cholangitis until stone extraction can be completed.

References

1. Everhart JE, Khare M, Hill M, Maurer KR. Prevalence and ethnic differences in gallbladder disease in the United States. *Gastroenterology*. 1999;117(3):632-639.
2. Williams E, Beckingham I, El Sayed G, et al. Updated guideline on the management of common bile duct stones (CBDS). *Gut*. 2017;66(5):765-782.
3. Maple JT, Ikenberry SO, Anderson MA, et al. The role of endoscopy in the management of choledocholithiasis. *Gastrointest Endosc*. 2011;74(4):731-744.
4. Staritz M, Ewe K, Meyer zum Büschenfelde KH. Endoscopic papillary dilation (EPD) for the treatment of common bile duct stones and papillary stenosis. *Endoscopy*. 1983;15:197-198.
5. Prat F, Fritsch J, Choury AD, et al. Endoscopic sphincteroclasy: a useful therapeutic tool for biliary endoscopy in Billroth II gastrectomy patients. *Endoscopy*. 1997;29(2):79-81.
6. Steiner R. *Laser Lithotripsy*: Clinical Use and Technical Aspects. Berlin: Springer-Verlag; 1988.
7. Andriulli A, Loperfido S, Napolitano G, et al. Incidence rates of post-ERCP complications: a systematic survey of prospective studies. *Am J Gastroenterol*. 2007;102(8):1781-1788.
8. Williams EJ, Taylor S, Fairclough P, et al. Risk factors for complication following ERCP; results of a large-scale, prospective multicenter study. *Endoscopy*. 2007;39(9):793-801.
9. Wang P, Li ZS, Liu F, et al. Risk factors for ERCP-related complications: a prospective multicenter study. *Am J Gastroenterol*. 2009;104(1):31-40.
10. Kapral C, Mühlberger A, Wewalka F, et al. Quality assessment of endoscopic retrograde cholangiopancreatography: results of a running nationwide Austrian benchmarking project after 5 years of implementation. *Eur J Gastroenterol Hepatol*. 2012;24(12):1447-1454.
11. Siiki A, Tamminen A, Tomminen T, Kuusanmäki P. ERCP procedures in a Finnish community hospital: a retrospective analysis of 1207 cases. *Scand J Surg*. 2012;101(1):45-50.
12. Glomsaker T, Hoff G, Kvaløy JT, et al. Patterns and predictive factors of complications after endoscopic retrograde cholangiopancreatography. *Br J Surg*. 2013;100(3):373-380.
13. Binmoeller KF, Brückner M, Thonke F, Soehendra N. Treatment of difficult bile duct stones using mechanical, electrohydraulic and extracorporeal shock wave lithotripsy. *Endoscopy*. 1993;25(3):201-206.

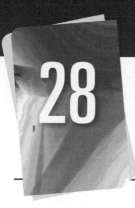

28

Management of Biliary and Pancreatic Ductal Obstruction: Endoprosthesis and Nasobiliary/Nasopancreatic Drain Placement

Nadav Sahar, MD
Richard A. Kozarek, MD, FACG, FASGE, AGAF, FACP

Therapeutic endoscopy has become the mainstay for treatment of biliary and pancreatic ductal obstruction and has acceptable complication rates in comparison to surgical or percutaneous drainage alternatives. Endoscopic placement of prostheses is useful in treating benign and malignant obstructions of the pancreaticobiliary tree, decompression of stone disease, prevention of post–endoscopic retrograde cholangiopancreatography (ERCP) pancreatitis, and closure of leakage and disruptions.

Biliary and pancreatic stents are now available in various designs and sizes and are either plastic or metal. Pancreatic stents generally differ from biliary stents by being of smaller diameter and having unique side holes that permit drainage of side branches.

INDICATIONS

As is the general rule for all ERCP cases, the indication for the procedure must be clear and not merely for diagnostic purposes (see Chapter 25). Of note, ductal drainage is often achieved by sphincterotomy alone, without the need for stenting (see Chapter 26). Common indications for endoscopic stenting include the following.

Biliary Endoprosthesis

1. Treatment of benign strictures (chronic pancreatitis, sclerosing cholangitis, posttransplant, post-sphincterotomy stenosis, etc.)
2. Malignant biliary obstruction (biliary, pancreatic, periampullary, or metastatic tumors)
3. Relief of obstructive jaundice
4. Closure of bile leaks or fistulae
5. Incomplete removal of bile duct stones
6. Trans-cystic duct gallbladder drainage in high-risk surgical patients

Pancreatic Endoprosthesis

1. Prevention of post-ERCP pancreatitis (usually reserved for high-risk patients—difficult cannulation, endoscopic ampullectomy, precut sphincterotomy, inadvertent repeated cannulation, etc.)
2. Treatment of pancreatic duct disruption or fistula
3. Drainage of pseudocysts
4. Pancreatic stones prior to endoscopic removal or extracorporeal shock-wave lithotripsy (ESWL)
5. Treatment of pancreatic strictures (such as seen in chronic pancreatitis)
6. Malignant pancreatic obstruction (more commonly for palliation)

Nasobiliary Drain

1. Palliation of malignant hilar strictures
2. Closure of bile leaks
3. Biliary obstruction secondary to difficult-to-treat bile duct stones
4. Post-ERCP when there is suspicion of incomplete stone removal, thereby enabling repeat cholangiogram

Nasopancreatic Drain

1. Similar to pancreatic endoprostheses when short-term drainage is desired or to aid targeting for ESWL
2. Pancreatic duct irrigation following ESWL

CONTRAINDICATIONS

Please refer to Chapter 25 for general contraindications to ERCP. Relative contraindications are few but may include placement of a covered metal stent across a compromised cystic duct in patients with an intact gallbladder or insertion of large pancreatic duct stents in patients with small-diameter ducts.

PREPARATION

Please also refer to general preparation before ERCP as detailed in Chapter 25 and the use of prophylactic antibiotics in Chapter 1.

EQUIPMENT, ENDOSCOPES, DEVICES, ACCESSORIES

1. The majority of therapeutic duodenoscopes have a 4.2 mm working channel enabling insertion of large endoprostheses up to 11.5 Fr in diameter. For pediatric patients or patients with high-grade luminal stenosis, smaller working channels may be required (i.e., pediatric colonoscopes, diagnostic

duodenoscopes, balloon enteroscopes, etc.), but these allow placement of stents up to 7 Fr in caliber. 7 mm duodenoscopes for neonates are variably available which allow placement of 5 Fr stents only.

2. Cannulation catheters range from 5 Fr standard-tip single channel to ultra-tapered 5-4-3 Fr and 6-7 Fr steerable ERCP catheters as well as dual-lumen ERCP catheters.

3. Guidewires range from 0.018″ to 0.035″ diameter and include hybrid and hydrophilic, straight, and angle-tips.

4. Sphincterotome (double or triple lumen to allow guidewire and contrast injection)
   a. Standard 6 Fr to 7 Fr diameter traction-type
   b. Small-caliber (5 Fr) wire-guided traction-type
   c. Billroth II sphincterotome designed for B-II and Roux anatomy
   d. Needle knife

5. Water-soluble contrast (standard plus nonionic contrast for patients allergic to iodinated contrast)

6. Electrocautery unit

7. Dilating catheter 3 Fr to 10 Fr diameter

8. Dilating balloons 4 mm to 20 mm

9. 5 Fr to 10 Fr screw-type dilators (or stent extractors)

10. Snares, rat-tooth grasping forceps, and stone-retrieval baskets

11. Sclerotherapy needles, thermocoagulation (bipolar or heater probe) probes, and endoscopic clips for hemostasis

12. Wire-guided cytology brush

13. Small biopsy forceps

BILIARY ENDOPROSTHESES

Plastic stents: These are composed of polyethylene, polyurethane, or polytetrafluoroethylene and range in diameter from 5 Fr to 11.5 Fr. Plastic biliary stents are available in lengths from 1 to 18 cm long, are straight (angled, curved) with internal and external flaps to preclude migration, or are pigtail shaped.

Self-expanding metallic stents (SEMS): These were designed in order to overcome early stent occlusion which can occur with plastic stents. They are available as uncovered, partially (PC-SEMS) or fully covered (FC-SEMS). Most SEMS are made of nitinol. They range in lengths from 4 to 12 cm and diameters from 6 to 10 mm.

PANCREATIC ENDOPROSTHESES

Plastic stents: Plastic pancreatic stents are available in diameters ranging from 3 Fr to 11.5 Fr and lengths ranging from 2 to 25 cm. The inner end is always straight with one, two, or no flanges.

In order to prevent inward migration, the outer end is either straight with two flanges or has a single partial pigtail. Most of these stents are deployed over a wire.

Self-expanding metallic stents (SEMS): Currently only one SEMS is specifically designed for drainage of the main pancreatic duct (Niti-S, TaeWoong, Seoul, South Korea). Other fully covered SEMS used off-label have shown promising results, to include the biliary WallFlex stent (Boston Scientific) and the Viabil stent (Gore Medical), although the smallest diameter of these stents is 8 mm. 4, 6, and 8 mm WallFlex stents designed for the pancreas are under study currently but have not been FDA approved.

PROCEDURE

Please refer to Chapter 2 for details on sedation and Chapter 25 addressing successful selective duct cannulation.

Biliary Stent Placement

1. Once the papillary orifice is cannulated and before stent placement, inject contrast under fluoroscopic guidance to visualize the anatomy and assess stricture/leak length and location.

2. Use a 0.025″ or 0.035″ guidewire with a hydrophilic tip to perform deep cannulation and traverse any stricture. Use caution when advancing proximally past the stricture to avoid perforating the duct.

3. When using stents up to 10 Fr in size, a biliary sphincterotomy is not mandatory. If multiple stent placement is planned or placement of stents of larger caliber, perform biliary sphincterotomy.

4. In cases involving tight strictures, predilation is required prior to stent placement. Using a dilating catheter to pass the stricture often obviates additional balloon dilation. When using hydrostatic, wire-guided balloon dilation, ideally dilate the stricture until a waist disappears on fluoroscopy. If a balloon cannot be passed through the stricture, use graduated dilators in increasing diameters from 3 Fr up to 7 to 10 Fr. If these cannot be passed, a corkscrew-type dilator or stent extractor can be used.

5. The choice of stent length is often based on endoscopist's experience. Some guidewires contain markers which are visible both endoscopically and fluoroscopically and facilitate measuring optimal stent length. Another method to approximate the desired stent length is to gently withdraw the catheter from the proximal end of the stricture to just outside the papilla while simultaneously grasping the catheter at its

entry point into the endoscope, thereby measuring the length of the catheter pulled out of the endoscope. Conversely, measure the length of guidewire pulled from the proximal to distal tip of the stricture. As a general rule, the length of the stent chosen should be at least 2 cm above the proximal end of the stricture and 1 cm above the papilla for plastic stents which are left completely intraductal, while metallic stents need to traverse the papilla for distal strictures. Use a longer initial stent when planning multiple stent deployments.

6. After stent selection, introduce the stent into the working channel and advance using a pusher catheter. Small stents up to 7 Fr in diameter are inserted tapered end first. Position the scope close to the papilla in a short configuration to avoid looping in the duodenal lumen. Close the endoscope elevator during initial stent advancement. Dialing the big wheel on the endoscope, gently lifting the elevator, and pulling back on the shaft of the endoscope in an anticlockwise fashion are all techniques that can aid in forward movement. Once the stent is out of the scope and in position, the assistant can pull back on the guidewire or guide catheter. Keep constant pressure on the pusher catheter while pulling back the guide catheter to prevent the stent from dislodging distally. If additional stents are needed, each should be deployed in the same manner. In cases with unsuccessful stent deployment, consider using a long endoscope positioning. Perform a definitive cholangiogram after stent placement to ensure contrast drains through the stent (Fig. 28.1).

7. For temporary drainage of unremovable bile duct stones, double-pigtail stents are preferable to straight stents with the goal of placing the upper pigtail above the most proximal stone. Placing two double-pigtail stents can help minimize distal migration. When placing pigtail stents, the endoscope is gradually pulled back during stent deployment to ensure that the stent can coil in the duodenum.

8. The use of SEMS is usually reserved for inoperable malignant obstruction with short-term life expectancy or for placement of covered SEMS for refractory bile duct stenoses. When choosing SEMS, it is important to consider that the initial length of stent shortens by up to 40% after deployment. A biliary sphincterotomy is not mandatory when using an uncovered SEMS. Deployment of SEMS is performed when the assistant slowly withdraws the outer sheath of the stent while the endoscopist simultaneously releases the elevator, withdraws the pushing catheter, and pulls back on the outer sheath. The SEMS begins to expand from its proximal end but when using reconstrainable SEMS, repositioning can be done

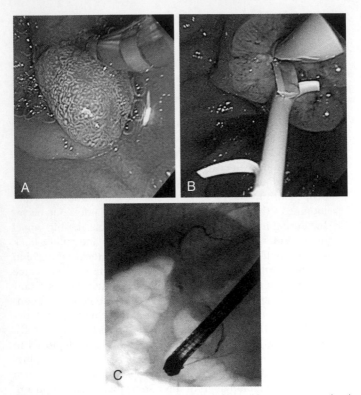

FIG. 28.1 A, Endoscopic view of a short-nosed traction sphincterotome cannulated alongside an ampullary adenoma. B, A 7 Fr by 5 cm plastic stent with a single external flap and a single internal flap in the bile duct alongside a 5 Fr by 3 cm plastic stent with two external flaps and two internal flaps in the ventral pancreatic duct. Both stents were placed following endoscopic papillectomy of the ampullary tumor. They were retrieved after 4 weeks with no residual neoplasm. C, Fluoroscopic view of deployment of the plastic stent into the common bile duct.

even after 80% of the stent has been deployed. After deployment of the outer sheath, the guidewire and push catheter can be removed. If the stent is positioned too far proximally, the stent can be repositioned from its distal end using a rattooth forceps or removed entirely. There are also laser-cut SEMS that have virtually no foreshortening with deployment. Laser-cut stents do not foreshorten and cannot be reconstrained during the delivery.

9. For treatment of hilar tumors, plastic stents or SEMS can be considered (or a combination of the two). SEMS are currently the prosthesis of choice in cases with an expected survival of more than 4 months, unless concomitant surgery or

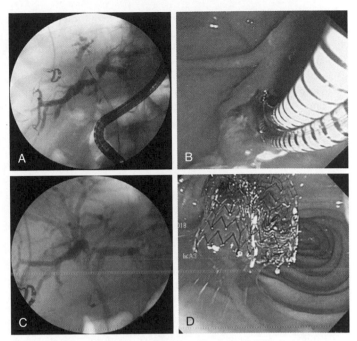

FIG. 28.2 A, Fluoroscopic view of 0.035 inch guidewire in the biliary tree demonstrating a malignant hilar obstruction with bilateral intrahepatic dilation. B, Endoscopic image of two 8 mm by 12 cm uncovered constrained biliary self-expanding metal stents (SEMS) being inserted in a side-by-side fashion after biliary sphincterotomy had been performed. C, Fluoroscopic view of the two biliary stents extending into each intrahepatic ductal system. D, Endoscopic image of the two SEMS, which drain the right and left systems, exiting the papilla.

photodynamic therapy is planned. Uncovered SEMS are used for hilar or intrahepatic obstruction to preclude occluding the contralateral intrahepatic system. The superiority of unilateral or bilateral stenting is still ill-defined, although recent studies suggest bilateral stenting is associated with better outcomes (Fig. 28.2).

10. Magnetic resonance cholangiopancreatography (MRCP) should be obtained prior to ERCP for hilar tumor staging and planning of segmental drainage. Cannulation should be initiated by injecting contrast only to the bottom of the stricture, minimizing injection into an obstructed duct to reduce the risk of cholangitis. Once the wire passes freely and deeply into the liver in the direction of the desired intrahepatic duct, advance the cannula deep into that lobe. Remove the guidewire and aspirate as much bile as possible to decompress the

duct. If at least 25% of the liver parenchyma appears to be drained, perform balloon dilation of the stricture, followed by placement of a single stent. If a large-caliber stent cannot be placed due to extreme stenosis or difficult angulation, consider placing a 5 Fr straight nasobiliary drain through the hilar stenosis for several days to decompress the duct and open up the stricture and assess for improvement in jaundice. This will usually allow subsequent placement of a larger stent at follow-up ERCP.

11. In cases where bilateral stents are indicated, attempt cannulating the left intrahepatic duct first which is usually more technically challenging. One technique is to place one guidewire into each intrahepatic ductal system and deploy the first stent into the side which was more difficult to cannulate. The second stent is then advanced along the second wire. The second technique involves deploying the first stent followed by inserting a guidewire alongside the stent into the opposite intrahepatic ductal system. The second stent is placed in a "Y" configuration. Often a temporary plastic stent is inserted alongside the first SEMS to facilitate deployment of the second SEMS. Stents of smaller diameter may need to be inserted initially and undergo upsizing at a subsequent ERCP session after 2 to 3 weeks. Alternatively, two laser-cut stents on 6 Fr delivery shafts can be inserted simultaneously through a 4.2 mm duodenoscope channel allowing placement of 2, 8 to 10 mm, 10 to 12 cm parallel SEMS whose distal ends exit the papilla.

Pancreatic Stent Placement

1. Pancreatic stent placement technique is similar to biliary stent placement, through either the major or minor papilla, except for a number of important differences: (1) the stents in use are generally much smaller (3 to 7 Fr); (2) they are deployed directly over the wire without a guide catheter; (3) pancreatic ducts are smaller and more tortuous than bile ducts and thus can be more difficult to pass a wire into deeply; (4) the pancreatic duct has side branches into which the tip of the guidewire is prone to enter; and (5) there is potential for pancreatic duct injury from a stent that is too large or malpositioned, especially in a normal small duct.

2. Stent diameter should be appropriate for the indication of the procedure and should not exceed maximal diameter of the pancreatic duct. Most small-diameter stents (3 to 4 Fr) are inserted over 0.018″ to 0.025″ guidewires, while a hydrophilic 0.035″ guidewire can be used for stents of larger diameters. The optimal diameter for prevention of post-ERCP

pancreatitis has yet to be defined; however, all stents placed for prophylaxis would ideally migrate spontaneously within several weeks of placement. Stents without a proximal barb are designed to ensure spontaneous distal migration, while those with a single pigtail are designed to anchor the stent in the duodenum and limit proximal migration.

3. Pancreatic sphincterotomy is usually unnecessary for placement of pancreatic stents. When performing dual sphincterotomy, such as after performing endoscopic papillectomy, pancreatic sphincterotomy is generally performed after biliary sphincterotomy as the pancreaticobiliary septum is well visualized and limits the extent of the incision. Pure cut current should be used in patients without chronic pancreatitis, whereas a blended or ERBE-type current can be used in patients with chronic pancreatitis.

4. When encountering tight strictures, as in chronic pancreatitis, balloon dilation may be indicated to allow subsequent stent placement.

5. Short, small-caliber pancreatic stents should be deployed slowly, thereby ensuring their distal end does not extend too far into the duct.

Nasobiliary Catheter Placement

1. Nasobiliary drains are used less frequently today in comparison to the past, partly due to patient discomfort and risk of dislodgement in uncooperative patients. These drains are still important options to consider when palliating malignant hilar strictures, closure of bile leaks, and in cases of incomplete removal of stones. They range in external diameter from 5 Fr to 10 Fr and are 250 cm long. The drains have either a straight or pigtail end.

2. Nasobiliary drain placement is initiated after standard biliary cannulation via ERCP followed by guidewire insertion. A biliary sphincterotomy is usually performed although not mandatory. Once the wire is in place, the nasobiliary catheter is advanced over the guidewire to the level of the hilum, maintaining endoscopic and fluoroscopic control for proper location. After the insertion of the nasobiliary catheter to its proper position, the endoscope is withdrawn with the aid of an assistant while simultaneously advancing the catheter shaft by the endoscopist. Once the endoscope is withdrawn from the mouth, it is crucial to hold the nasobiliary catheter in place during the endoscope removal.

3. The nasobiliary drain needs to then be transferred from the mouth to the nose. This is done with the help of a nasal transfer tube that is inserted in similar fashion to a nasogastric

tube, into the patient's nose up to the posterior pharynx. It is then retrieved by extending a finger deep into the patient's mouth or with the aid of the endoscope. The transfer tube is pulled out of the mouth, then the endoscopist feeds the tip of the guidewire and nasobiliary catheter through the tube and gently pulls the tube back through the nose. The transfer tube is then removed, and the nasobiliary catheter is pulled back until the pharyngeal loop is straightened, without pulling the distal end in the biliary tree. The nasobiliary drain should be secured to the patient's nose. Contrast is injected through the catheter to reconfirm the position of the catheter in the biliary system.

Nasopancreatic Drain Placement

Nasopancreatic drains are no longer frequently in use unless placed after ESWL and pancreatic stone extraction for saline irrigation or to irrigate areas of walled-off pancreatic necrosis. In the latter situation these irrigations are usually done through drains placed transmurally as opposed to transpapillary. The technique of placement is similar to that of the nasobiliary drain. They are commonly 5 Fr to 7 Fr in diameter, except that straight-type 4 Fr or 5 Fr drains with one or two inner retention flanges are generally used; a guidewire must be passed to at least the mid-body of the pancreas and the drain passed over the guidewire.

ADVERSE EVENTS

Please refer to Chapter 25 for a detailed review of typical adverse events related to ERCP, such as hemorrhage or perforation as a consequence of sphincterotomy or adverse events related to sedation. This chapter will focus on adverse events related directly to placement of endoprostheses. The relevant adverse events to consider include:

1. Occlusion of a biliary endoprosthesis—this leads to malfunction of the stent, usually manifesting as cholestasis or cholangitis. Early occlusion, up to 4 weeks from the procedure, is more common with plastic stents than with metal stents, which tend to occlude after 3 to 9 months. Occluded stents are treated by stent replacement with a new stent or placement of a new stent through the indwelling stent.

2. Biliary stent migration—also more common with the use of plastic stents or fully covered SEMS, can occur in up to 5% of cases, either proximally or distally. Treatment is stent removal or exchange.

3. Occlusion/migration of a pancreatic endoprosthesis—inward migration can be minimized by using single pigtail stents.

Migrated stents should be retrieved endoscopically. Use of large-diameter pancreatic stents may lead to chronic ductal stenosis and relapsing pancreatitis. Plain abdominal x-ray performed within 2-3 weeks of placement is important in documenting spontaneous migration of stents placed for prevention of post-ERCP pancreatitis.

4. Cholecystitis—usually a result of cystic duct obstruction with retained gallbladder stones. Treatment is surgical cholecystectomy, with endoscopic or percutaneous interventions reserved for high-risk surgical patients.

5. Perforation of the lateral duodenal wall is very uncommon but may occur as a result of distal stent migration. Such perforations may often be diagnosed at time of stent removal/replacement and may beinnocuous or catastrophic.

6. Aspiration pneumonia has been reported with the use of a nasobiliary drain; hence patient cooperation is crucial prior to lavage of the drain.

Bibliography

1. Krishnamoorthi R, Jayaraj M, Kozarek R. Endoscopic stents for the biliary tree and pancreas. *Curr Treat Options Gastroenterol.* 2017;15:397-415.
2. Khan MA, Baron TH, Kamal F, et al. Efficacy of self-expandable metal stents in management of benign biliary strictures and comparison with multiple plastic stents: a meta-analysis. *Endoscopy.* 2017;49:682-694.
3. Lee TH, Kim TH, Moon JH, et al. Bilateral versus unilateral placement of metal stents for inoperable high-grade malignant hilar biliary strictures: a multicenter, prospective, randomized study (with video). *Gastrointest Endosc.* 2017;86:817-827.
4. Srinivasan I, Kahaleh M. Metal stents for hilar lesions. *Gastrointest Endosc Clin N Am.* 2012;22:555-565.
5. Coté GA, Slivka A, Tarnasky P, et al. Effect of covered metallic stents compared with plastic stents on benign biliary stricture resolution: a randomized clinical trial. *JAMA.* 2016;315:1250-1257.
6. Dumonceau JM, Tringali A, Blero D, et al. Biliary stenting: indications, choice of stents and results: European Society of Gastrointestinal Endoscopy (ESGE) clinical guideline. *Endoscopy.* 2012;44:277-298.
7. Pfau PR, Pleskow DK, Banerjee S, et al. ASGE technology assessment committee: pancreatic and biliary stents. *Gastrointest Endosc.* 2013;77:319-327.
8. Price LH, Brandabur JJ, Kozarek RA, et al. Good stents gone bad: endoscopic treatment of proximally migrated pancreatic duct stents. *Gastrointest Endosc.* 2009;70:174-179.
9. Itoi T, Sofuni A, Itokawa F, et al. Role of endoscopic nasobiliary drainage indication and basic technique. *Dig Endosc.* 2006;18:S105-S109.

PART SIX

Endoscopic Ultrasound

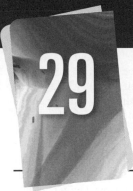

Basics of Endoscopic Ultrasound

Monique T. Barakat, MD
Subhas Banerjee, MD

Endoscopic ultrasound (EUS) is a procedure which allows sonographic imaging of the luminal gastrointestinal (GI) tract together with surrounding structures and organs. The procedure has revolutionized the diagnosis and management of cancer by facilitating enhanced loco-regional imaging, ultrasound-guided fine-needle aspiration (FNA) and biopsy (FNB), placement of fiducials in tumor masses to guide delivery of radiation therapy, and injection of neurolytic agents to address cancer-associated pain. Rapidly evolving therapeutic EUS techniques and supporting devices now facilitate drainage of pancreatic pseudocysts and walled-off pancreas necrosis, bile duct and gallbladder drainage, and hemostasis for both variceal and nonvariceal hemorrhage.

Endoscopic ultrasound relies upon emission of high-frequency sound waves from the EUS probe. These sound waves travel freely through fluid and soft tissues; however, they are reflected back (as "echoes") when they encounter a more solid (dense) structure. For example, the ultrasound waves will travel freely through bile (liquid) in the gallbladder, then echo back when the waves encounter a gallstone within the gallbladder. In this way, as ultrasound waves encounter structures of variable density within the body, echoes of varying strength result in an image of structures surrounding the ultrasound probe, with each exhibiting a unique density.

The echoendoscope is similar to a standard endoscope, but has oblique-viewing optics and an ultrasound transducer at its tip, together with a water inflatable balloon to enhance acoustic coupling. Dual purpose buttons on the endoscope handle allow for air insufflation and suctioning of the gastrointestinal lumen, as well as inflation and deflation of the balloon. The ultrasound transducer at the tip of the EUS scope emits high-frequency sound waves which travel through the tissue being evaluated.

A proportion of these transmitted waves are also reflected, refracted, scattered, and absorbed. The reflected waves are received by the same transducer as "echoes" and are processed to form an image of the area being evaluated. The whiteness or blackness of each point of the image on the gray scale depends on the amplitude of the echo, which in turn depends on the density of the tissue. EUS processors incorporate Doppler technology, which allows identification of blood vessels within the field of imaging and allows differentiation from other tubular structures such as the bile and pancreatic ducts. Doppler technology allows for identification of a safe pathway which avoids blood vessels for FNA, thereby minimizing the risk of bleeding as a procedural complication.

Obtaining an optimal image requires modulation of several factors. Sound waves travel best through water, whereas air creates noise and reverberations resulting in EUS image degradation. Optimal endosonographic images are therefore attained either by filling the gastrointestinal lumen with water, or by suctioning air out of the lumen and filling the echoendoscope balloon with water to improve acoustic coupling with the structure of interest. When imaging a wall lesion, the ultrasound beam should ideally be perpendicular to the lesion to avoid imaging artifacts that arise from tangential views. The area of interest should be in the focal zone of the ultrasound probe, usually about 1.5 cm from the probe.

There are two types of echoendoscopes: radial and linear. The radial echoendoscope scans in a plane perpendicular to the axis of the endoscope to produce an axial image similar to that of a computed tomography (CT) scan. The linear echoendoscope scans in a plane parallel to the axis of the endoscope shaft. This plane of imaging allows visualization of needles as they are advanced beyond the tip of the echoendoscope, thereby facilitating sampling of tissue or cystic fluid (FNA/FNB), and visualization of devices advanced through the echoendoscope channel (e.g., stents, coils, fiducials, neurolytic agents).

Ultrasound mini-probes that can be advanced through the accessory channel of standard endoscopes, either alone or over a guidewire, are available and may offer advantages in certain clinical scenarios. These include immediate assessment of subepithelial nodules incidentally noted during standard endoscopy, and assessment of lesions out of the reach of a standard echoendoscope (e.g., cecal lesions) and lesions where adequate alignment with a standard echoendoscope is difficult to achieve.

INDICATIONS FOR EUS

1. For diagnostic tissue acquisition in the setting of known or suspected malignancy (e.g., mediastinal/abdominal masses, subepithelial nodules, or lymph nodes).

2. For evaluation of known or suspected biliary or pancreatic ductal obstruction (e.g., stone, mass lesion, stricture).

3. For identification and characterization of pancreatic cystic lesions (e.g., pseudocyst/cystic neoplasm) and for FNA to obtain cyst fluid for analysis (carcinoembryonic antigen [CEA], cytology, amylase, lipase).

4. To discern the layer of origin of subepithelial nodules identified by other modalities (e.g., CT, magnetic resonance imaging [MRI], standard endoscopy).

5. To diagnose/localize small neuroendocrine tumors of the pancreas (e.g., insulinoma, gastrinoma), as EUS is superior to CT/MRI for identification of small lesions.

6. For diagnosis of early chronic pancreatitis where diagnostic changes may not be evident on CT imaging. Additionally, EUS-guided FNB may facilitate diagnosis of IgG4-associated pancreatitis.

7. For staging of esophageal, pancreatic, and rectal malignancy. However, with improvements in noninvasive imaging, requests for staging of pancreatic and rectal malignancy are gradually declining.

8. For fiducial placement in tumors to guide radiation oncology therapy.

9. For celiac plexus nerve block (chronic pancreatitis) or celiac plexus neurolysis (malignancy) to manage pain.

10. For transluminal pancreatic pseudocyst drainage (e.g., establishment of cyst-gastrostomy or cyst-duodenostomy tract).

11. For management of walled-off pancreatic necrosis (typically cyst drainage followed by serial procedures for endoscopic necrosectomy, to debride and facilitate resolution).

12. To enable gallbladder drainage when other management options such as surgery or transpapillary gallbladder drainage are not considerations.

13. To achieve hemostasis in variceal bleeding (e.g., glue/coil injection into gastric varices) and occasionally for intractable nonvariceal bleeding which is not amenable to standard endotherapy.

14. To evaluate internal and external anal sphincter integrity in the setting of defecatory dysfunction.

CONTRAINDICATIONS

In addition to the specific contraindications listed below, general absolute and relative contraindications that apply to all endoscopic procedures also apply to EUS.

Absolute Contraindications

1. Large esophageal perforation
2. Untreated esophageal stricture (though some dilation can be performed to facilitate EUS)
3. Cardiopulmonary instability

Relative Contraindications

1. Coagulopathy (Diagnostic EUS may be performed in coagulopathic/anticoagulated patients; however, coagulopathy should be corrected in patients who are undergoing FNA/FNB or EUS-based intervention.)

PREPARATION

1. The procedure should be explained to the patient in simple terms and alternatives discussed. The patient should be informed of possible complications (bleeding, infection, pancreatitis, and perforation) and the potential for missed or misdiagnosed lesions. Risks of sedation or general anesthesia as planned should also be discussed.
2. The patient should have nothing by mouth for 6 to 8 hours prior to the procedure, as presence of food may interfere with transmission of ultrasound and thereby imaging, in addition to increasing procedure-related aspiration risk. Aspiration risk is relatively higher in EUS patients with achalasia, in patients with delayed gastric emptying/gastric outlet obstruction, and when upper gastrointestinal water insufflation is planned. General anesthesia should be considered for these procedures.
3. For anorectal ultrasound, a sigmoid colon and rectum free of stool is necessary. Enema administration prior to the procedure or complete bowel preparation may be administered. Anorectal ultrasound may be performed with sedation or as an unsedated procedure in the appropriate clinical context.

EQUIPMENT

1. Appropriate echoendoscope for indication (radial or linear).
2. Echoendoscope balloon for acoustic coupling
3. Ultrasound processor and light source
4. Water pump to instill water into the gastrointestinal lumen to enhance acoustic coupling

5. Ancillary equipment such as FNA/FNB needles, fiducials, nerve block/neurolysis solutions etc.
6. Personal protective equipment (e.g., gloves, gowns, masks)

PROCEDURE

Performing EUS in the Upper Gastrointestinal Tract

Advancing the Echoendoscope

1. EUS may be performed under general anesthesia, monitored anesthesia care, or sedation. It is increasingly being performed with anesthesia support. If performed under monitored anesthesia care or sedation, a topical anesthetic agent such as viscous lidocaine is usually administered to minimize irritation to the patient's pharynx (gag reflex) during echoendoscope advancement. The patient is typically positioned in the left lateral decubitus position. However, this procedure may be performed in the supine or semiprone position depending on other factors such as whether ERCP is also planned. A bite block is placed to protect the teeth.
2. With the patient's neck partially flexed, the lubricated echoendoscope is advanced through the hypopharynx. Visualization should be maintained, with care to avoid advancing the scope against fixed resistance. The scope should be advanced past the epiglottis to the cricopharyngeus, and then into the esophageal lumen. The echoendoscope should be advanced under direct vision at all times with enough air insufflation to permit visualization.

Visualization of Esophagus, Stomach, and Duodenum

1. An overview of key structures imaged at each anatomical location is included in Table 29.1. As the echoendoscope is advanced into the esophagus, the thyroid gland, trachea and bronchi, and cardiac chambers are visualized. The aorta serves as a landmark and is best kept at the 5-o'clock position on the video monitor. On entering the stomach, the celiac trunk is seen emerging from the aorta and subsequently bifurcating into the hepatic and splenic arteries. With slight further advancement of the echoendoscope, the pancreatic body and tail come into view (homogenous "salt and pepper" echo-texture). Examination of the pancreatic body and tail is typically performed using a transgastric approach (gastric body). The gallbladder is often best evaluated in the prepyloric region or duodenal bulb. While in the stomach, the five layers of the gastric wall can be identified (Fig. 29.1).

TABLE 29.1	EUS Stations
Anatomical Position	**Key Structures Imaged**
Esophagus	Mediastinal structures including the aorta, pulmonary artery, azygous vein, trachea and bronchi, thoracic duct, subcarinal space, aortopulmonary window
Stomach	Vascular structures such as the aorta, celiac artery, splenic vessels, superior mesenteric vessels and portal vein, pancreas neck/body/tail, spleen, liver, left kidney, adrenal gland, gallbladder
Duodenal bulb	Pancreas head/neck, bile duct, gallbladder, right lobe of liver
Second portion of duodenum	Pancreas head/uncinate, right kidney
Rectum	Prostate, seminal vesicles, uterus, perirectal space, internal/external anal sphincters

2. The remainder of the pancreaticobiliary evaluation is best accomplished in the duodenum—typically at three positions (the apex of the duodenal bulb, in the ampullary region, and distal to the ampulla). In these positions, torque, endoscope advancement/withdrawal, and tip inflection are utilized to identify and complete the evaluation of the pancreas, the pancreas duct, bile duct, and portal/splenic vasculature (Figs. 29.2 and 29.3).

Performing EUS in the Lower Gastrointestinal Tract
Advancing the Echoendoscope

1. The patient is typically positioned in the left lateral decubitus position. The lubricated echoendoscope is advanced through the anal canal into the rectum. Air is then suctioned and water instilled within the rectum to optimize echoendoscopic views.

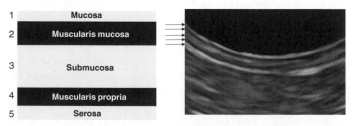

1	Mucosa
2	Muscularis mucosa
3	Submucosa
4	Muscularis propria
5	Serosa

FIG. 29.1 Wall layers of the digestive tract as seen by EUS.

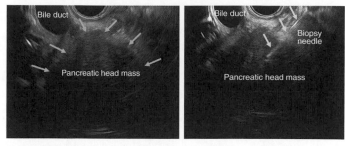

FIG. 29.2 Biliary dilation terminating in pancreatic head mass as seen by EUS.

Visualization of Sigmoid Colon and Rectum

1. Water insufflation of the rectal/sigmoid lumen can provide excellent acoustic coupling, obviating the need for inflation of the echoendoscope balloon. This is especially helpful for smaller lesions that would otherwise be compressed by a balloon. The patient may be tilted in the anti-Trendelenburg position to maintain rectal insufflation with water. Where limited bowel prep has been performed, care must be taken to minimize the amount of fluid instilled, as large amounts of fluid may stimulate colonic motility and thereby promote transit of stool from the colon into the rectum.

2. An overview of key structures imaged at each anatomical location is included in Table 29.1. Identification of regional anatomic landmarks such as the bladder, uterus, prostate, seminal vesicles (anterior), and spine (posterior) can facilitate relative localization of lesions. Anterior structures (e.g., prostate, bladder) should be positioned at 12-o'clock position for consistency. Tangential views are difficult to avoid in the distal rectum and at the rectosigmoid junction due to angulation.

3. Evaluation of the integrity and diameter of the internal and external anal sphincters is best achieved by slow echoendoscope withdrawal across the length of the sphincters with the balloon inflated.

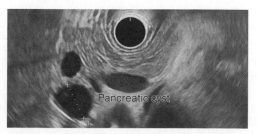

FIG. 29.3 Pancreatic cyst and dilated pancreatic duct as seen by EUS.

COMPLICATIONS

Adverse event rates associated with EUS are similar to those of standard upper/lower endoscopy procedures (approximately 0.1% overall adverse event rate, <0.01% mortality rate). The most common adverse events can be grouped into four categories:

1. Cardiopulmonary: The most common EUS complications are related to the cardiopulmonary system, including aspiration events/pneumonia, bradycardia, hypotension, and adverse sedative medications reactions. The risk of aspiration can be decreased by using general anesthesia for procedures in which insufflation of water into the gastric lumen is anticipated.

2. Infection: Aspiration/drainage of fluid from cystic lesions may potentially seed bacteria into these sterile environments and cause infection. Transrectal tissue sampling of solid lesions may also be associated with an increased risk of infection. Administration of antibiotics during and following these specific procedures may decrease this risk, although antibiotic prophylaxis is typically not utilized prior to diagnostic EUS, FNA, or FNB of solid lesions and fiducial placement.

3. Bleeding: Bleeding occurs at a rate of <0.05% and is typically associated with biopsies (FNA/FNB), Mallory-Weiss tears induced by retching during EUS, or mucosal injury due to endoscope trauma.

4. Perforation: Perforation occurs in up to 0.1% of patients undergoing echoendoscopy. The most common sites of perforation are the pharynx/upper esophagus and duodenum. As the echoendoscope's distal tip tends to be longer and stiffer than that of standard endoscopes, it is more likely to cause trauma or result in perforation during endoscope passage through the pharynx. Similarly, impaired visualization during echoendoscope advancement into the second part of the duodenum may result in trauma/perforation of the duodenal wall.

CPT CODES

43231—Esophagoscopy with endoscopic ultrasound examination.
43232—Esophagoscopy with transendoscopic ultrasound-guided intramural or transmural fine-needle aspiration/biopsy(s).
43237—Esophagogastroduodenoscopy with endoscopic ultrasound examination limited to the esophagus, stomach or duodenum, and adjacent structures.

43238—Esophagogastroduodenoscopy with transendoscopic ultrasound-guided intramural or transmural fine-needle aspiration/biopsy(s), esophagus (includes endoscopic ultrasound examination limited to the esophagus, stomach or duodenum, and adjacent structures).

43240—Esophagogastroduodenoscopy with transmural drainage of pseudocyst (includes placement of transmural drainage catheter(s)/stent(s) and endoscopic ultrasound, when performed).

43242—Esophagogastroduodenoscopy with transendoscopic ultrasound-guided intramural or transmural fine-needle aspiration/biopsy(s), esophagus (includes endoscopic ultrasound examination of the esophagus, stomach, and either the duodenum or a surgically altered stomach where the jejunum is examined distal to the anastomosis).

43253—Esophagogastroduodenoscopy with transendoscopic ultrasound-guided transmural injection of diagnostic or therapeutic substance(s) (e.g., anesthetic, neurolytic agent) or fiducial marker(s) (includes endoscopic ultrasound examination limited to the esophagus, stomach, and either the duodenum or a surgically altered stomach where the jejunum is examined distal to the anastomosis).

43259—Esophagogastroduodenoscopy, flexible, transoral; with endoscopic ultrasound examination, including the esophagus, stomach, and either the duodenum or a surgically altered stomach where the jejunum is examined distal to the anastomosis.

45341—Sigmoidoscopy with endoscopic ultrasound examination.

45342—Sigmoidoscopy with transendoscopic ultrasound-guided intramural or transmural fine-needle aspiration/biopsy(s).

Sedation: If a procedure is performed with endoscopist-prescribed moderate sedation, then separate sedation billing codes should be entered (99151, 99152, 99153, 99155, 99156, 99157, and G0500).

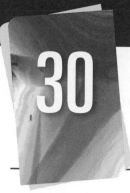

30

Endoscopic Ultrasound-Guided Fine Needle Aspiration and Biopsy

Melinda C. Rogers, MD
V. Raman Muthusamy, MD

Endoscopic ultrasound (EUS) was first introduced in 1980 as a transluminal imaging modality and has evolved to include therapeutic interventions such as fluid sampling and tissue acquisition of lesions in and adjacent to the gastrointestinal tract. Tissue acquisition has advanced from fine needle aspiration (FNA) for cytology to include fine needle biopsy (FNB) for histology with the development of new tools that allow for the capture of a piece of core tissue with preserved architecture and morphology. These techniques reliably give the ability to sample lesions that conventional cross-sectional imaging (computed tomography or magnetic resonance imaging) cannot identify due to their small size and may be inaccessible by percutaneous techniques. Additionally EUS can achieve a tissue diagnosis less invasively than procedures such as mediastinoscopy, diagnostic laparoscopy, laparotomy, and thoracotomy. It is important to note that the sensitivity and specificity are practitioner dependent and competency requires focused training to achieve technical mastery of this skill set. Additional factors, such as the presence of on-site cytopathology and the specific characteristics of the lesion, can influence the accuracy of EUS-guided tissue acquisition. EUS with FNA/FNB has become the standard of care for many conditions of the gastrointestinal tract and adjacent structures due to its high diagnostic accuracy as well as the minimal invasiveness and safety of this procedure.

INDICATIONS

Endosonography-guided tissue acquisition can be safely performed from the esophagus, stomach, duodenum, and rectosigmoid colon. Indications for EUS include the following:

1. Primary diagnosis of lesions within the gastrointestinal tract (esophagus, stomach, duodenum, and rectosigmoid), adjacent

organs (pancreas, liver, kidneys, adrenals, spleen, gallbladder, bile duct), and spaces (mediastinal, pleural, peritoneal, and pelvic)
2. Staging of metastatic disease
3. Evaluation of unexplained lymphadenopathy in the mediastinum, abdomen, or retroperitoneum
4. Sampling of peritoneal or pleural fluid
5. Liver biopsy for unexplained liver test abnormalities or presence of fibrosis
6. Prior nondiagnostic biopsy

RELATIVE CONTRAINDICATIONS

1. Altered anatomy prohibiting access
2. Vessel present in between the needle and target lesion
3. Mediastinal cystic lesions
4. Lymph node or other lesion biopsy in which the primary tumor is within the needle path
5. Small lesions (<5 mm)
6. Active use of antithrombotic or anticoagulant medications (with the exception of low-dose aspirin and nonsteroidal anti-inflammatories).[1] In select cases, the benefit of performing FNA with a 25 G needle may outweigh the risk of bleeding in select patients requiring the use of antithrombotic or anticoagulant medications

ABSOLUTE CONTRAINDICATIONS

1. Uncorrectable bleeding diathesis (international normalized ratio [INR] >1.5, platelets <50,000)
2. Unacceptable sedation risk

PREPARATION

EUS with FNA can be performed in both the ambulatory and inpatient settings. Initial patient evaluation should include a history, physical examination, and review of the pertinent medical records, including available imaging. Informed consent must be obtained and should include a thorough discussion of the indication, risks, benefits, alternatives, and timing of the EUS procedure. Consent must also be obtained for the administration of the appropriate level of sedation. It is our practice to perform most diagnostic EUS procedures with monitored anesthesia care; however, general anesthesia may be most appropriate if the patient is at risk for sedation-related complications, airway obstruction, aspiration, or in the setting of combined procedures, such as EUS and endoscopic retrograde cholangiopancreatography (ERCP).

Patients are required to fast for a stated period of time prior to EUS of the upper GI tract. This practice is to allow for sufficient gastric emptying to occur before the procedure so as to reduce the risk of aspiration and also to allow for adequate endoscopic visualization. There is currently no universally accepted standard for the time frame that a patient must be fasting prior to the procedure. Our practice follows the American Society of Anesthesiologists (ASA) guidelines, which indicate that patients should be fasting a minimum of 2 hours after ingestion of clear liquids and 6 hours after ingestion of a light meal before sedation is administered.[2] Patients with a documented history of delayed gastric emptying may require longer periods of fasting. For patients undergoing EUS of the lower GI tract, a full colonoscopy prep is also recommended. In select cases of distal lesions (rectal) or the inability to tolerate an oral preparation, a series of enemas may be administered to cleanse the distal colon.

EUS with FNA has a higher risk of procedure-related bleeding compared with diagnostic upper endoscopy.[1] As such, patients on anticoagulants and antithrombotic medications should be instructed to discontinue these medications at an appropriate interval (depending on the medication) prior to their procedure.[3] In certain patients with high-risk cardiac and/or hypercoagulable conditions, the risk of discontinuing these medications may outweigh the risk of bleeding. In such a situation, using the smallest FNA needle (25 G) with a limited number of passes and avoidance of suction would seem appropriate.

The risk of bacteremia related to EUS with FNA of solid lesions of the upper GI tract is low (0% to 5.8%) and comparable to that of diagnostic endoscopy.[4-6] Similarly, rates of bacteremia or clinically significant infectious complication associated with aspiration of rectal or perirectal lesions are low, and routine antibiotic prophylaxis for these indications is not recommended. The risk of infectious complication related to aspiration of pancreatic and peripancreatic cysts varies in published reports, ranging from 0.6% to 14% but is generally considered to be very low.[7,8] In one large retrospective study, there was no difference in infectious complications after EUS-FNA of cystic lesions with or without antibiotic prophylaxis. Additionally, there were reports of adverse events related to antibiotic usage, including allergic reaction and *Clostridium difficile* diarrhea.[9] There are currently no prospective studies examining the effectiveness of periprocedural antibiotics in reducing procedure-related infectious complications. It is the recommendation of the American Society for Gastrointestinal Endoscopy (ASGE) to administer prophylactic antibiotics before and for 3 to 5 days after aspiration of pancreatic and peripancreatic cysts.[10] Additionally, there are limited data available on the risk of infectious complication associated with aspiration of fluid compartments. It is reasonable to consider periprocedural antibiotics when aspirating fluid compartments, such as ascites, especially in patients with cirrhosis so as to reduce the risk of spontaneous bacterial peritonitis. There is a significant risk of infectious complications related to aspiration of mediastinal cysts with reports of mediastinitis even with the use of periprophylaxis. Thus, we would advise avoiding aspiration of mediastinal cysts.

EQUIPMENT

EUS is currently available in two primary imaging planes; radial and curved linear array. EUS with FNA and/or FNB is performed using a linear-array echoendoscope since the imaging transducer is oriented parallel to the long axis of the endoscope, allowing for clear visualization of the biopsy needle as it exits the therapeutic channel of the echoendoscope and into the target lesion in real time (Fig. 30.1). Doppler and/or power flow imaging–equipped echoendoscopes allow for easy identification of vascular structures.

EUS-FNA needles are available in multiple sizes including a 19, 22, and 25 gauge. Most aspiration needles have a handle assembly for the controlled advancement of the needle, an attachment for a vacuum syringe, a protective sheath, a stylet to avoid damage

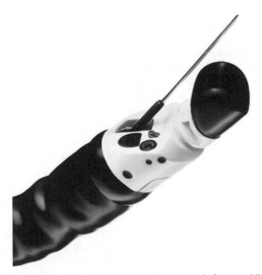

FIG. 30.1 Echogenic needle tip exiting the working channel of a curved linear-array echoendoscope (Boston Scientific Expect needle). (Permission for use granted by Boston Scientific Corporation.)

to the working channel, and a hollow needle in one of the above sizes. The primary aim of FNA is to acquire an adequate tissue sample with minimal number of passes while avoiding injury to the surrounding tissue. Studies comparing 22 G and 25 G aspiration needles for histology did not show a significant difference between the two, while several studies and a meta-analysis comparing 22 G and 25 G aspiration needles for cytology from solid pancreatic lesions show a higher diagnostic accuracy with the 25 G needle.

FNB needles also come in a 19-, 22-, and 25-gauge size (Fig. 30.2). The bevel of the needle is variably shaped depending on the manufacturer to allow for shearing of the target lesion in order to acquire a histologic sample (Figs. 30.3 and 30.4). FNB needles are a relatively new development in the field and an area of ongoing clinical research. Initial studies of core biopsy needles failed to show a significant difference with regard to sample adequacy, diagnostic accuracy, or acquisition of a histologic core tissue sample compared to a standard aspiration needles.[11] Some studies have shown an improved sample cellularity and fewer passes required to obtain an adequate sample when using a core biopsy needle. A recent study looking at core biopsy of multiple types of solid lesions showed a diagnostic adequacy of 98.5% with a mean of three needle passes[12] through the target lesion. A prospective randomized controlled trial comparing FNA and FNB in patients referred for EUS with tissue acquisition showed significantly higher specimen adequacy with FNB

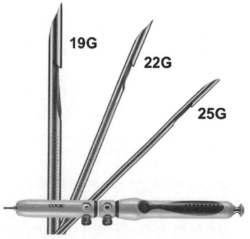

FIG. 30.2 Cook19-, 22-, and 25-gauge ProCore needle with core trap cut out. (Image used with permission of Cook Medical Incorporated.)

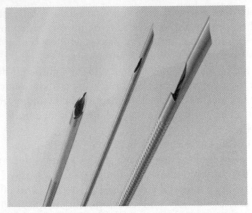

FIG. 30.3 Cook Medical 22-gauge Ultra-aspiration needle (left), 25-gauge Procore biopsy needle (middle), and 20-gauge ProCore biopsy needle (right). (Permission for use granted by Cook Medical Inc.)

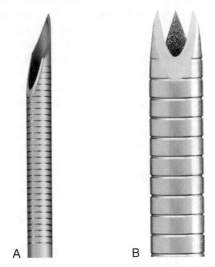

FIG. 30.4 A, Boston Scientific Expect aspiration needle and (B) Boston Scientific Acquire biopsy needle. (Permission for use granted by Boston Scientific Corporation.)

needles for all solid lesions. There was no difference in diagnostic yield in the two groups for pancreatic masses, and primary advantage observed with FNB needles was for subepithelial lesions and lymphadenopathy.[13] Importantly, these studies have not demonstrated an increased rate of complications with the use of core biopsy needles.

The role of EUS-guided liver biopsy for parenchymal disease has emerged along with the advances in technology of the core biopsy needle. While the safety and efficacy of FNA for focal liver lesions is well established, there is now emerging data to support the safety and efficacy of EUS core biopsy as an alternative to per-cutaneous or transjugular liver biopsy in the evaluation of paren-chymal liver disease. Both 19 G and 22 G core biopsy needles have been shown to yield samples adequate for histologic diagnosis in all cases, with a median number of complete portal tracts rang-ing from 17 to 18 in each sample.[14,15] There were no major adverse events in either study.

The choice of needle type and size is complex and is impacted by multiple factors including the type of lesion, location, bleeding risk of the patient, suspected pathology, presence of on-site cytol-ogy, as well as practitioner preference. It is common practice to use a core biopsy needle to obtain histologic (tissue) specimens and a 22 or 25 G FNA needle for cytologic evaluations. When immunohistochemistry testing may be needed (i.e., subepithelial lesions, suspected lymphoma), it is beneficial to use a core biopsy needle to provide additional tissue and architecture for evalua-tion/testing. When performing FNA of lesions in the pancreatic head or uncinate, a 25G needle may be beneficial due to its flexi-bility in accessing these areas.

PROCEDURE

1. The procedure is typically performed with the patient in the left lateral position, however, can also be performed supine or prone, particularly if being combined with ERCP.
2. As appropriate, consider performing a standard forward-viewing endoscopic evaluation prior to EUS to identify any anatomic abnormalities and note any important landmarks such as with tumor staging.
3. A radial EUS evaluation should be performed in select situa-tions such as with luminal tumor staging if the linear imaging plane is insufficient.
4. As able, place the target lesion in the center of the field and along the projected plane of the needle. If this is not possible, the echoendoscope should be adjusted to place the lesion within the deflection range of the elevator. Care should be taken to minimize the acuity of the elevator angle as this can impede easy passage of the needle. The distance between the probe and the target lesion should be minimized so as to reduce the risk of injury to adjacent structures. This mea-surement can also be used to set the needle actuation lock (if present) on the needle handle to avoid advancing beyond the intended target.

5. Perform a Doppler evaluation to exclude the presence of any intervening vessels along the projected needle path. If a vessel cannot be avoided, FNB should not be performed due to the increased risk of bleeding from the shearing force produced by the bevel. It may be appropriate to use a 25 G aspiration needle in select cases where the risk of bleeding is deemed acceptable.

6. Remove the rubber valve from the working channel port. Advance the needle catheter device with the stylet in place and the needle in the fully withdrawn and locked position through the working channel. Secure the handle of the needle to the working channel port. In some situations, it may be beneficial to insert the needle device prior to scope positioning, as it may be difficult or impossible to advance the needle if the echoendoscope is not sufficiently straight.

7. Most needle devices may contain a sheath that can be advanced out of the luminal end of the working channel. Extending the sheath can aid with needle puncture in cases of mobile subepithelial lesions and in some situations when trying to perform needle puncture through the bulb or second portion of the duodenum.

8. After the needle is secured in the working channel and scope position is achieved, advance the needle, approximately 1 cm, into the ultrasound view without puncturing through the lumen to ensure a proper trajectory. The elevator or big knob of the echoendoscope may be adjusted to alter the needle tract, if necessary.

9. Once proper positioning is confirmed, briskly advance the needle with the stylet slightly withdrawn (if the stylet has a blunt tip), in a controlled manner, under clear visualization into the target lesion. If available, use the lock on the handle, as needed, to control the depth of needle advancement.

    a. Fluid
        i. Advance the stylet to remove any contaminant tissue obtained during needle advancement.
        ii. Remove the stylet and attach a syringe under negative pressure.
        iii. Negative pressure can be increased if little or no fluid is obtained. It may be necessary to increase the size of the aspiration needle if minimal fluid is retrieved.
        iv. Carefully monitor needle position during fluid aspiration to ensure the needle does not exit the target lesion. The needle may be moved in a gradual, to-and-fro movement, within the lesion while taking care not to exit the lesion into the lumen. It should remain in the center of the lesion in cases where a cyst is collapsing. When aspiration is complete, release the negative pressure prior to removing the needle.
            • If bloody return is visualized, immediately close the syringe as this can contaminate cytology results.

- If the needle is inadvertently withdrawn into the lumen under negative pressure, the sample may become contaminated with epithelium and luminal contents.
- Multiple syringes may be required to fully aspirate larger lesions, especially if cytology is desired.

b. Solid lesions

   i. Advance the stylet to remove any contaminant tissue obtained during needle advancement.

   ii. Gradually withdraw and advance the needle through the entire length of the lesion, taking care not to exit the lesion. If the needle is inadvertently withdrawn into the lumen, remove the needle, as further passes will result in luminal contamination of the sample.

  iii. Tissue acquisition may be performed using the standard suction, "slow pull"/"capillary" method, or "wet suction" technique.

- For standard suction, a 10 mL syringe is attached to the needle hub and 5 mL of suction is applied as the needle is moved in a to-and-fro manner (typically 10 to 20 passes are performed). The suction catheter is slow released and the entire needle assembly removed.
- The "slow pull" technique involves the assistant slowly withdrawing the stylet while simultaneously the needle is moved back and forth within the lesion. The stylet should be withdrawn the same distance as the throw of the needle. This is typically continued until approximately two-thirds of the stylet has been withdrawn from the needle. The entire needle apparatus is then removed.
- "Wet suction" technique involves removing the stylet from the needle and flushing the needle with saline to replace the column of air with saline. The needle is then passed into the target lesion and suction applied as a to-and-fro motion is performed within the lesion. Suction is released prior to the needle exiting the lesion and the specimen placed on a glass side using the stylet. The use of suction when sampling solid lesions is somewhat controversial. It has been proposed that this may lead to dilution or contamination of the sample with blood. A randomized controlled trial demonstrated that "wet suction" technique lead to increased specimen cellularity and diagnostic yield of solid lesions as compared to standard suction technique.[16]
- When performing standard suction or wet suction, the stylet can be removed prior to advancing the needle into the lesion. The stylet should remain in the core of the needle when performing "slow pull"/"capillary" technique.

iv. The most common method to ensure sampling of the entire lesion is termed "fanning" or "multipass" technique. After introducing the needle into the target lesion, make 6 to 10 gradual, to-and-fro movements within the lesion, while simultaneously adjusting the needle trajectory with manipulation of the elevator or up/down scope tip deflection to orient the needle into a different tract within the lesion. If the lesion is not amenable to fanning, a multiple pass technique can be performed where the needle is advanced to-and-fro in a single plan, withdrawn, and then advanced again into different areas of the target lesion. This may be necessary for firm lesions or if scope position does not allow for adequate elevator or tip deflection to change the trajectory of the needle.

v. Additional techniques to maximize diagnostic yield include minimizing needle dwell time within the lesion to reduce risk of bleeding, thus improving sample quality on subsequent passes, and avoiding needle passes through cystic and necrotic (usually centrally located) areas within the lesion.

c. Liver biopsy
i. Studies have demonstrated tissue adequacy for both the 19 G and 22 G core biopsy needles. There are several techniques described in the literature including a single pass technique using wet suction, slow pull method, and more recently reports of using heparin-primed needles.[14,17]

10. Rapid on-site evaluation (ROSE)
a. This requires the presence of a cytopathologist in the endoscopy suite to perform immediate feedback to the endosonographer regarding the quality of the aspirates and/or tissue. Rapid on-site cytologic analysis has been shown in multiple studies to reduce the number of passes needed to obtain an adequate tissue sample and decrease the need for repeat procedures due to nondiagnostic tissue samples.[18] However, given the improved diagnostic yield and specimen adequacy with FNB needles, this may no longer hold true in the future.

b. If on-site cytopathology is not available, the number of needle passes required to obtain an adequate sample varies by size, type, and location of the lesion. A recent prospective study in the United States demonstrated no increase in diagnostic sensitivity beyond four passes with an FNA needle for pancreatic malignancy.[19] Currently, the European Society of Gastrointestinal Endoscopy (ESGE) recommends performing three needle passes for sampling lymph nodes and liver lesions, five passes for solid pancreatic masses, and a single pass when sampling pancreatic cysts due to the potential for introducing an infection.[20]

11. Specimen preparation

  a. There are different types of tissue specimen preparation, including tissue smear, liquid-based cytologic preparation, cell block, and formalin fixation. The choice of preparation depends on the type of tissue specimen being analyzed, institutional practices, staff training, and the time and/or distance between the endoscopy suite and the pathology laboratory.

  b. Slides and specimen containers should be labeled individually with the patient name or medical record number as well as the pass number.

  c. For FNA, there is a significant variety in how these specimens are processed. Generally, for cytology specimens, the aspirated material is expressed onto glass slides using either an air-filled syringe or the stylet. The slides are subsequently fixed using either air dry, spray fix, or alcohol fixation. Residual material may then be expressed into the appropriate specimen container. The needle should then be flushed with air to purge the contents of any remaining specimen and saline, then the stylet reinserted.

  d. For cystic lesions, leave the entire specimen in the syringe and label appropriately. Do not dilute with saline if performing biochemical analysis (e.g., carcinoembryonic-antigen, amylase).

  e. For histologic analysis, glass slides may be prepared by slowly reintroducing the stylet into the needle so as to express a small amount of tissue onto the slide. A second slide is then to create a smear, after which the slide is fixed (air dry, spray fix, or alcohol fix). The remainder of the tissue is then expressed directly into formalin by fully inserting the stylet. The stylet is then removed and a saline flush used to express any residual material directly into formalin.

POSTPROCEDURE

1. Patients should be monitored in an appropriately staffed recovery area until discharge criteria for standard endoscopic procedures are met.

2. Liver biopsy patients may be placed on 2 hours bed rest post procedure. This theoretically reduces the risk of postprocedure bleeding, but there is little evidence to support this practice.

3. Patients are encouraged to take clear liquids for their first meal in the recovery area. If this is well tolerated, they may resume the diet tolerated prior to the procedure. For patients, undergoing sampling of a pancreatic lesion, we encourage a low-fat diet for 3 days to minimize the risk of pancreatitis.
4. All patients are encouraged to contact their endoscopist for pain, fever, or any distressing symptoms.
5. Patients who undergo core biopsy may be advised to continue withholding antiplatelet or anticoagulant medications for any additional 48 to 72 hours.

ADVERSE EVENTS

1. Perforation can occur, most commonly of the cervical esophagus, due to the blind intubation with the echoendoscope or in the presence of malignant strictures, especially at the superior duodenal angle.
2. Infectious complications have been described when performing EUS with FNA. The current ASGE guidelines recommend administration of prophylactic antibiotics before and for 3 to 5 days after aspiration of pancreatic and peripancreatic cysts. It is recommended to avoid the aspiration of mediastinal cysts due to reports of mediastinitis even with the use of prophylactic antibiotics.
3. Bleeding is an infrequent complication of EUS with FNA. Importantly, rates do not seem to increase with FNB, as initially feared.
4. Pancreatitis has been reported in 1% to 2% of patients undergoing FNA of pancreatic masses, cysts, or the pancreatic duct.
5. Bile duct peritonitis has been described with FNA of the gallbladder and pancreatic head masses.
6. Tumor seeding has been described in few case reports. This is a very rare, but serious, potential adverse event when sampling malignant lesions.

CPT CODES FOR EUS FINE NEEDLE ASPIRATION PROCEDURES
Upper Gastrointestinal Procedures

43232—Esophagoscopy, flexible, transoral; with transendoscopic ultrasound-guided intramural or transmural fine needle aspiration/biopsy(s).

43238—Esophagogastroduodenoscopy, flexible, transoral; with transendoscopic ultrasound-guided intramural or transmural fine needle aspiration/biopsy(s), (includes endoscopic ultrasound examination limited to the esophagus, stomach or duodenum, and adjacent structures).

43242—Esophagogastroduodenoscopy, flexible, transoral; with transendoscopic ultrasound-guided intramural or transmural fine needle aspiration/biopsy(s) (includes endoscopic ultrasound examination of the esophagus, stomach, and either the duodenum or a surgically altered stomach where the jejunum is examined distal to the anastomosis).

Lower Gastrointestinal Procedures

44407—Colonoscopy through stoma; with transendoscopic ultrasound-guided intramural or transmural fine needle aspiration/biopsy(s), includes endoscopic ultrasound examination limited to the sigmoid, descending, transverse, or ascending colon and cecum and adjacent structures.

45342—Sigmoidoscopy, flexible; with transendoscopic ultrasound-guided intramural or transmural fine needle aspiration/biopsy(s)

45392—Colonoscopy, flexible; with transendoscopic ultrasound-guided intramural or transmural fine needle aspiration/biopsy(s), includes endoscopic ultrasound examination limited to the rectum, sigmoid, descending, transverse, or ascending colon and cecum and adjacent structures.

References

1. Acosta RD, Abraham NS, Chandrasekhara V, et al. The management of antithrombotic agents for patients undergoing GI endoscopy. *Gastrointest Endosc.* 2016;83(1):3-16.
2. Practice guidelines for preoperative fasting and the use of pharmacologic agents to reduce the risk of pulmonary aspiration: application to healthy patients undergoing elective procedures: an updated report by the American Society of Anesthesiologists Committee on Standards and Practice Parameters. *Anesthesiology.* 2011;114:495-511.
3. Baron TH, Kamath PS, McBane RD, Management of antithrombotic therapy in patients undergoing invasive procedures. *N Engl J Med.* 2013;368:2113-2124.
4. Levy MJ. Norton ID, Wiersema MJ, et al. Prospective risk assessment of bacteremia and other infectious complications in patients undergoing EUS-guided FNA. *Gastrointest Endosc.* 2003;57(6):672-678.
5. Eloubeidi MA, Tamhane T, Varadarajulu S, Wilcox CM, Frequency of major complications after EUS-guided FNA of solid pancreatic masses: a prospective evaluation. *Gastrointest Endosc.* 2006;63:622-629.
6. Early DS, Acosta RD, Chandrasekhara V, et al. Adverse events associated with EUS ad EUS-FNA. *Gastrointest Endosc.* 2013;77:839-843.
7. Wiersema MJ, Vilmann P, Giovannini M, Chang KJ, Wiersema LM, Endosonography-guided fine-needle aspiration biopsy: diagnostic accuracy and complication assessment. *Gastroenterology.* 1997;112:1087-1095.
8. Lee LS, Saltzman J, Bounds B, Poneros J, Brugge W, Thompson C, EUS-guided fine needle aspiration of pancreatic cysts: a retrospective analysis of complications and their predictors. *Clin Gastroenterol Hepatol.* 2005;3:231-236.
9. Guarner-Argente C, Shah P, Buchner A, Ahmad NA, Kochman ML, Ginsberg GG, Use of antimicrobials for EUS-guided FNA of pancreatic cysts: a retrospective, comparative analysis. *Gastrointest Endosc.* 2011;74:81-86.

10. Khashab MA, Chithadi KV, Acosta RS, et al. Antibiotic prophylaxis for GI endoscopy. *Gastrointest Endosc.* 2015;81(1):81-89.

11. Bang JY, Hawes R, Varadarajulu S. A meta-analysis comparing ProCore and standard fine-needle aspiration needles for endoscopic ultrasound-guided tissue acquisition. *Endoscopy.* 2016;48(4):339-349.

12. Adler DG, Muthusamy VR, Ehrlich DS, et al. A multicenter evaluation of a new EUS core biopsy needle: experience in 200 patients. *Endosc Ultrasound.* 2019;8(2):99-104.

13. Aadam AA, Wani S, Amick A, et al. A randomized controlled cross-over trial and cost analysis comparing endoscopic ultrasound fine needle aspiration and fine needle biopsy. *Endosc Int Open.* 2016;4:497-505.

14. Nieto J, Khaleel H, Challita Y, et al. EUS-guided fine-needle core liver biopsy sampling using a novel 19-gauge needle with modified 1-pass, 1 actuation wet suction technique. *Gastrointest Endosc.* 2018;(2):469-475.

15. Hasan MK, Idrisov E, Kadkhodayan K, et al. Endoscope ultrasound guided liver biopsy using a 22 gauge fine needle biopsy needle: a prospective study. *Gastrointest Endosc.* 2018;87(6):AB75-AB76.

16. Attam R, Arain MA, Bloechl SJ, et al. "Wet suction technique (WEST)": a novel way to enhance the quality of EUS-FNA aspirate. Results of a prospective, single-blind, randomized, controlled trial using a 22-gauge needle for EUS-FNA of solid lesions. *Gastrointest Endosc.* 2015;81(6):1401-1407.

17. Mok SRS, Diehl DL, Johal AS, et al. A prospective pilot comparison of wet and dry heparinized suction for EUS-guided liver biopsy (with videos). *Gastrointest Endosc.* 2018;(18):32924-32929.

18. Matynia AP, Schmidt RL, Barraza G, Layfield LJ, Siddiqui AA, Adler DG, Impact of rapid on-site evaluation on the adequacy of endoscopic-ultrasound guided fine-needle aspiration of solid pancreatic lesions: a systematic review and meta-analysis. *J Gastroenterol Hepatol.* 2014;29:697-705.

19. Mohamadnejad M, Mullady D, Early DS, et al. Increasing number of passes beyond 4 does not increase sensitivity of detection of pancreatic malignancy by endoscopic ultrasound-guided fine-needle aspiration. *Clin Gastroenterol Hepatol.* 2017;(7):1071-1078.

20. Savides TJ. Tricks for improving EUS-FNA accuracy and maximizing cellular yield. *Gastrointest Endosc.* 2009;69(2 suppl):S130-S133.

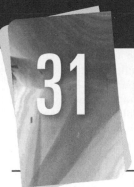

31

Endoscopic Ultrasound-Guided Liver Biopsy

Enad Dawod, MD
Jose M. Nieto, DO, AGAF, FACP, FACG, FASGE

Liver pathology falls on a very wide spectrum, which makes it difficult to distinguish specific pathologies based on clinical presentation, serologic markers, or imaging alone. Liver biopsy (LB) plays a vital role in liver disease management through establishing a specific underlying etiology, determining the severity of liver damage, determining prognosis, and preventing missing fibrosis or cirrhosis that would be otherwise missed on laboratory or imaging evaluation. The need for LB also varies by the etiology of liver disease as the emergence of noninvasive markers for hepatitis C and fibrosis decreased the need for histological evaluation. However, with other etiologies such as autoimmune hepatitis and nonalcoholic hepatosteatosis, the need for liver sampling still persists.[1-3] More importantly, LB has a role in altering treatment in many patients based on histopathological findings.[4]

Percutaneous liver biopsy (PC-LB) is the conventional and most commonly used method for liver sampling. This method, however, does come with its own set of limitations, high cost, and procedure-related adverse events, which makes PC-LB an unfeasible method of monitoring patients in the long run.[5] PC-LB is limited by the absence of mass visualization, high rates of sampling error, and failure to obtain samples adequate enough for histological evaluation.[6] The high rate of procedural-related adverse events is attributed to the invasive nature of the procedure and they include severe pain, intraperitoneal and subcapsular hemorrhage, unintentional sampling of adjacent organs, pneumothorax, marked hypotension, and discomfort to the patient.[7,8] The rate of adverse events in the PC method may be up to 60% in the first 2 hours after the procedure.[4,9] When there are contraindications for the PC method, such as ascites or coagulopathy, a transjugular fluoroscopy-guided approach is used.[10]

Endoscopic ultrasound (EUS)-guided LB is an emerging approach that provides an alternative to the conventional method. The EUS-guided approach could be utilized during the evaluation of both focal and parenchymal liver disease. Several studies have been published that have demonstrated safety and efficacy of EUS in liver sampling in addition to its ability to obtain tissue adequate for establishing histopathological diagnosis.[8,11-13] EUS-LB could decrease the time to diagnosis and help avoid the need for a second procedure to reach a diagnosis when an EUS is performed in the evaluation of abnormal imaging, unexplained liver tests, or other pancreatobiliary disease.

TECHNIQUE
EUS-FNA and EUS-FNB for Focal Liver Lesions

1. EUS examinations are usually performed in the left lateral decubitus position with a linear echoendoscope.
2. All patients undergo moderate/deep sedation, which in the United States is administered by a staff anesthesiologist or a registered nurse.
3. The cytology aspiration is performed using an EUS-FNA needle and for tissue acquisition, an EUS-FNB needle (25G and 22G are more commonly used, than 19G FNA/FNB needles for focal lesions).
4. The left lobe of the liver is accessed with the echoendoscope in the proximal stomach, distal to the gastroesophageal junction. The right lobe of the liver is accessed with the echoendoscope positioned in the duodenal bulb and torqued counterclockwise, beyond the view of the portal vein and the gallbladder (if present).
5. Doppler is used to identify an area of liver parenchyma in the expected trajectory of the needle that is clear of blood vessels or bile ducts.
6. After initial puncture is made into the lesion or liver parenchyma, 7 to 14 actuations (back-and-forth motions of the needle) are made per pass and a "fanning" technique is used to maximize tissue sampling. This technique involves changing the trajectory of the needle with each back-and-forth movement. Negative pressure can be applied using suction with a 10 to 20 mL syringe or the stylet can be slowly withdrawn from the needle after it enters the target lesion. Suction is released by closing the syringe lock, and the needle could then be finally removed. Aspiration specimens are expelled onto glass slides by reinserting the stylet. The aspiration could be repeated until enough specimens are obtained, as deemed adequate by gross inspection (Fig. 31.1).

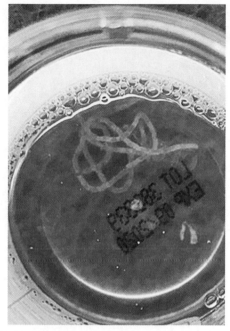

FIG. 31.1 Live view of parenchymal tissue obtained via EUS.

7. When on-site evaluation is performed, the specimen samples are smeared on glass slides for cytological examination, fixed in 95% ethanol, and stained with hematoxylin and eosin stain (Fig. 31.2).
8. After completion of the EUS-FNA, the patient is observed in the endoscopic recovery unit for 30 to 60 minutes, depending on the endoscopist's preference, and discharged if no immediate complications are noted.[13,14]

EUS for Parenchymal Disease

The use of EUS is more established in focal liver lesions than in parenchymal liver disease. However, the use of a newer flexible core needles have made it possible to obtain parenchymal cores.[11,15] Quick-Core (Cook Medical Inc, Bloomington, IN) was the first FNB needle designed for obtaining core biopsy specimens by means of a spring-loaded tru-cut mechanism.[16] EUS-modified liver biopsy sampling (EUS-MLB) for obtaining a parenchymal core uses a novel 19-gauge needle (Sharkcore; Medtronic, Sunnyvale, CA) or the Acquire (Franseen tip Needle, Boston, MA) with a modified 1-pass 1-actuation wet suction technique. The 19-gauge needle has a modified tip design containing

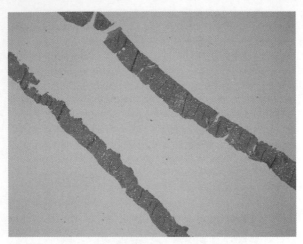

FIG. 31.2 Histological view of the parenchymal tissue sampled via EUS.

six cutting edge surfaces and an opposing bevel to catch tissue as it is sheared off.[11] The introduction of other biopsy needles into the market place is expected.

EUS-Modified Liver Biopsy Sampling

1. All patients undergo moderate/deep sedation, which in the United States is administered by a staff anesthesiologist or a registered nurse. A complete EUS examination for the primary procedure indication is performed.

2. Echoendoscopy is performed using a standard linear-array echoendoscope. In addition, complete EUS surveillance of the visualized liver and upper abdominal region was done to ensure the absence of varices or tumor.

3. EUS-MLB under real-time US guidance is performed by using a 19-gauge needle (Sharkcore; Medtronic) or (Acquire, Boston Scientific). Although FNB needles are used, 19G FNA needles can also be used.

4. The needle is primed with saline solution, and maximal suction is applied via a syringe after 7 cm of the needle had entered the liver under direct US guidance, being careful to avoid large vessels using Doppler.

5. A rapid-puncture one 7-cm actuation technique is used to sample each lobe for a total of 1 actuation per lobe. The 8-cm 19-gauge core needle is then passed into the liver and approximately 1 cm passed through stomach or duodenal wall. The other 7 cm was passed into the liver parenchyma. The left lobe is accessed by the transgastric route and the right lobe by the transduodenal route.

6. Wet suction is used to indicate tissue acquisition into the bore of the needle by displacing the saline solution into the syringe; this notifies the endoscopist to turn off the suction[11](Figs. 31.1 to 31.4).

7. Some endoscopists employ a slow-pull capillary suction technique and multiple passes for FNB as per solid lesions.[15]

ADVERSE EVENTS

In terms of adverse events, the most common adverse events encountered in the PC method include hypotension, hemothorax, biliary peritonitis, pneumothorax, tumor seeding, hemorrhage, and mostly pain.[4] In regard to EUS-LB, the most reported adverse events are pain and hemorrhage, but the rate of these adverse events remains low. The abdominal pain is usually subsided within 1 hour after the procedure, and hematomas are usually self-subsiding as well.[11] A 1-hour recovery time after the EUS-LB has been shown to be sufficient in almost all cases.[17] In a recently published meta-analysis involving 437 patients who undergone EUS-LB, the pooled rate of adverse events with EUS-guided LB was 2.3%. Subanalysis showed that rate of adverse events with the 19-gauge FNA needle is not significantly different than the rate of adverse events with other biopsy needles.[18]

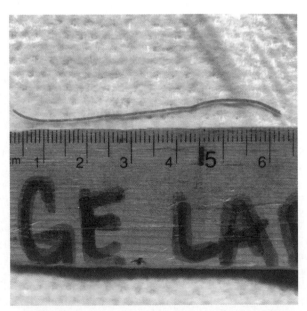

FIG. 31.3 Endoscopic live view sampling. (Courtesy of Jose Nieto.)

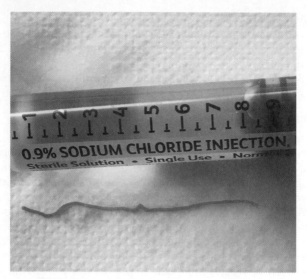

FIG. 31.4 Endoscopic live view. (Courtesy of Jose Nieto.)

EUS-LB is unique in its ability to avoid sampling errors encountered with the PC method, which is due to the quick and safe sampling of both lobes of liver. Given the fact the patient is usually sedated, this allows the endoscopist more attempts at obtaining enough tissue for diagnosis as opposed to the PC method where patient discomfort might limit the amount of times a tissue could be obtained.

EUS-LB uses real-time live endoscopic and sonographic visualization simultaneously, which prevents undesirable sampling of adjacent organs and blood vessels. EUS-LB allows clear and accurate visualization of the liver and the adjacent organs, due to the close the proximity of the transducer to the liver through the transgastric and transduodenal routes.[19]

EUS-LB has shown excellent histological yield. Many factors come into play in producing an adequate histological yield. Firstly, the sample size must be large enough to provide a good representation of the parenchyma. Secondly, there is the specimen length in which there is discordance in recommended length based on the etiology.[9,20] Another parameter is the number of complete portal tracts (CPTs), which have been used to assess the quality of specimen and to compare different needle types used in EUS-LB.[21] In a recently published metanalysis involving 437 patients who undergone EUS-LB, the histological yield was 93.9%. On further subgroup analysis, the rate of diagnostic yield was better with the 19-gauge FNA needle compared to other core needles. FNA needle had a significantly lower rate of insufficient specimen than core biopsy needles (QuickCore and ProCore).[18] A recent prospective crossover study involving 125 patients showed that the use heparinized suction provide the best specimens with the least amount of fragmentation compared to other dry suction methods.[22]

Since EUS-LB is done under deep sedation, the problem of the significant patient discomfort is avoided as opposed to with the PC method. The clinical factor that affect EUS-LB is operator's experience as EUS-LB is a fairly new procedure and could only be performed at tertiary centers by experienced endoscopists. Patient factors also are important, such as the presence of altered anatomy. In patients with history of Roux-EN-Y, the EUS-LB is performed through the transgastric approach.[13]

In patients with international normalized ratio > 1.5 and thrombocytopenia (platelets < 50,000/μL), EUS-LB should be avoided as there is a risk of bleeding.[19]

The role of EUS-LB in nonalcoholic fatty liver disease (NAFLD) is particularly important as EUS-LB is essential in detecting the progression of NAFLD to nonalcoholic steatohepatitis, which has significant implications on morbidity and mortality.[12]

Concomitant EUS-LB is a feasible, cost-effective, safe, and accurate method of obtaining LB when EUS is indicated for the evaluation of other hepatobiliary disease.[12,13]

In the management of focal liver lesions, the role of EUS-LB in the management of incidentally found liver lesions on CT and MR has evolved rapidly. EUS-LB can be used in further characterization of the lesion and establishing the diagnosis. EUS-LB has demonstrated superior ability in being able to detect smaller lesions that were not previously detected on imaging.[14,23] The detection of previously not seen lesions often alters the course of management of patients as EUS-LB not only could establish the diagnosis, but also could play a role in staging of the lesion and potentially impact the decision to undergo surgery. EUS-LB could also be used in obtaining biopsy of lesion not previously seen on imaging.

EUS-LB could also prove critical in the management of metastatic liver disease given the fact that pancreatic and liver lesions could be evaluated simultaneously. The ability of EUS to detect smaller lesions and metastasis to liver is also critical in deeming the malignancy operable or not. Additionally, to date there are no reports of malignancy seeding as a result of EUS.[14]

While there are many retrospective studies that compared EUS-LB to the PC method and few studies that compared different needles used in EUS-LB, there is a need for studies of prospective nature with bigger number of patients to establish efficacy of EUS-LB. We anticipate that further technological advancements will provide more tools that will further increase the safety and effectiveness of EUS-LB.

TABLE 31.1   EUS-Guided Liver Biopsy of Parenchymal Disease

Authors	Number of Patients	Median Complete Portal Tracts (CPTs)	Median Total Specimen Length (TSL)	Adverse Events
Nieto et al[24]	210 (Franseen)	24	6.5	0
	210 (Fork-Tip)	19.5	6	1
Nieto et al[11]	165	18	6	1.8%
Nieto et al[11]	116	18	6	2
Shah et al[15]	24	32	6.5	2
Saab et al[25]	47	18 (14-24)	6.5 (4.6-8)	2
Sey et al[26]	45 (QC) 30 (PC)	5 (QC) 2 (PC)	20 (PC) 9 (QC)	2
Diehl et al[13]	110	14 (range, 0-203)	3.8 (0-68)	1
Stavropoulos et al[27]	31	9	36.9	0
Dewitt et al[28]	21	2 (total) 3 (partial)	9	0

PC, reverse bevel needle; QC, Quick-core needle.

The potential for EUS-LB is huge. As we edge closer to more widespread use of EUS-LB, the focus should be on perfecting the technique and in establishing superiority of one technique over the other. Rapid improvement in needle technology has resulted in significant improvement in outcomes, so we would expect continuous improvement in histological yield as the needle technology evolves further.

EUS-LB is a promising and rapidly evolving approach in the management of liver disease. When EUS is performed for another indication, concomitant EUS-LB is a safe, feasible, cost-effective

TABLE 31.2   EUS-Guided Biopsy of Liver Lesions

Authors	Number of Patients	Overall Cytologic Diagnosis	Number of Passes (Median)	Adverse Events
DiMaio et al[29]	250	81%	3	10
Fujii-Lau et al[30]	322	73%	3.4 (mean)	10
Lee et al[31]	21	90.5	2	0
Prachayakul et al[32]	14	78%	N/A	0
DeWitt et al[33]	77	91%	N/A	0
Hollerbach et al[34]	41	94	1.4	2
tenBerge et al[35]	167	89%	N/a	6

way of obtaining liver tissue with excellent histological yield (Table 31.1). As new treatments for diseases like NAFLD emerge, the utility of EUS-LB will definitely increase. For focal lesions, EUS-LB offers more targeted approach. For unexplained parenchymal disease, EUS-LB provides a safe modality that reduces sample variability encountered with other methods of obtaining LB (Table 31.2).

References

1. Rockey DC, Caldwell SH, Goodman ZD, Nelson RC, Smith AD, American Association for the Study of Liver Diseases. Liver biopsy. *Hepatology.* 2009;49:1017-1044.

2. Cross TJ, Calvaruso V, Maimone S, et al. Prospective comparison of Fibroscan, King's score and liver biopsy for the assessment of cirrhosis in chronic hepatitis C infection. *J Viral Hepat.* 2010;17:546-554.

3. Sheen V, Nguyen H, Jimenez M, et al. Routine laboratory blood tests may diagnose significant fibrosis in liver transplant recipients with chronic hepatitis C: a 10 Year experience. *J Clin Transl Hepatol.* 2016;4:20-25.

4. Parth J, Parekh RM, Diehl DL, Baron TH. Endoscopic ultrasound-guided liver biopsy. *Endosc Ultrasound.* 2015;4:85-91.

5. Schulman AR, Lin MV, Rutherford A, Chan WW, Ryou M. A prospective blinded study of endoscopic ultrasound elastography in liver disease: towards a virtual biopsy. *Clin Endosc.* 2018;51:181-185.

6. Dumonceau JM, Deprez PH, Jenssen C, et al. Indications, results, and clinical impact of endoscopic ultrasound (EUS)-guided sampling in gastroenterology: European Society of Gastrointestinal Endoscopy (ESGE) Clinical Guideline – updated January 2017. *Endoscopy.* 2017;49:695-714.

7. Pineda JJ, Diehl DL, Miao CL, et al. EUS-guided liver biopsy provides diagnostic samples comparable with those via the percutaneous or transjugular route. *Gastrointest Endosc.* 2016;83:360-365.

8. Saraireh HA, Bilal M, Singh S. Role of endoscopic ultrasound in liver disease: where do we stand in 2017? *World J Hepatol.* 2017;29:1013-1021.

9. Bravo AA, Sheth SG, Chopra S. Liver biopsy. *N Engl J Med.* 2001;15(344):495-500.

10. Shiha G, Ibrahim A, Helmy A, et al. Asian-Pacific Association for the Study of the Liver (APASL) consensus guidelines on invasive and non-invasive assessment of hepatic fibrosis: a 2016 update. *Hepatol Int.* 2017;11:1-30.

11. Nieto J, Khaleel H, Challita Y, et al. EUS-guided fine-needle core liver biopsy sampling using a novel 19-gauge needle with modified 1-pass, 1 actuation wet suction technique. *Gastrointest Endosc.* 2018;87(2):469-475.

12. Saab SPJ, Jimenez MA, Grotts JF, et al. Endoscopic ultrasound liver biopsies accurately predict the presence of fibrosis in patients with fatty liver. *Clin Gastroenterol Hepatol.* 2017;15:1477-1478.

13. Diehl DL, Johal AS, Khara HS, et al. Endoscopic ultrasound-guided liver biopsy: a multicenter experience. *Endosc Int Open.* 2015;3:E210-E215.

14. Oh D, Seo DW, Hong SM, et al. Endoscopic ultrasound-guided fine-needle aspiration can target right liver mass. *Endosc Ultrasound.* 2017;6:109-115.

15. Shah ND, Sasatomi E, Baron TH. Endoscopic ultrasound-guided parenchymal liver biopsy: single center experience of a new dedicated core needle. *Clin Gastroenterol Hepatol.* 2017;15:784-786.

16. Schulman AR, Thompson CC, Odze R, Chan WW, Ryou M. Optimizing EUS-guided liver biopsy sampling: comprehensive assessment of needle types and tissue acquisition techniques. *Exp Endoscopy.* 2017;85:419-426.

17. Mok SRS, Diehl DL. The role of EUS in liver biopsy. *Curr Gastroenterol Rep.* 2019;21:6.

18. Mohan BP, Shakhatreh M, Garg R, Ponnada S, Adler DG. Efficacy and safety of EUS-guided liver biopsy: a systematic review and meta-analysis. *Gastrointest Endosc.* 2019;89:238-246.e3.

19. Magalhães J, Monteiro S, Xavier S, Leite S, de Castro FD, Cotter J. Endoscopic ultrasonography – emerging applications in hepatology. *World J Gastrointest Endosc.* 2017;9:378-388.

20. Gleeson FC, Clayton AC, Zhang L, et al. Adequacy of endoscopic ultrasound core needle biopsy specimen of nonmalignant hepatic parenchymal disease. *Clin Gastroenterol Hepatol.* 2008;6:1437-1440.

21. Lee WJ, Uradomo LT, Zhang Y, Twaddell W, Darwin P. Comparison of the diagnostic yield of EUS needles for liver biopsy: ex vivo study. *Diagn Ther Endosc.* 2017:2017.

22. Mok SRS, Diehl DL, Johal AS, et al. A prospective pilot comparison of wet and dry heparinized suction for EUS-guided liver biopsy (with videos). *Gastrointest Endosc.* 2018;88:919-925.

23. Singh P, Mukhopadhyay P, Bhatt B, et al. Endoscopic ultrasound versus CT scan for detection of the metastases to the liver: results of a prospective comparative study. *J Clin Gastroenterol.* 2009;43:367-373.

24. Nieto J, Penn E, Lankarani A, et al. Su1419 A multi-center retrospective study of 336 eus-guided fine needle core liver biopsy with A modified 1-pass 1-actuation wet suction technique comparing two types of eus core needles. *Gastrointest Endosc.* 2018;87:AB348-AB349.

25. Saab S, Phan J, Jimenez MA, et al. Endoscopic ultrasound liver biopsies accurately predict the presence of fibrosis in patients with fatty liver. *Clin Gastroenterol Hepatol.* 2017;15:1477-1478.

26. Sey MS, Al-Haddad M, Imperiale TF, et al. EUS-guided liver biopsy for parenchymal disease: a comparison of diagnostic yield between two core biopsy needles. *Gastrointest Endosc.* 2015;83:347-352.

27. Stavropoulos SN, Im GY, Jlayer Z, et al. High yield of same-session EUS-guided liver biopsy by 19-gauge FNA needle in patients undergoing EUS to exclude biliary obstruction. *Gastrointest Endosc.* 2012;75:310-318.

28. Dewitt J, McGreevy K, Cummings O, et al. Initial experience with EUS-guided Tru-cut biopsy of benign liver disease. *Gastrointest Endosc.* 2009;69:535-542.

29. DiMaio CJ, Kolb JM, Benias PC, et al. Initial experience with a novel EUS-guided core biopsy needle (SharkCore): results of a large North American multicenter study. *Endosc Int Open.* 2016;4:E974-E979.

30. Fujii-Lau LL, Abu Dayyeh BK, Bruno MJ, et al. EUS-derived criteria for distinguishing benign from malignant metastatic solid hepatic masses. *Gastrointest Endosc.* 2015;81:1188-1196.

31. Lee YN, Moon JH, Kim HK, et al. Usefulness of endoscopic ultrasound-guided sampling using core biopsy needle as a percutaneous biopsy rescue for diagnosis of solid liver mass: combined histological-cytological analysis. *J Gastroenterol Hepatol.* 2015;30:1161-1166.

32. Prachayakul V, Aswakul P, Kachintorn U. EUS guided fine needle aspiration cytology of liver nodules suspicious for malignancy: yields, complications and impact on management. *J Med Assoc Thai.* 2012;95(suppl 2):S56-S60.

33. DeWitt J, LeBlanc J, McHenry L, et al. Endoscopic ultrasound-guided fine needle aspiration cytology of solid liver lesions: a large single-center experience. *Am J Gastroenterol.* 2003;98:1976-1981.

34. Hollerbach S, Willert J, Topalidis T, Reiser M, Schmiegel W. Endoscopic ultrasound-guided fine-needle aspiration biopsy of liver lesions: histological and cytological assessment. *Endoscopy.* 2003;743-749.

35. tenBerge J, Hoffman BJ, Hawes RH, et al. EUS-guided fine needle aspiration of the liver: indications, yield, and safety based on an international survey of 167 cases. *Gastrointest Endosc.* 2002;55:859-862.

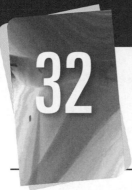

32 | EUS-Guided Drainage of Pancreatic Collections and Necrosectomy

Ryan Law, DO
Todd H. Baron, MD

Injury to the pancreas regardless of the etiology results in parenchymal inflammation, often leading to disruption of the main pancreatic duct and/or secondary branches. Following ductal injury, leakage of pancreatic contents may lead to formation of fluid-filled pancreatic or peripancreatic collections with or without the presence of solid debris. Clinically severe acute pancreatitis evolves over several weeks culminating in walled-off necrosis (WON) in many cases (Fig. 32.1). The aim of endoscopic therapy is to provide drainage of liquid contents and mechanical removal of necrotic tissue, if necessary. Endoscopic intervention remains the current standard of care for patients with pancreatic fluid collections. This chapter will focus on the indications, techniques, and outcomes of endoscopic therapy and management of pancreatic fluid collections.

IMAGING

1. CT or MRI should be performed before endoscopic intervention to assess the size, shape, wall thickness, and contents, discern adjacent relevant vascularity, and ascertain the relationship between the cavity and gastrointestinal lumen, presence of gas, and solid material.
2. CT and MRI appearance of PFCs can vary widely. CT showing nondependent air within a cavity is indicative of the presence of solid debris.
3. Understanding the burden of necrosis, the presence or absence of extension into the paracolic gutters and interactions between multiple cavities, if present, will guide the index procedure and streamline subsequent interventions.

INDICATIONS FOR AND TIMING OF ENDOSCOPIC DRAINAGE

1. Gastric outlet obstruction due to compression
2. Biliary obstruction due to compression

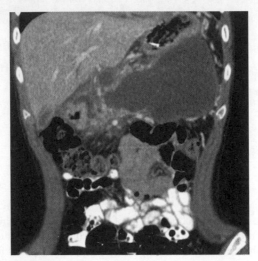

FIG. 32.1 Coronal image of abdominal CT findings of walled-off pancreatic necrosis abutting the stomach. Note heterogeneity within the collection.

3. Abdominal pain
4. Failure to thrive (fatigue, anorexia, weight loss)
5. Infection

CONTRAINDICATIONS
1. Uncontrolled coagulopathy
2. Overt luminal perforation

PREPROCEDURAL CONSIDERATIONS
1. Ensure adequate international normalized ratio (INR) and platelet count
2. Administration of broad-spectrum antibiotics
3. Anesthesia support
4. Carbon dioxide for insufflation

ENDOSCOPIC DRAINAGE
1. Endoscopic ultrasound (EUS)-guided access is superior and should be used whenever available (Fig. 32.2).
2. Assessment prior to puncture: extent, volume, and density of material within the collection.
3. Transmural puncture. Choice of device includes electrocautery-based instruments such as biliary needle knives and specialized cystenterostomy devices (Cystotome, Cook Endoscopy, Winston-Salem, NC) and electrocautery-enhanced delivery tips of luminal apposing metal stents (LAMSs). Noncautery puncture employs EUS-FNA (fine needle aspiration) needles.

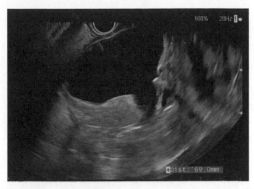

FIG. 32.2 Endoscopic ultrasound (EUS) image of collection shown in Figure 1 just prior to drainage, shown in Fig. 32.1.

4. Stents. Traditional plastic double pigtails, traditional covered biliary and esophageal self-expandable metal stents (SEMSs), and LAMSs are available. The latter has simplified the management of PFCs.

5. Fluoroscopy is not mandatory but can be helpful to guide drainage.

6. If an FNA needle is used for puncture, a 19G needle should be chosen to allow a long-length (450 cm), 0.025 to 0.035" wire. Fluid can be aspirated for analysis. Contrast can be injected if fluoroscopy is used. The guidewire is advanced into the collection and coiled at least once. If cautery is used, it is passed over the wire. For traditional stent placement, the tract will need to be dilated to allow passage of the stent delivery system. If plastic stents are placed, the tract should be dilated to 6, 8 or 10 mm depending on diameter and number of stents (usually two) being placed. For SEMS with delivery systems of 7 to 10Fr, dilation of 4 to 6 mm is adequate.

7. For drainage of purely liquid collections (pancreatic pseudocysts), balloon dilate tract to 8 to 10 mm followed by placement of two 10Fr double-pigtail stents (length of 3 to 5 cm) to mitigate concerns for stent migration into or out of the cavity. Place an endoscopically visible, indelible mark at the midpoint of the stent prior to placement, if markers are not present on the stent.

8. Small-bore (10 mm), fully covered, biliary SEMS or small-diameter LAMS (10 mm) can be placed for management of collections which are predominately liquid.

9. For collections with solid debris (WON), placement of a large-caliber (16 to 23 mm midbody diameter) esophageal stent (6 to 7 cm length) or large-diameter LAMS (15 or 20 mm) is recommended (Fig. 32.3A).

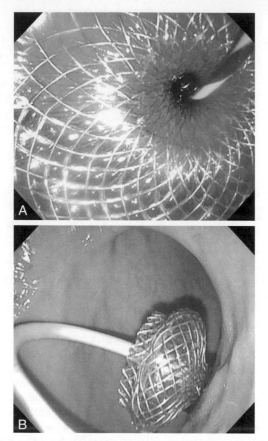

FIG. 32.3 Endoscopic image of large-diameter luminal apposing stent (A) immediately after deployment and (B) after placement of 10Fr double-pigtail stent within it (same patient as Figs. 32.1 and 32.2).

10. A double-pigtail plastic stent can also be placed within the deployed SEMS to serve as a buffer between the stent flange and the lumen/cavity wall and to inhibit necrotic debris from occluding the SEMS (Fig. 32.3B).
11. When cautery-enhanced LAMS are placed, puncture with the delivery system is done either without a guidewire ("freehand") or over a guidewire that had been passed through an FNA needle followed by stent deployment without need for tract dilation. A 10Fr double-pigtail stent is subsequently placed within the LAMS to maintain stent patency, prevent stent impaction, facilitate removal if a buried stent occurs, and leave room for plastic pigtail stents to treat disconnected ducts as the cavity resolves.

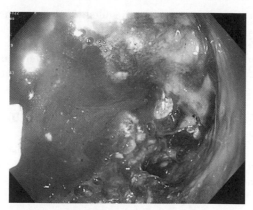

FIG. 32.4 Endoscopic view of necrotic cavity several weeks after placement of large-diameter a lumen-apposing metal stent (LAMS). Direct endoscopic necrosectomy was performed using cold polypectomy snare.

12. For patients with WON, removal of solid debris is often needed. A 7Fr nasocystic irrigation tube can be placed into the cavity, adjacent to transmural stents, to permit irrigation. Up to 200 mL of normal saline (±3% hydrogen peroxide) is vigorously infused through the tube every 2 to 4 hours initially to lavage debris from the cavity.

13. Direct endoscopic necrosectomy (DEN) allows removal of solid debris. DEN is performed by passing an endoscope transmurally into the collection using diagnostic or therapeutic endoscopes (Fig. 32.4). Mechanical debridement is accomplished with various endoscopic accessories (i.e., stone retrieval baskets, polypectomy snares, polyp retrieval nets, grasping forceps, etc.). Once the necrotic tissue is freed, it is extracted from the cavity and deposited in the lumen. Larger pieces may be cut into smaller pieces using a polypectomy snare with or without electrocautery, then cleared from the collection to avoid unnecessary transmural passage into and out of the cavity.

POSTPROCEDURE CARE

1. Patients may resume (or initiate) oral intake the day of the procedure assuming clinical stability and absence of intraprocedural adverse events.
2. Continue peroral antibiotics for several weeks until the cavity completely resolves as determined by cross-sectional imaging.
3. Repeat DEN is almost universally necessary for WON when plastic stents are used and requires tract dilation to reenter the collection.

4. Future procedures can be scheduled if solid remains or performed as determined by clinical status and/or cross-sectional imaging.
5. Patients requiring ongoing hospitalization often require frequent procedures (every 1 to 2 days), while stable outpatients can generally tolerate 1 to 2 weeks between DEN.

ADJUNCTIVE TREATMENT STRATEGIES (IF NEEDED) FOR WALLED-OFF NECROSIS

1. Nutritional support with parenteral or enteral supplementation
2. Percutaneous drainage and surgical drainage (when endoscopy alone fails)

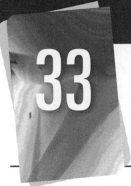

33   EUS-Guided Biliary Drainage

Woo Hyun Paik, MD, PhD
Do Hyun Park, MD, PhD

Endoscopic ultrasound (EUS)-guided biliary drainage (EUS-BD) has emerged as an alternative to percutaneous transhepatic biliary drainage (PTBD), particularly after failed endoscopic retrograde cholangiopancreatography (ERCP).[1,2] EUS-BD has some advantages over ERCP and PTBD.[3,4] ERCP is not technically feasible when the papilla is not endoscopically accessible, while EUS-BD is possible in surgically altered anatomy or inaccessible papilla. One of the most common adverse events of ERCP is postprocedure pancreatitis. In EUS-BD, papillary manipulation is avoided, thus eliminating the risk of acute pancreatitis. Stent patency may be longer in EUS-BD than in ERCP since the stents do not cross a stricture and instead reside in healthy tissue. When performed by experienced endoscopists, EUS-BD provides similar efficacy to PTBD and is more comfortable and physiologic because of avoidance of external drains and restoration of internal drainage. However, EUS-BD has not become widely adopted because of the complexity of the procedure and relative lack of dedicated devices and accessories.[5]

EUS-BD is classified into three categories: rendezvous technique, antegrade stenting, and transmural stenting.[2] The EUS-BD approach taken is determined by accessibility to the duodenum and papilla. When the papilla is endoscopically accessible, the rendezvous technique may be preferred as an approach when ERCP and selective cannulation of the bile duct fail. However, guidewire manipulation traversing through the ampulla can be challenging. Antegrade stenting may be suitable when a guidewire can be passed through the papilla from an EUS transgastric intrahepatic approach. Antegrade stenting is useful especially when the papilla is inaccessible endoscopically. Transmural stenting is the most widely performed form of EUS-BD. Transmural stenting is performed in one of the two ways: EUS-guided hepaticogastrostomy (EUS-HGS) and EUS-guided choledochoduodenostomy

(EUS-CDS). EUS-CDS may be technically easier than EUS-HGS. EUS-HGS has more adverse events than EUS-CDS, with potential risks of life-threatening adverse events including mediastinitis and pneumomediastinum.[6] EUS-CDS is more likely to cause bile leak than EUS-HGS. In cases of surgically altered anatomy or duodenal obstruction, hepaticogastrostomy is preferred as the duodenum cannot be reached. In patients with acute cholecystitis and high risk of surgery, EUS-guided gallbladder drainage (EUS-GBD) may be considered. In addition, EUS-GBD can be used for decompression of malignant distal bile duct obstruction when ERCP fails and the biliary ducts proximal to the obstruction are not dilated.[7]

INDICATIONS

1. Failed deep biliary cannulation during ERCP
2. Surgically altered anatomy
3. Duodenal obstruction or prior duodenal metal stent placement across the papilla
4. Unavailability of PTBD or refusal of PTBD and surgical bypass

CONTRAINDICATIONS

1. Patients with coagulopathy
2. Multifocal intrahepatic ductal obstruction

EQUIPMENT

1. Conventional EUS-guided fine needle aspiration needle (FNA) (usually 19-gauge) or novel needle for EUS-BD (EUS access needle, Cook Medical, Bloomington, USA); it has blunt needle tip that can prevent shearing of guidewires
2. A curvilinear array echoendoscope
3. Fluoroscopy system
4. A guidewire; a 0.025-inch VisiGlide guidewire (Olympus America, San Jose, USA) is preferred in EUS-BD because of its adequate stiffness and improved negotiation capability. 0.035-inch guidewires (Jagwire, Boston Scientific, Natick, USA; Tracer, Cook Medical) may be useful
5. Diluted contrast media
6. 4F cannula for difficult guidewire manipulation
7. Devices for fistula dilation: 4F cannula, 6F, and 7F bougie catheters, 4-mm balloon catheter (Hurricane RX, Boston Scientific), needle knife, and 6F cystotome (Cook Medical). The use of a needle knife for fistula dilation is not recommended for the risk of adverse events including pneumoperitoneum and bleeding[8]
8. Biliary stents: fully covered or partially covered self-expandable metal stents are superior to plastic stents in

preventing bile leak. To prevent stent migration, several types of metal stents with flared end, uncovered portion at the bile duct side, flaps, or flanges have been developed but are not available in the United States. Lumen-apposing metal stents (LAMSs) for EUS-CDS and EUS-GBD are commonly used (off-label). The addition of novel dedicated devices that combine electrocautery with a LAMS or a tapered metal tip introducer as a push-type dilator with a preloaded metallic stent for one-step EUS-BD without additional fistula dilation has been introduced, which can shorten procedural times and decrease procedure-related adverse events.[9,10]

PREPARATION

1. Obtain informed consent.
2. Administer prophylactic antibiotics before EUS-BD.
3. There is no consensus about fasting time in EUS-BD; however, we recommend fasting time as for other upper endoscopic procedures and per anesthesia guidelines.
4. EUS-BD can be performed under moderate/deep sedation or general anesthesia.
5. CO_2 insufflation during the procedure is recommended to reduce the risk of pneumoperitoneum.

PROCEDURES

Rendezvous Technique

1. The extra- or intrahepatics are accessed with an EUS-FNA needle. The extrahepatic approach may be preferred because the intrahepatic approach requires more difficult guidewire manipulation that has to pass through the stricture site as well as the papilla. The extrahepatic bile duct can be assessed by two methods: push and pull methods. Although pull methods have a more unstable endoscope position than push methods, negotiation of guidewire across the papilla is easier with pull methods. The intrahepatics can be approached via puncture of liver segment 2 (B2) or segment 3 (B3). B2 duct is less angulated than B3 and is preferred (Fig. 33.1).
2. After puncturing the bile duct, aspiration is used to confirm bile duct access (Fig. 33.2A).
3. Contrast is injected to obtain cholangiography, and a guidewire is negotiated across the stricture and through the papilla in an antegrade manner. Coiling of the guidewire inside the duodenum is necessary to prevent loss of guidewire during withdrawal of the needle and the echoendoscope (Fig. 33.2B).
4. After removal of the EUS needle and then the echoendoscope, a conventional duodenoscope is passed into the duodenum.

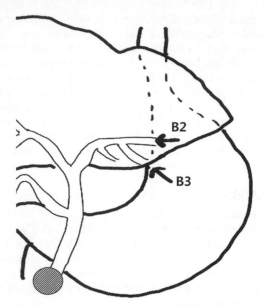

FIG. 33.1 Schematics of endoscopic ultrasound (EUS)-guided approach to the intrahepatics.

5. Selective deep biliary cannulation is possible by cannulating alongside the existing guidewire. When this approach fails, the guidewire is grasped with a biopsy forceps or snare, and then the guidewire is pulled through the working channel out of the endoscope (Fig. 33.2C). A catheter or sphincterotome is inserted over the guidewire. The rendezvous technique may be the safest EUS-BD approach; however, it is cumbersome and time consuming.

Antegrade Stenting

1. With a 19-gauge EUS needle, the intrahepatics are punctured and cholangiography is obtained (Fig. 33.3A).
2. B2 may be preferred over B3 since B2 is usually less angulated.
3. After guidewire manipulation across the stricture site and the papilla, the guidewire is looped in the duodenum, and then the needle is withdrawn (Fig. 33.3B).
4. A 4-mm balloon catheter is useful for dilatation of the papilla and stricture site to facilitate advancement of the stent delivery system.
5. The biliary stents are deployed over the guidewire in an antegrade manner (Fig. 33.3C).
6. To minimize bile leak at the puncture site, a 5Fr nasobiliary catheter is placed over the wire and remains temporarily.

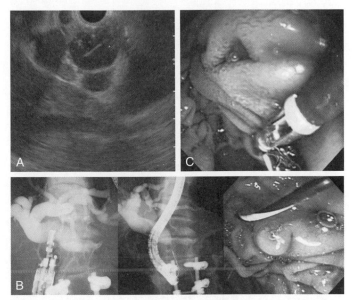

FIG. 33.2 Endoscopic ultrasound (EUS)-guided rendezvous technique. A, EUS-guided puncture of the common bile from the duodenal bulb position. B, An EUS-guided cholangiogram is obtained followed by antegrade guidewire passage through the ampulla and into the duodenum. The echoendoscope is then carefully removed leaving the guidewire in place. C, A duodenoscope is placed alongside the guidewire and the guidewire is grasped with forceps. The guidewire is withdrawn through the working channel of the duodenoscope to allow for subsequent retrograde biliary interventions. (From Paik WH, Park DH. Endoscopic ultrasound-guided biliary access, with focus on technique and practical tips. *Clin Endosc.* 2017;50:104-111. With permission.)

Transmural Drainage

As previously mentioned, EUS-CDS (Fig. 33.4A) and EUS-HGS (Fig. 33.4B) are two main methods in EUS-guided transmural drainage. EUS-GBD (Fig. 33.4C) can be performed in patients with acute cholecystitis and high risk of surgery. The basic steps of EUS-guided transmural drainage are as follows: accessing the biliary system with EUS needle, injection of contrast media for cholangiography, guidewire manipulation, fistula dilatation, and stent deployment.

ENDOSCOPIC ULTRASOUND–GUIDED CHOLEDOCHODUODENOSTOMY

1. The long scope position is preferred because it directs the needle toward the hilum of the liver and facilitates guidewire manipulation. Since the common bile duct runs parallel to the portal vein, it is easy to identify the common bile duct on

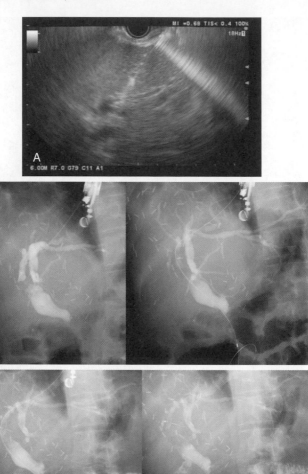

FIG. 33.3 Endoscopic ultrasound (EUS)-guided antegrade stenting. A, Under EUS-guidance a left intrahepatic bile duct is punctured with and FNA-needle. B, A cholangiogram is obtained and a distal common bile duct stricture is defined. A guidewire is passed antegrade through the common bile duct stricture and into the duodenum. C, Following tract dilation, a stent insertion catheter is passed antegrade across the distal bile duct stricture and the stent is released. (From Paik WH, Park DH. Endoscopic ultrasound-guided biliary access, with focus on technique and practical tips. *Clin Endosc.* 2017;50:104-111. With permission.)

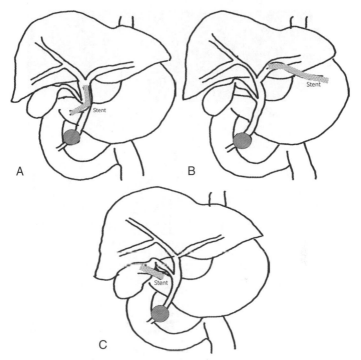

FIG. 33.4 Schematics of endoscopic ultrasound (EUS)-guided choledochoduodenostomy (A), hepaticogastrostomy (B), and gallbladder drainage (C).

EUS real-time image. Before puncturing the bile duct, color Doppler imaging can be used to identify regional vasculature (Fig. 33.5A).

2. After confirming access of the common bile duct by aspiration of bile, radiocontrast is administered to obtain cholangiography (Fig. 33.5B).

3. A guidewire is passed through the needle into the intrahepatics, and EUS needle is removed gently (Fig. 33.5C). During guidewire negotiation, excessive manipulation may cause shearing of the guidewire coating.

4. The fistula tract is dilated to facilitate the advancement of stent delivery system. Mechanical dilation is preferred over cautery dilation due to safety issue. A 4-mm Hurricane balloon catheter is preferred over sequential dilatation with a 4F cannula and bougie catheter since sequential dilatation lengthens procedural time and may cause separation between the bile duct and the duodenum (Fig. 33.5D).

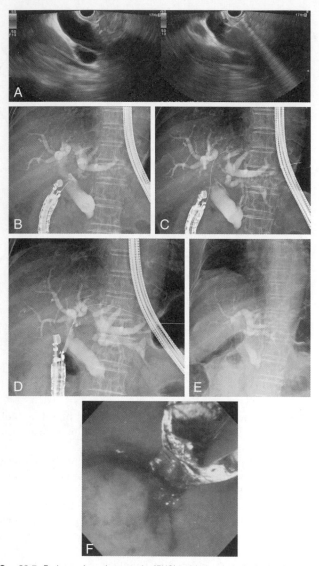

FIG. 33.5 Endoscopic ultrasound (EUS)-guided choledochoduodenostomy. A, Endosonographic identification and FNA needle puncture of the common bile duct from the duodenal bulb position. B, EUS-guided cholangiogram is obtained. C, Retrograde guidewire passage into the left biliary system. D, Tract dilation is performed with a balloon dilator to allow passage of the stent insertion catheter. E, The fully-covered self-expandable metal stent is deployed to create a choledochoduodenostomy. F, Drainage of bile and contrast into the duodenum following stent deployment.

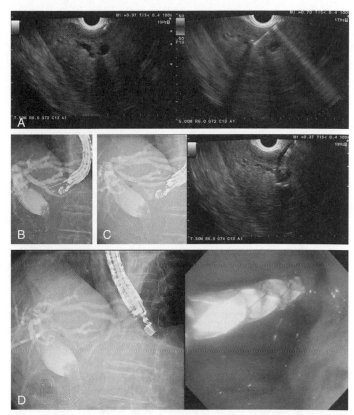

FIG. 33.6 Endoscopic ultrasound (EUS)-guided hepaticogastrostomy. A, Endosonographic identification and puncture with an FNA needle of a dilated left intrahepatic bile duct. B, Following EUS-guided cholangiogram, a guidewire is passed antegrade and coiled within the common bile duct. C, Tract dilation of liver parenchyma, liver capsule, and gastric wall is performed with a balloon dilator. D, A fully-covered self-expandable metal stent is placed to complete the hepaticogastrostomy.

5. In EUS-CDS, the length of metal stent is 4 to 6 cm. After inserting the stent delivery system, stent deployment should be performed under EUS and fluoroscopic guidance rather than endoscopic view (Fig. 33.5E).

6. Flow of bile from the stent can be seen by endoscopic view (Fig. 33.5F).

ENDOSCOPIC ULTRASOUND–GUIDED HEPATICOGASTROSTOMY

1. For successful EUS-HGS, the puncture site should be selected carefully. At the optimal access point, the intrahepatics run from the upper left to the lower right on EUS

imaging, and the diameter of the intrahepatics is more than 5 mm and the length is more than 1 cm (Fig. 33.6A).[11] B3 is preferred over B2 to prevent puncturing from the esophagus. B3 puncture is usually achieved in the lesser curvatures of stomach body; thus, during deployment, the tip of the stent in the stomach can be verified and stent migration prevented.

2. A guidewire is negotiated toward the liver hilum (Fig. 33.6B). When the guidewire is advanced into the peripheral biliary tract on fluoroscopic finding, liver impaction method that slightly withdraws the EUS needle into the hepatic parenchyma on EUS can prevent guidewire kinking or shearing with the EUS needle.[12]

3. Fistula dilation is performed as for EUS-CDS (Fig. 33.6C).

4. The distal half of a metal stent is deployed under EUS and fluoroscopic guidance, and then the remaining is deployed inside the working channel to stabilize the position of the echoendoscope. Finally, the scope is gently withdrawn, and

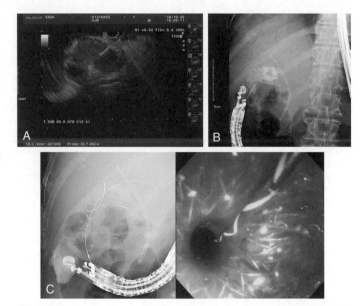

FIG. 33.7 Endoscopic ultrasound (EUS)-guided gallbladder drainage. A, The gallbladder is punctured with an EUS FNA needle under endosonographic visualization. B, Contrast is injected under fluoroscopy and a cholecystogram is obtained. C, Following tract dilation, a stent insertion catheter is passed into the gallbladder and a fully-covered self-expandable metal stent is deployed to complete creation of a cholecystoenterostomy.

the stent deployment technique allows a secure and stable position and decreases the distance between the liver parenchyma and the stomach (Fig. 33.6D).[13]

5. To prevent stent migration by shortening of the stent, a stent length of 8 to 10 cm or more is recommended.

ENDOSCOPIC ULTRASOUND–GUIDED GALLBLADDER DRAINAGE

1. Visualize the distended gallbladder with EUS at the duodenum or the antrum of the stomach (Fig. 33.7A).
2. The neck or body of the gallbladder is preferred for access with EUS needle (Fig. 33.7B).
3. After puncturing the gallbladder, a guidewire is inserted into the gallbladder and coiled.
4. Fistula dilation is performed along the guidewire.
5. A self-expandable metal or plastic stent is placed between the gallbladder and the duodenum or the stomach (Fig. 33.7C). For the transient relief of acute cholecystitis, a 5F nasobiliary tube can be placed. When a metal stent is used, the above stent deployment technique described in EUS-HGS is useful to prevent intraperitoneal stent migration.
6. When intraperitoneal migration develops, the guidewire should be kept in position, and a second overlapping metal stent can be inserted over the existing guidewire as a bridging method.

References

1. Giovannini M, Moutardier V, Pesenti C, et al. Endoscopic ultrasound-guided bilioduodenal anastomosis: a new technique for biliary drainage. *Endoscopy*. 2001;33:898-900.
2. Paik WH, Park DH. Endoscopic ultrasound-guided biliary access, with focus on technique and practical tips. *Clin Endosc*. 2017;50:104-111.
3. Lee TH, Choi JH, Park do H, et al. Similar efficacies of endoscopic ultrasound-guided transmural and percutaneous drainage for malignant distal biliary obstruction. *Clin Gastroenterol Hepatol*. 2016;14:1011-1019.
4. Paik WH, Lee TH, Park DH, et al. EUS-guided biliary drainage versus ERCP for the primary palliation of malignant biliary obstruction: a multicenter randomized clinical trial. *Am J Gastroenterol*. 2018;113:987-997.
5. Yoon WJ, Park DH, Choi JH, et al. The underutilization of EUS-guided biliary drainage: perception of endoscopists in the East and West. *Endosc Ultrasound*. 2019;8:188-193.
6. Ogura T, Higuchi K. Technical tips for endoscopic ultrasound-guided hepaticogastrostomy. *World J Gastroenterol*. 2016;22:3945-3951.
7. Imai H, Kitano M, Omoto S, et al. EUS-guided gallbladder drainage for rescue treatment of malignant distal biliary obstruction after unsuccessful ERCP. *Gastrointest Endosc*. 2016;84:147-151.

8. Park DH, Jang JW, Lee SS, et al. EUS-guided biliary drainage with transluminal stenting after failed ERCP: predictors of adverse events and long-term results. *Gastrointest Endosc.* 2011;74:1276-1284.

9. Park DH, Lee TH, Paik WH, et al. Feasibility and safety of a novel dedicated device for one-step EUS-guided biliary drainage: a randomized trial. *J Gastroenterol Hepatol.* 2015;30:1461-1466.

10. El Chafic AH, Shah JN, Hamerski C, et al. EUS-guided choledochoduodenostomy for distal malignant biliary obstruction using electrocautery-enhanced lumen-apposing metal stents: first US, multicenter experience. *Dig Dis Sci.* 2019;64(11):3321-3327.

11. Oh D, Park DH, Song TJ, et al. Optimal biliary access point and learning curve for endoscopic ultrasound-guided hepaticogastrostomy with transmural stenting. *Therap Adv Gastroenterol.* 2017;10:42-53.

12. Ogura T, Masuda D, Takeuchi T, et al. Liver impaction technique to prevent shearing of the guidewire during endoscopic ultrasound-guided hepaticogastrostomy. *Endoscopy.* 2015;47:e583-e584.

13. Paik WH, Park DH, Choi JH, et al. Simplified fistula dilation technique and modified stent deployment maneuver for EUS-guided hepaticogastrostomy. *World J Gastroenterol.* 2014;20:5051-5059.

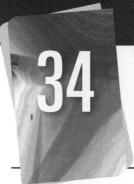

34

EUS-Guided Pancreatic Duct Drainage

Manuel Perez-Miranda, MD, PhD

Endoscopic ultrasound (EUS)-guided pancreatic duct drainage (EUS-PD) is a second-line procedure that allows drainage of the pancreatic duct when ERCP, the primary endoscopic procedure for pancreatic duct drainage, is either not feasible or unsuccessful.[1] EUS-PD is performed in the fluoroscopy room by an experienced operator assisted by well-trained personnel in properly sedated and monitored patients at a facility with multidisciplinary backup. The availability of appropriate equipment and a wide array of devices cannot be overemphasized. EUS-PD complements pancreatic ERCP making endotherapy available to complex patients who would otherwise have to undergo surgery or percutaneous procedures for duct decompression or would have to face the suboptimal prospect of medical treatment. Depending on patient anatomy, operator expertise, and predictability of ERCP difficulty, EUS-PD can be performed within the same session of failed ERCP.[2] Alternatively, EUS-PD can be scheduled in the future. Following transgastric or transduodenal EUS-guided pancreatography, drainage is established by means of transmural, transpapillary (either retrograde or antegrade), or a combined approach.[1,2] A successful index EUS-PD may need follow-up procedures for stent revision, which no longer require an EUS endoscope.[3]

INDICATIONS

The triad of (1) typical clinical manifestations, associated with (2) imaging evidence of pancreatic duct obstruction/disruption, in the setting of (3) established pancreatic disease, warrant EUS-PD whenever ERCP is unsuccessful, with the possible exception of known resectable pancreatic malignancy. There are three main reasons for failure of pancreatic ERCP: difficulty in access to the papilla (as in surgically altered upper GI anatomy

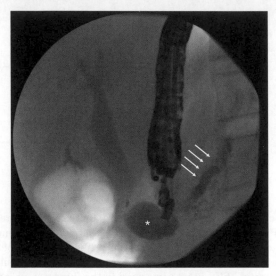

FIG. 34.1 Disconnected pancreatic duct syndrome as a late sequela of acute necrotizing pancreatitis. An intervening pseudocyst (*) is located between the pancreatic duct in the head and the dilated upstream pancreatic duct in the body and tail (arrows). The patient is having acute relapsing pancreatitis. Transgastric puncture of the pancreatic duct in the body of the pancreas, with the scope oriented toward the tail. The two-stage treatment plan involves pancreaticogastrostomy to temporary decompress the duct, followed by rendezvous reconnection of the disconnected pancreatic duct at a follow-up procedure through the mature pancreatogastric fistula.

or in duodenal strictures), in cannulation (as in minor papilla or in prior biliary sphincterotomy) or in guidewire access to blocked duct segments (as in transected or disrupted ducts). Therefore, ERCP failure can often be anticipated prior to undertaking ERCP (e.g., acute relapsing pancreatitis post-Whipple[4]; disconnected pancreatic duct syndrome [Fig. 34.1]; history of previous failed pancreatic ERCPs). However, on other occasions the indication for EUS-PD may arise during ERCP (e.g., failed guidewire passage across tortuous chronic pancreatitis strictures or impacted pancreatic duct stones; failed minor papilla cannulation of newly diagnosed divisum). As in the examples above, all indications for EUS-PD include varying combinations of the following triad elements.

Clinical Manifestations

1. Severe, persistent pancreatic-type abdominal pain
2. Acute relapsing pancreatitis
3. Refractory pancreatic fistula

Background Diagnoses

1. Chronic pancreatitis
2. Pancreatico-enterostomy stricture (most commonly, post-Whipple)
3. Pancreas divisum
4. Pancreatic trauma (including surgery)
5. Pancreatic cancer[5,6]
6. Acute necrotizing pancreatitis

Underlying Pancreatic Duct Anatomy

1. Pancreatic strictures
   a. Ductal (e.g., chronic pancreatitis or pancreatic duct adenocarcinoma)
   b. Papillary (e.g., minor papilla or major papilla after biliary sphincterotomy)
   c. Anastomotic (e.g., pancreato-jejunostomy)
2. Pancreatic duct stones
3. Pancreatic duct disruption
4. Disconnected pancreatic duct

CONTRAINDICATIONS

Absolute

1. Active, uncontrolled perforation
2. Inability to undergo sedation
3. Uncorrectable coagulopathy

Relative

1. Nondilated pancreatic duct (<2 mm)
2. Altered upper GI anatomy precluding EUS imaging of the pancreas (e.g., Roux-en-Y gastric bypass)
3. Transient inflammatory changes (e.g., pseudocyst) potentially interfering with optimal EUS access to the pancreatic duct
4. Known resectable pancreatic malignancy

PREPARATION

1. Patient evaluation and consent: Thorough clinical evaluation, including cross-sectional imaging and MRI pancreatography (ideally with IV secretin), is essential to establish the indication and to define procedural approach. Depending on anticipated likelihood of ERCP failure and on institutional policy, informed consent is obtained for both ERCP and EUS-PD.
2. Periprocedural medications: Antiplatelet/anticoagulation agents and antibiotic prophylaxis should be managed per American Society for Gastrointestinal Endoscopy guidelines.[7]

The value of rectal nonsteroidal anti-inflammatory drugs and of intravenous hydration in decreasing the risk of postprocedural pancreatitis has not been established for EUS-PD, but are reasonable to consider.

3. Sedation: The level of sedation required for EUS-PD is comparable to that of complexity level IV ERCP. Monitored anesthesia care or general endotracheal intubation are most common in the United States; however, nurse- or endoscopist-administered propofol can also be used to provide optimal sedation.

EQUIPMENT AND DEVICES

Equipment

1. Therapeutic channel (3.8 or 4.0 mm) linear-array echoendoscope (forward or forward-oblique viewing)
2. A duodenoscope (or colonoscope/enteroscope in cases of surgically altered upper GI anatomy) may be required for certain procedural approaches (i.e., rendezvous)
3. High-quality fluoroscopy
4. Image and ultrasound processors
5. Carbon dioxide insufflation
6. Patient monitoring equipment
7. Radiation protection measures
8. Personal protective equipment for universal precautions

Devices

1. EUS-fine-needle aspiration needles, most commonly 19G (21 or 22G may be considered for smaller ducts)
2. Injectate: contrast material and saline solution
3. Guidewires: typically angled-tip 0.025-inch high-performance hydrophilic long (420 cm) guidewires (for 19G needles). Thinner (0.018-inch or 0.021-inch) guidewires are required for 22G needles. Thicker (0.35-inch) and/or stiffer guidewires may be required for additional support during dilation or for better luminal coiling during the endoscope exchange phase of rendezvous. Guidewires of different tip configurations or hydrophilic coatings may have to be tried throughout the same procedure
4. Low profile steering catheters commonly used for percutaneous interventional angiography or low profile (3.5 French) taper-tipped ERCP cannulas
5. Mechanical dilating catheters: stepped axial dilators of 3-5-7 French diameter and balloon dilators of 4 to 6 mm diameter (less commonly, screw-type metal dilators; mechanical dilation is preferred over cautery dilation)

6. Cautery dilating catheters: small caliber (6 French) cysto-tome is preferable to needle knife, if locally available

7. Plastic stents: standard biliary (without side holes) or pancre-atic (with side holes) 5 to 8.5 French, 7 to 20 cm long, straight or double pigtail stents are used (typically, straight 7 French)

8. Grasping devices (i.e., polypectomy snare, forceps)

9. Sphincterotomes: either standard double or triple lumen (for antegrade guidewire steering) or dedicated (to facilitate par-allel rendezvous cannulation)[8]

10. Over-the-wire stone retrieval balloons: these allow occlusion antegrade pancreatography after fistula dilation and might be used to facilitate antegrade or retrograde pancreatic stone retrieval

PROCEDURE

Transmural EUS-PD (i.e., pancreaticogastrostomy and pancreati-coduodenostomy) can be broken down into six procedural steps. The initial three steps are EUS-related: target identification, duct puncture, and guidewire access. The last three steps are ERCP-related: guidewire manipulation, track dilation, and stent placement.[9] Antegrade transpapillary EUS-PD entails the same six steps; however, guidewire manipulation is more demanding than in transmural EUS-PD. In retrograde transpapillary EUS-PD (i.e., rendezvous), track dilation (step number 5) is replaced by endoscope exchange, and stent insertion (step number 6) is per-formed via ERCP. The success-limiting steps of EUS-PD are 4 to 6[9]; however, steps 1 to 3 provide the best needle access site and may greatly facilitate subsequent limiting steps.

Step 1: Location of Entry Point

A dilated segment of pancreatic duct close to the transducer from a stable echoendoscope position is sought under EUS. Color Doppler helps to identify and avoid puncturing interposed vessels. The orientation of the scope tip and projected needle trajectory are assessed on fluoroscopy prior to puncture (Figs. 34.1-34.3). The echoendoscope is more stable in the long (duo-denal) position (Fig. 34.2), but this approach is only possible in patients with native GI anatomy and pancreatic duct strictures within the pancreas head.

Step 2: Puncture and Ductography

Needle size is tailored to the pancreatic duct diameter. 19G nee-dles are preferable but require ducts >4 mm, whereas 21 or 22G needles are required in ducts <2 mm.[10] Pancreatic duct puncture requires a fast, hard needle thrust. This may result in the needle

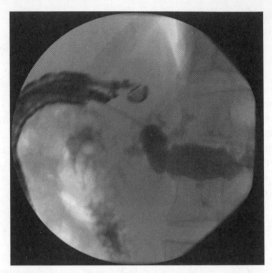

FIG. 34.2 Transduodenal EUS-guided pancreatography in a patient with severe chronic pancreatitis, dominant head stricture, massive dilatation of the upstream pancreatic duct, and refractory pain. Echoendoscope in the bulb in the long route. Retrograde puncture aiming to bypass the stricture by means of pancreaticobulbostomy eventually creating a stent-free permanent fistula.

"piercing" the duct. When piercing occurs, the needle is slowly pulled backward under EUS. Once the needle is seen under EUS inside the duct, contrast injection and pancreatography ultimately confirm access and provide a road map for subsequent guidewire placement.

Step 3: Initial Guidewire Access

Following pancreatography, the preloaded (or newly introduced) guidewire is advanced under fluoroscopy into the pancreatic duct. The endoscopist manipulates the guidewire while an assistant holds the echoendoscope in position, keeping the guidewire in sonographic view, indicating that access plane and axis are maintained.[1] Advancement of 0.025-inch angle-tip hydrophilic guidewires through 19G needles causes less friction than 0.035 guidewires. 22G needles usually only allow passage of 0.018 guidewires, which can be used for rendezvous. Backward guidewire movements should be very gentle and be stopped if any resistance is noted to prevent guidewire shearing. On occasion, a guidewire may go with surprising ease through a tight stricture which was impossible to canalize from a retrograde approach (Fig. 34.3).

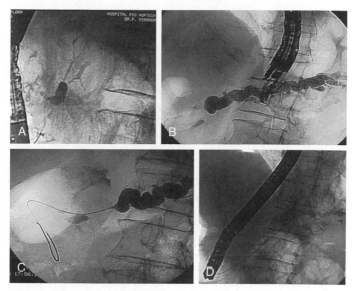

FIG. 34.3 High-grade pancreatic stricture secondary to pancreatic head adenocarcinoma causing pancreatic-type abdominal pain. At ERCP no pancreatic duct filling upstream the stricture is obtained (A). Transgastric EUS-guided puncture with the echoendoscope oriented toward the head (B) subsequently results in smooth antegrade guidewire passage across the stricture and the papilla into the duodenum (C). After endoscope exchange, the guidewire is retrieved with a snare up the working channel of a duodenoscope (classic rendezvous), allowing retrograde pancreatic stent placement for pain control under dual guidewire traction (D).

Step 4: Guidewire Manipulation

This step defines the final drainage route (transpapillary or transmural) and is critical to procedural success. The manipulation of guidewires afforded by needles is limited. Flexible catheters are often required to overcome strictures. The needle is carefully removed over-the-wire under fluoroscopy taking care to prevent guidewire dislodgment and is then replaced for a tapered tip catheter or stepped axial dilator. These catheters can occasionally be advanced directly over-the-wire into the duct. Alternatively, special steering catheters—borrowed from interventional radiology[11] or designed ad hoc[3]—may allow transmural noncautery access into the pancreatic duct. If antegrade guidewire passage across the stricture/papilla is achieved, coiling the guidewire within the small bowel with two or three loops is advisable to prevent guidewire dislodgment during endoscope exchange for subsequent rendezvous (usually in patients with native anatomy) or, alternatively, to provide support for track dilation during antegrade stenting (usually in patients with altered anatomy).

Step 5A: Puncture Tract Dilation

This step is required for antegrade and transmural stent placement, whereas it is skipped for rendezvous EUS-PD. Cautery
dilation of the puncture track is most often necessary to advance
a flexible catheter into the pancreatic duct. Thin caliber cysto-
tomes are preferable to needle knives for cautery dilation but
are not universally available. For smooth transmural stent insertion, additional balloon dilation up to 4 or 6 mm is also required.
Again, fluoroscopic monitoring and careful coordination with
the assistant is mandatory during these two exchanges to prevent guidewire dislodgment from the pancreatic duct. Keeping
the elevator in the closed (or up) position may also help stabilize
the guidewire in place during serial dilator exchanges.

Step 5B: Guidewire Rendezvous

Antegrade exit of the guidewire from the pancreatic duct through
the papilla or the pancreatico-enterostomy can be used to facilitate retrograde cannulation via a rendezvous technique. The
echoendoscope is removed leaving the guidewire in place. A
duodenoscope (or colonoscopy/enteroscope in altered GI anatomy) is advanced toward the papilla or pancreatico-enterostomy
anastomosis alongside the guidewire. Guidewire position is monitored under fluoroscopy throughout endoscope exchange. Upon
reaching the ampulla, rendezvous cannulation of the pancreatic
duct can be achieved in two ways: (1) the guidewire is retrieved
with a snare or forceps and gradually withdrawn through the
working channel of the endoscope while an assistant feeds
additional guidewire via the mouth (classic rendezvous); or (2)
a sphincterotome or cannula loaded with a second guidewire is
placed alongside the EUS-delivered guidewire (parallel rendezvous). Classic rendezvous allows dual traction from both ends of
the guidewire, which greatly facilitates stent placement across
tight strictures. Parallel rendezvous avoids endoscope exchange
and risk of guidewire dislodgment. A common practice is to start
by parallel and cross over to classic rendezvous if unsuccessful.

Step 6: Stent Placement

Straight plastic stents, usually 7F, are placed into the upstream
pancreatic duct across the pancreatic parenchyma and GI wall
to effectively decompress the pancreas duct. Tapered single pigtail plastic stents appear to be easier to insert than double pigtail
plastic stents. During transmural stent insertion, the axis and
plane of access are monitored under EUS, the position of the first
end of the stent (intraductal in transmural and intraluminal in
antegrade EUS-PD) is monitored under fluoroscopy, and the position of the second end of the stent is monitored endoscopically.

POSTPROCEDURE

Following sedation, patients should be monitored for 2 to 3 hours for any anesthesia-related or immediate postprocedure adverse events. Depending on practice settings, EUS-PD can be performed as an outpatient or inpatient procedure. Follow-up procedures are typically scheduled as outpatient procedures.

FOLLOW-UP

Duration of follow-up, interventions performed (stent removal, exchange, or upsizing), and their time intervals after index EUS-PD are not standardized. Follow-up of rendezvous EUS-PD mirrors the pattern of pancreatic ERCP, ranging from just one follow-up procedure for stent removal, to several stent exchanges until duct remodeling is achieved. Transmural EUS-PD can be converted to transpapillary (antegrade or retrograde) EUS-PD at a follow-up procedure, in some cases. Alternatively, a permanent fistula can be created by periodic exchange and/or upsizing of transmural stents at 3- to 8-month intervals over 12 to 24 months.[3,12] Although periodic stent exchange is the most common management approach, it is unclear if stents can be indefinitely left in situ in select patients.[13]

ADVERSE EVENTS

1. Severe self-limiting (24 hours) abdominal pain requiring IV analgesia without overt pancreatitis or perforation is common (10% to 20%).
2. Perforation, pancreatic duct leak with pseudocyst formation or pancreatic ascites, abscess, and severe acute pancreatitis remain a possibility (1%).
3. Bleeding.
4. Stent migration occurs in approximately 10%, most commonly outward stent migration; however, stent passage is usually asymptomatic. Inward stent migration occurs rarely.

References

1. Perez-Miranda M, de la Serna C, Diez-Redondo P, et al. Endosonography-guided cholangiopancreatography as a salvage drainage procedure for obstructed biliary and pancreatic ducts. *World J Gastrointest Endosc.* 2010;2:212-222.
2. Shah JN, Marson F, Weilert F, et al. Single-operator, single-session EUS-guided anterograde cholangiopancreatography in failed ERCP or inaccessible papilla. *Gastrointest Endosc.* 2012;75:56-64.
3. Matsunami Y, Itoi T, Sofuni A, et al. Evaluation of a new stent for EUS-guided pancreatic duct drainage: long-term follow-up outcome. *Endosc Int Open.* 2018;6:E505-E512.
4. Kinney TP, Li R, Gupta K, et al. Therapeutic pancreatic endoscopy after Whipple resection requires rendezvous access. *Endoscopy.* 2009;41:898-901.

5. Wehrmann T, Riphaus A, Frenz MB, et al. Endoscopic pancreatic duct stenting for relief of pancreatic cancer pain. *Eur J Gastroenterol Hepatol.* 2005;12:1395-1400.

6. Oh D, Park DH, Cho MK, et al. Feasibility and safety of a fully covered self-expandable metal stent with antimigration properties for EUSguided pancreatic duct drainage: early and midterm outcomes (with video). *Gastrointest Endosc.* 2016;83:366-373.

7. ASGE Standards of Practice Committee. Adverse events associated with ERCP. *Gastrointest Endosc.* 2017;85:32-47.

8. Nakai Y, Isayama H, Matsubara S, et al. A novel "hitch-and-ride" deep biliary cannulation method during rendezvous endoscopic ultrasound-guided ERCP technique. *Endoscopy.* 2017;49:983-988.

9. Vila JJ, Pérez-Miranda M, Vazquez-Sequeiros E, et al. Initial experience with EUS-guided cholangiopancreatography for biliary and pancreatic duct drainage: a Spanish national survey. *Gastrointest Endosc.* 2012;76:1133-1141.

10. Barkay O, Sherman S, McHenry L, et al. Therapeutic EUS-assisted endoscopic retrograde pancreatography after failed pancreatic duct cannulation at ERCP. *Gastrointest Endosc.* 2010;71:1166-1173.

11. Vila J, Huertas C, Gonçalves B, et al. A novel method for endoscopic ultrasound-guided pancreatic rendezvous with a microcatheter. *Endoscopy.* 2015;47:E575-E576.

12. Tessier G, Bories E, Arvanitakis M, et al. EUS-guided pancreatogastrostomy and pancreatobulbostomy for the treatment of pain in patients with pancreatic ductal dilatation inaccessible for transpapillary endoscopic therapy. *Gastrointest Endosc.* 2007;65:233-241.

13. Kahaleh M, Artifon ELA, Perez-Miranda M, et al. Endoscopic ultrasonography guided biliary drainage: summary of consortium meeting, May 7th 2011, Chicago. *World J Gastroenterol.* 2013;19:1372-1379.

PART SEVEN

Endoscopic Therapy for Hemostasis

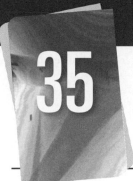

35 Injection Therapy for Hemostasis

Jessica X. Yu, MD, MS

Injection therapy in the field of gastroenterology is the directed delivery of a liquid agent into the wall of the gastrointestinal (GI) tract or adjacent structures.[1] This is utilized for a variety of indications including, but not limited to, the following: to treat GI bleeding from lesions in the upper and lower GI tract; to deliver medications such as botulinum toxin to the lower esophageal sphincter to treat achalasia, corticosteroids for esophageal strictures; to inject tattooing agents such as India ink submucosally to mark an area; and to inject saline submucosally to lift a lesion prior to endoscopic removal.[1] This chapter will focus on applications of injection therapy for nonvariceal bleeding.

Endoscopic injection is used for the treatment of actively bleeding lesions and to prevent rebleeding from lesions with high-risk stigmata. Dilute epinephrine is most commonly used and works through a combination of tamponade by volume effect, vasoconstriction, and direct effect on clotting cascade.[2] Epinephrine injection is highly effective for achieving hemostasis and has been found to decrease the rebleeding rate, need for surgery, and mortality rate for peptic ulcer bleeding.[3] Epinephrine injection with a second modality such as clipping or cautery further reduces these risks compared to epinephrine injection alone[4] and is thus recommended for definitive therapy.[5-8] Other injection agents such as sclerosants and glues work through direct tissue effect; however, they are less well studied and associated with higher adverse events rates compared to epinephrine.[9] Details of the injection procedure are described below.

INDICATIONS

1. Treat actively bleeding lesions and prevent rebleeding of lesions with high-risk stigmata.

CONTRAINDICATIONS

1. See contraindications to upper (Chapter 5) and lower endoscopy (Chapters 8 and 9)
2. Known hypersensitivity to hemostatic agent

PREPARATION

1. See upper endoscopy (Chapter 5) or lower endoscopy (Chapters 8 and 9).
2. Assess hemodynamics and resuscitate. Blood transfusion target Hgb >7 (higher if other comorbidities such as coronary artery disease).[10]
3. Risk stratification should be performed to determine timing of endoscopic evaluation.
4. Initiate adjunctive medical therapy for nonvariceal upper GI bleeding. Intravenous proton pump inhibitor has been shown to decrease the rate of high-risk stigmata on endoscopy.[11] Promotility agents (intravenous erythromycin) can be given preendoscopy and has been shown to decrease the need for repeat endoscopies.[12]
5. Correct coagulopathy or thrombocytopenia. Consider hemostasis if international normalized ratio (INR) is between 1.5 and 2.5 with or without concomitant reversal. Reversal should be attempted for patients with INR > 2.5.[13] Platelet transfusion should be given for patients with active bleeding and platelets <50,000. Platelet transfusion has not been found to be beneficial in patients who are on antiplatelet agents (aspirin, clopidogrel) but do not have thrombocytopenia.[14]

EQUIPMENT

1. Appropriate endoscope, lubricant, personal protective equipment (gown, gloves, mask with visor), working intravenous (IV) equipment, sedation medications.
2. Disposable injection needle within sheath (21- to 25-g, 4- to 6-mm needle, various sheath lengths available) (Fig. 35.1). These are supplied by a variety of manufacturers. There are no published studies comparing different injection needles.[1,15]
3. A variety of agents are available (Table 35.1). For nonvariceal GI bleeding, dilute epinephrine (1:10,000, 1:20,000) is commonly used. Epinephrine may be used in combination with another agent. The agent of choice is drawn up in 5- to 10-mL syringes.

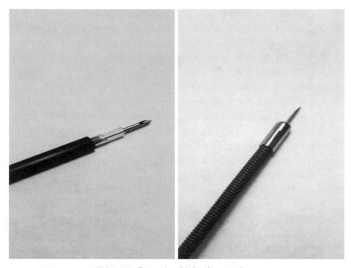

FIG. 35.1 Example of injection needles.

PROCEDURE

1. Perform diagnostic endoscopy to locate the source of bleeding.
2. Have the assistant attach the syringe with the hemostatic agent of choice to the end of the injection device, and prime the device with the hemostatic agent until a few drops of fluid are seen to exit the needle.

TABLE 35.1	Strength and Dosages of Hemostatic Agents for Gastrointestinal Bleeding		
Hemostatic Agent	**Strength**	**Standard Dose/Site**	**Maximal Total Dose**
Epinephrine	1 mg/mL diluted 1:10,000 or 1:20,000 in normal saline	0.5-2 mL	Unknown, up to 25 mL safe
Ethanol	98%	0.1- 0.5 mL	2 mL
Ethanolamine oleate	5%	1-2 mL	20 mL
Morrhuate sodium	50 mg/mL	1-5 mL	20 mL
Sodium tetradecyl sulfate	1%	0.5-2 mL	10 mL
Polidocanol	1%	0.5-1 mL	5 mL
N-butyl cyanoacrylate	1:1 with Lipiodol	1 mL	6 mL

Data from Bucci C, Rotondano G, Marmo R. Injection and cautery methods for nonvariceal bleeding control. *Gastrointest Endosc Clin N Am.* 2015;25:509-522; Park WG, Yeh RW, Triadafilopoulos G. Injection therapies for nonvariceal bleeding disorders of the GI tract. *Gastrointest Endosc.* 2007;66:343-354; and Croffie J, Somogyi L, Chuttani R, et al. Sclerosing agents for use in GI endoscopy. *Gastrointest Endosc.* 2007;66:1-6.

3. Pass the injection device through the working channel until the tip of the sheath comes into endoscopic view. Difficulty may be encountered if the endoscope is in a looped or retroflexed position, and the endoscope may need to be repositioned to allow for advancement of the device.[1]

4. Select the site around the bleeding lesion for injection.

5. Have the assistant advance the tip of the needle beyond the sheath. The assistant, via appropriate mechanism (varies by brand) on the device handle, can adjust the length of the needle protruding from the sheath. The endoscopist then advances the sheath to place the needle tip into the submucosa at the site chosen for injection.

6. Have the assistant push the end of the syringe to deliver the hemostatic agent. If the needle tip is placed appropriately in the submucosa, elevation of the mucosa will be noted. If the needle is too deep, no change will be observed. If the needle is too shallow, liquid will run onto the mucosa. Adjust the needle tip location accordingly and have the assistant push the desired volume (Table 35.1).

7. Have the assistant retract the needle into the sheath.

8. Repeat steps 4 to 7 until either hemostasis is achieved or a maximum volume of hemostatic agent felt to be safe has been delivered (Table 35.1). Four-quadrant injection of 0.5 to 2.0 mL each are delivered. Repeat injection until blanching of the tissue and bleeding cessation is achieved. Smaller volumes (5 to 10 mL) are generally used to limit systemic side effects.[9] Larger volumes (>30 mL) have been reported in small studies to have lower rates of rebleeding compared to smaller volumes but were not associated with no difference in need for surgery, hospital length of stay, or mortality.[16,17] Moreover, larger volumes have been associated with cardiovascular and hemodynamic effects, though this is mainly seen with esophageal injections.[18,19]

9. Retract the needle into the sheath prior to removing the entire injection device from the endoscope to avoid damaging the working channel of the scope with the needle.

10. A second modality of hemostasis should be applied for certain indications[5-8](see Chapters 36 and 37).

POSTPROCEDURE

1. Monitor vital signs.

2. Follow hemoglobin and hematocrit to evaluate efficacy of treatment.

3. If evidence of rebleeding is observed, the endoscopist may need to repeat the procedure or obtain intervention by a surgeon and/or an interventional radiologist.

ADVERSE EVENTS

The following are potential adverse events:
1. Allergic reaction
2. Perforation
3. Laceration
4. Rebleeding

Adverse event rates are low and vary by agent and site of injection.[1] For example, sclerosant and ethanol injection can cause tissue damage and lead to necrosis and perforation. Cyanoacrylate injection has been associated with arterial embolization.[2,9]

Other uses for this technique include:
1. To tattoo lesion or site
2. To lift lesion prior to endoscopic mucosal resection
3. To inject botulinum toxin for patients with achalasia, gastroparesis, or anal fissure
4. To inject steroids into refractory strictures
5. To treat varices

CPT CODES

43236—Upper gastrointestinal endoscopy including esophagus, stomach, and either the duodenum and/or jejunum as appropriate; diagnostic, with submucosal injection

43255—Upper gastrointestinal endoscopy including esophagus, stomach, and either the duodenum and/or jejunum as appropriate; with control of bleeding, any method

45334—Sigmoidoscopy, flexible; with control of bleeding, any method

45335—Sigmoidoscopy, flexible; with submucosal injection

45381—Colonoscopy, flexible, proximal to splenic flexure; with submucosal injection

45382—Colonoscopy, flexible, proximal to splenic flexure; with control of bleeding, any method

64640—Destruction by a neurolytic agent; other peripheral nerve or branch

References

1. Nelson DB, Bosco JJ, Curtis WD, et al. ASGE technology status evaluation report. Injection needles. February 1999. American Society for Gastrointestinal Endoscopy. *Gastrointest Endosc*. 1999;50:928-931.
2. Bucci C, Rotondano G, Marmo R. Injection and cautery methods for nonvariceal bleeding control. *Gastrointest Endosc Clin N Am*. 2015;25:509-522.
3. Chung SC, Leung JW, Steele RJ, et al. Endoscopic injection of adrenaline for actively bleeding ulcers: a randomised trial. *Br Med J (Clin Res Ed)*. 1988;296:1631-1633.
4. Vergara M, Bennett C, Calvet X, et al. Epinephrine injection versus epinephrine injection and a second endoscopic method in high-risk bleeding ulcers. *Cochrane Database Syst Rev*. 2014;(10):CD005584.

5. Strate LL, Gralnek IM. ACG clinical guideline: management of patients with acute lower gastrointestinal bleeding. *Am J Gastroenterol*. 2016;111:755.

6. Laine L, Jensen DM. Management of patients with ulcer bleeding. *Am J Gastroenterol* 2012;107:345-360; quiz 361.

7. Hwang JH, Fisher DA, Ben-Menachem T, et al. The role of endoscopy in the management of acute non-variceal upper GI bleeding. *Gastrointest Endosc*. 2012;75:1132-1138.

8. Pasha SF, Shergill A, Acosta RD, et al. The role of endoscopy in the patient with lower GI bleeding. *Gastrointest Endosc*. 2014;79:875-885.

9. Park WG, Yeh RW, Triadafilopoulos G. Injection therapies for nonvariceal bleeding disorders of the GI tract. *Gastrointest Endosc*. 2007;66:343-354.

10. Villanueva C, Colomo A, Bosch A, et al. Transfusion strategies for acute upper gastrointestinal bleeding. *N Engl J Med*. 2013;368:11-21.

11. Sreedharan A, Martin J, Leontiadis GI, et al. Proton pump inhibitor treatment initiated prior to endoscopic diagnosis in upper gastrointestinal bleeding. *Cochrane Database Syst Rev*. 2010:CD005415.

12. Barkun AN, Bardou M, Martel M, et al. Prokinetics in acute upper GI bleeding: a meta-analysis. *Gastrointest Endosc*. 2010;72:1138-1145.

13. Acosta RD, Abraham NS, Chandrasekhara V, et al. The management of antithrombotic agents for patients undergoing GI endoscopy. *Gastrointest Endosc*. 2016;83:3-16.

14. Zakko L, Rustagi T, Douglas M, et al. No benefit from platelet transfusion for gastrointestinal bleeding in patients taking antiplatelet agents. *Clin Gastroenterol Hepatol*. 2017;15:46-52.

15. Conway JD, Adler DG, Diehl DL, et al. Endoscopic hemostatic devices. *Gastrointest Endosc*. 2009;69:987-996.

16. Park CH, Lee SJ, Park JH, et al. Optimal injection volume of epinephrine for endoscopic prevention of recurrent peptic ulcer bleeding. *Gastrointest Endosc*. 2004;60:875-880.

17. Lin HJ, Hsieh YH, Tseng GY, et al. A prospective, randomized trial of large- versus small-volume endoscopic injection of epinephrine for peptic ulcer bleeding. *Gastrointest Endosc*. 2002;55:615-619.

18. Schlag C, Karagianni A, Grimm M, et al. Hemodynamics after endoscopic submucosal injection of epinephrine in a porcine model. *Endoscopy*. 2012;44:154-160.

19. von Delius S, Thies P, Umgelter A, et al. Hemodynamics after endoscopic submucosal injection of epinephrine in patients with nonvariceal upper gastrointestinal bleeding: a matter of concern. *Endoscopy*. 2006;38:1284-1288.

20. Croffie J, Somogyi L, Chuttani R, et al. Sclerosing agents for use in GI endoscopy. *Gastrointest Endosc*. 2007;66:1-6.

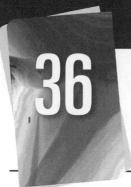

36

Bipolar Probe, Heater Probe, and Argon Plasma Coagulation

Anoop Prabhu, MD

THERMAL THERAPIES—BIPOLAR PROBE AND HEATER PROBE

Thermal therapy remains a cornerstone in the endoscopic management of gastrointestinal bleeding. The mechanism by which thermal therapy achieves hemostasis is related to multiple factors, including coagulation of tissue protein, contraction of vessels, edema, coaptation, and indirect activation of the coagulation cascade with promotion of intravascular fibrin thrombi.[1] Thermal devices deliver heat to tissues in one of two ways: (1) indirectly by passage of electric current through tissue (i.e., bipolar probe, Fig. 36.1) also called electrosurgery or (2) via direct heat transfer (i.e., heater probe, Fig. 36.2), also called electrocautery.

Bipolar electrosurgery delivers thermal energy by completion of an electrical circuit between two electrodes via non-desiccated tissue. As the bipolar probe contains the ground terminal within the probe, a grounding pad is not needed. As the treated tissue desiccates, the resistance increases, thereby limiting the breadth and depth of tissue injury.[2] Some versions of the probe come with both irrigation as well as an injection needle for application of epinephrine. Optimal technique employs lower power settings (i.e., 15 W) for longer durations (10 to 12 seconds).[3]

The heater probe consists of a Teflon-coated hollow aluminum cylinder with an irrigation port, an inner heating coil, and a distal thermal couple, with the latter maintaining a constant temperature.[4] The Teflon is designed to prevent probe adherence to the developing coagulum. Once treatment is initiated with a foot pedal, the duration of activation cannot be stopped until the entire amount of preselected joules is delivered.[5]

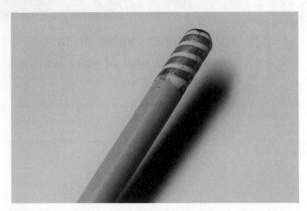

FIG. 36.1 Image of a bipolar probe. (Permission for use granted by Boston Scientific Corporation.)

Both bipolar and heater probe require application of pressure to the target tissue to ensure coaptive sealing of the vessel walls to obliterate the lumen.

ARGON PLASMA COAGULATION

The argon plasma coagulation (APC) delivery catheter is a monopolar, noncontact probe which both emits inert argon gas and contains an electrode that ionizes this gas flow. When inert argon is ionized, it is converted to argon plasma which is conducted by an "arc" to the nearest tissue, producing coagulation necrosis to a depth of penetration of approximately 2 to 3 mm. The directionality of the argon plasma flow can be axial, circumferential (Fig. 36.3), or perpendicular ("side fire"). In the

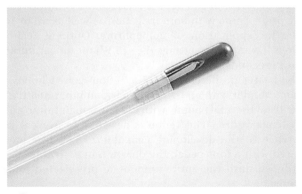

FIG. 36.2 Image of a heater probe. (Image Courtesy of Olympus America Inc.)

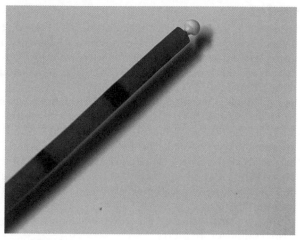

FIG. 36.3 Image of a circumferential APC probe. (© Erbe Elektromedizin GmbH.)

application of APC, carbonization (or "char") should be kept to a minimum. Inadvertent contact with tissue can cause pneumatosis as a result of intramural dissection of argon gas.

INDICATIONS

1. To treat actively bleeding lesions or lesions at high risk for future bleeding including ulcers, arteriovenous malformations (AVM)s, Dieulafoy lesions, Mallory-Weiss tears, gastric antral vascular ectasia (GAVE), and culprit lesions associated with diverticular haemorrhage
2. To accomplish tissue ablation (primarily with APC) for management of residual abnormal tissue (such as Barrett esophagus or residual adenomas) or prior to endoscopic closure of chronic fistulae/defects

CONTRAINDICATIONS

1. See contraindications to upper endoscopy or colonoscopy (Chapters 5 and 19)
2. Ineffective sedation with inability of patient to remain still during endoscopy
3. Uncorrectable coagulopathy

PREPARATION

1. See preparation for upper endoscopy or colonoscopy (Chapter 5)
2. Correct coagulopathy or thrombocytopenia. Goal of international normalized ratio <1.5, platelet count >50,000
3. Pretest all electrical equipment

EQUIPMENT

1. Appropriate endoscope (if 10-Fr probe to be used, then endoscope must have therapeutic-sized channel), lubricant, personal protective equipment (gown, gloves, mask with visor), working intravenous (IV) equipment, sedation medications
2. Device of choice: 7- or 10-Fr heater probe (Heat Probe, Olympus America, Center Valley, PA) bipolar probe with integrated irrigation (e.g., Gold Probe, Boston Scientific, Natick, MA; Bicap Superconducter, ConMed, Chelmsford, MA; Quicksilver, Cook Medical, Winston-Salem, NC; SolarProbe, Olympus America, Center Valley, PA; or Bipolar probe, US Endoscopy, Mentor, OH), or argon plasma catheter (APC or FiAPC, ERBE USA, Marietta, GA)
3. Appropriate electrosurgical generator with foot pedal control
4. Normal saline for irrigation

PROCEDURE

1. Perform diagnostic endoscopy to locate the source of bleeding or lesion to treat. The endoscopist may choose to use thermal monotherapy or injection therapy prior to thermal therapy.
2. Remove adherent blood clots to optimize visualization of the exact bleeding site. If there is concern for provocation of bleeding with clot removal, injection of 1:10,000 epinephrine around the site prior to clot removal can be considered.

Bipolar Probe

1. Attach a bipolar probe to both the electrosurgical unit and irrigation system filled with normal saline.
2. Turn on the electrosurgical device, and set the power to: 12 to 16 W for active bleeding, visible vessel, Dieulafoy lesion, postpolypectomy ulcer, and bleeding diverticulum; 10 to 14 W for bleeding and nonbleeding AVMs; 12 to 14 W for a bleeding Mallory-Weiss tear.
3. Advance the bipolar probe through the working channel of the endoscope.
4. The tip may be applied directly or tangentially to the lesion, but good apposition of the tip to tissue is necessary.
5. Depress the foot pedal to deliver current, and keep the tip in place with firm pressure for 5 to 10 seconds depending on the type, size, and depth of the lesion. Good therapy for visible vessels is indicated by a depression (or "footprint") at the site suggesting coaptation.

6. Either directly remove the probe or use irrigation to remove the tip from the tissue if the coagulum from the tissue is adherent to the probe.
7. Repeat steps 4 through 6 until coagulation/hemostasis is achieved.

Heater Probe

1. Attach both the heater probe and irrigation bottle to the generator.
2. Set the generator to deliver the appropriate amount of energy (20 to 30 J/pulse for visible vessels, 5 to 10 J/pulse for AVMs).
3. Advance the heater probe through the working channel of the endoscope.
4. The tip may be applied directly or tangentially to the lesion, but good apposition of the tip to tissue is necessary.
5. Repeat step 4 until coagulation/hemostasis is achieved. Previous studies have suggested a total of four 30 J pulses per tamponade station.[6]

Argon Plasma Coagulation

1. Attach the APC catheter to the argon plasma source.
2. Set the generator to deliver the appropriate amount of argon gas flow rate and wattage (1.4 L/min, 40 to 50 W for stomach and rectum, 0.8 L/min, 20 to 30 W for right colon and small bowel, respectively).
3. Advance the APC catheter through the working channel of the endoscope.
4. The catheter may be directed immediately in front (with axial probe) or tangentially to (with sidefire or circumferential probe) the lesion, but direct tissue contact with the probe should be avoided.
5. Depress the foot pedal to deliver the argon plasma to achieve coagulation and dessication. Care should be taken to keep carbonization (or "charring") to a minimum.
6. Suction should be used intermittently as argon gas accumulation within the lumen can predispose to barotrauma and even perforation.
7. Repeat steps 4 through 6 until coagulation/hemostasis is achieved.

POSTPROCEDURE

1. Monitor vital signs.
2. For inpatients, if the lesion has been actively bleeding or remains at high risk for rebleeding, follow the hemoglobin and

hematocrit trend every 6 to 12 hours to evaluate treatment efficacy.

3. If there is evidence of rebleeding, the procedure may need to be repeated or may require consultation with interventional radiology or surgery.

ADVERSE EVENTS

1. Precipitation of bleeding: up to 5% with heater probe and 18% with bipolar electrocautery.[4]

2. Perforation: 1.8% to 3% with heater probe; rarely in upper gastrointestinal lesions and up to 2.5% in right-colon AVMs with bipolar electrocautery.[4] For APC, rates have been reported anywhere from 0.2% to 3.7%.[7,8]

3. Bowel explosion: a rare complication reported with APC use, thought to be related to probe contact with mucosa combined with poor colon prep.[9]

CPT CODES

43227—Esophagoscopy, flexible, transoral; with control of bleeding, any method

43258—Esophagogastroduodenoscopy, flexible, transoral; with control of bleeding, any method

44366—Small intestinal endoscopy, enteroscopy beyond second portion of duodenum, not including ileum; with control of bleeding (e.g., injection, bipolar cautery, unipolar cautery, laser, heater probe, stapler, plasma coagulator)

44378—Small intestinal endoscopy, enteroscopy beyond second portion of duodenum including ileum; with control of bleeding (e.g., injection, bipolar cautery, unipolar cautery, laser, heater probe, stapler, plasma coagulator)

44391—Colonoscopy through stoma; with control of bleeding, any method

45334—Sigmoidoscopy, flexible; with control of bleeding, any method

45382—Colonoscopy, flexible; with control of bleeding, any method

References

1. Wara P, Berg V, Jacobsen NO, Casalnuovo C, Amdrup E. Possible mechanism of hemostasis effected by electrocoagulation. *Endoscopy*. 1984;16(2):43-46.
2. Laine L. Therapeutic endoscopy and bleeding ulcers. Bipolar/multipolar electrocoagulation. *Gastrointest Endosc*. 1990;36(5 suppl):S38-S41.
3. Morris ML, Tucker RD, Baron TH, Song LM. Electrosurgery in gastrointestinal endoscopy: principles to practice. *Am J Gastroenterol*. 2009;104(6):1563-1574.
4. Asge Technology C, Conway JD, Adler DG, et al. Endoscopic hemostatic devices. *Gastrointest Endosc*. 2009;69(6):987-996.

5. Fullarton GM, Birnie GG, Macdonald A, Murray WR. Controlled trial of heater probe treatment in bleeding peptic ulcers. *Br J Surg*. 1989;76(6):541-544.
6. Jensen DM. Heat probe for hemostasis of bleeding peptic ulcers: technique and results of randomized controlled trials. *Gastrointest Endosc*. 1990;36(5 suppl):S42-S49.
7. Herrera S, Bordas JM, Llach J, et al. The beneficial effects of argon plasma coagulation in the management of different types of gastric vascular ectasia lesions in patients admitted for GI hemorrhage. *Gastrointest Endosc*. 2008;68(3):440-446.
8. Peng Y, Wang H, Feng J, et al. Efficacy and safety of argon plasma coagulation for hemorrhagic chronic radiation proctopathy: a systematic review. *Gastroenterol Res Pract*. 2018;2018:3087603.
9. Ben Soussan E, Mathieu N, Roque I, Antonietti M. Bowel explosion with colonic perforation during argon plasma coagulation for hemorrhagic radiation-induced proctitis. *Gastrointest Endosc*. 2003;57(3):412-413.

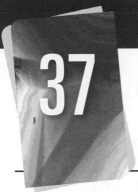

Clips and Loops

Hiroyuki Aihara, MD, PhD

The use of clip in endoscopy was first reported by Hayashi et al in 1975.[1] Currently, clips are used for multiple indications including hemostasis for active bleeding, prophylactic mucosal defect closure after endoscopic mucosal resection (EMR), perforation closure, and preoperative marking.

The use of endoscopic loop was first reported by Hachisu et al[2] in 1991 for the removal of large pedunculated polyps.

INDICATIONS
Endoclips (Fig. 37.1)
1. Hemostasis for active bleeding (ulcers, diverticula, etc.)
2. Prophylactic mucosal defect closure after polypectomy or EMR
3. Closure of small gastrointestinal (GI) tract luminal perforations
4. Endoscopic preoperative marking to assist surgical identification

Endoloops (Fig. 37.2)
1. Prevention of post-polypectomy bleeding for pedunculated polyps (Paris Ip)
2. Removal of subepithelial tumors (SETs) with or without retrieval of specimens[3]

CONTRAINDICATIONS
Endoclips
Any GI varices with or without bleeding.

Endoloops
Lesions without enough stalk length for polypectomy (Paris Isp, Is, IIa, IIc, or SETs showing extraluminal growth pattern).

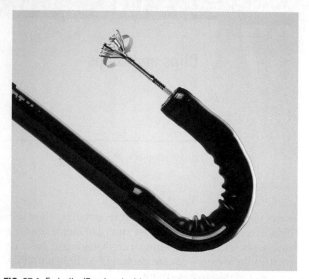

FIG. 37.1 Endoclip. (Reprinted with permission from Olympus America, Inc.)

PREPARATION

1. The patient should be kept nil per os (NPO) for 4 to 6 hours prior to the procedure.
2. Patients with gastrointestinal bleeding should be adequately resuscitated.

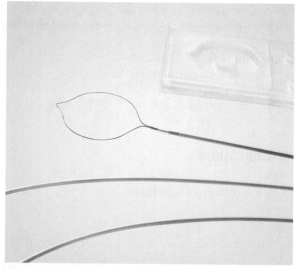

FIG. 37.2 Endoloop. (Reprinted with permission from Olympus America, Inc.)

3. The operator of endoclips and endoloops must be physician or medical personnel under the supervision of a physician and must have received sufficient training in the maneuver of these devices.

EQUIPMENT

1. An endoscope with at least a 2.8 mm accessory channel
2. Choose an appropriate-length loading device depending on whether a gastroscope or a colonoscope is used

PROCEDURE

Endoclips

1. Identify the lesion to be clipped. If a large amount of blood is obscuring visualization, consider repositioning the patient for a better visualization of the area. If the area is not fully visualized because of gastric or colonic folds, consider using an attachment cap.
2. Position the target lesion enface.
3. Advance the clipping device through the accessory channel of the endoscope. Do not force the instrument if resistance to insertion is encountered. Reduce the angulation of the endoscope until the instrument passes smoothly. Attempting to force the instrument could cause injury in the GI tract, such as perforation, bleeding, or mucosal damage. It could also damage the endoscope and/or clip.
4. Bring the clip into endoscopic view, and advance the endoscope toward the target lesion. Place it at 6-o'clock position in the endoscopic field by applying torque to the scope.
5. Have the assistant open the clip arms to their maximum width. Then have the assistant to rotate the clip to a best position. Reposition the sheath and the endoscope to the optimal position.
6. Advance the entire device to allow the fully extended clips to surround the target lesion, and gently press against the surrounding tissue.
7. Ask the GI assistant to close and deploy the clip around the lesion.
8. Evaluate the target lesion and the site of clip deployment, and repeat this sequence as needed.

Endoloops (Fig. 37.3)

1. Identify the pedunculated lesion that will be snared, and place it at the 6-o'clock position in the endoscopic field.
2. Advance the preassembled loop-loading device with the attached loop through the accessory channel of the endoscope. Do not insert the instrument into the endoscope if the loop is not completely retracted into the tube sheath.

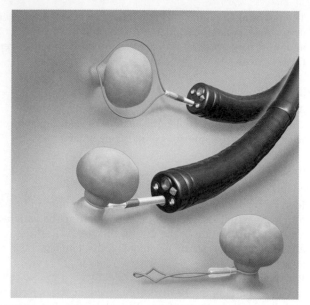

FIG. 37.3 Maneuver of endoloop. (Reprinted with permission from Olympus America, Inc.)

3. Once the sheath with retracted loop is in endoscopic view, advance the endoscope toward the target lesion.

4. Ask the assistant to slowly extend the loop out of the sheath until the size of the loop reaches optimal size in relation to the lesion.

5. Maneuver the nylon loop and the endoscope so that the loop fully surrounds the lesion. Carefully bring down the loop so it rests around the stalk of the lesion.

6. Ask the assistant to close the loop by pulling on the slider of the loading device until resistance is felt. It is important not to apply excessive force when ligating the lesion stalk, as this can inadvertently cut the stalk of the lesion and result in arterial bleeding.

7. Ask the assistant to push the slider until it touches the clamping ring. This will extend the hook from the sheath.

8. Ask the assistant to detach the loop from the hook to deploy the loop.

9. After adequate ligation pressure is seen, as evidenced by bluish discoloration of the lesion, use a standard polypectomy snare to remove the lesion.

10. Place the polypectomy snare around the stalk a few millimeters above the previously placed endoloop. The snare should not contact the endoloop, as this can lead to their becoming

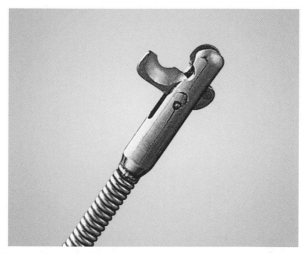

FIG. 37.4 Loop cutter. (Reprinted with permission from Olympus America, Inc.)

fused. This may produce difficulty disengaging the snare or lead to premature cutting of the endoloop with resultant bleeding. This step can be skipped if retrieval of specimen is not planned, especially for SETs.

11. Any unnecessary part of the loop can be cut using the loop cutter (Fig. 37.4).

POSTPROCEDURE PATIENT OBSERVATION

1. Resuscitation and supportive care should continue in cases of GI bleeding.
2. Patients with perforations successfully closed with clipping should be watched for signs of peritonitis or clinical deterioration. These symptoms indicate failure of the clipping to seal the perforation and would necessitate prompt surgical evaluation. Prophylactic antibiotics and NPO should be instituted to assist in sealing the perforation and to prevent peritoneal infection.
3. Loops placed prophylactically on large lesions can prematurely dislodge; therefore, patients should be instructed to contact the endoscopist for any signs of lower GI bleeding.

References

1. Hayashi T, Yonezawa M, Kuwabara T, Kudoh I. The study on staunch clip for the treatment by endoscopy. *Gastroenterol Endosc.* 1975;17:92-101.
2. Hachisu T. A new detachable snare for hemostasis in the removal of large polyps or other elevated lesions. *Surg Endosc.* 1991;5:70-74.
3. Lee SH, Park JH, Park DH, et al. Endoloop ligation of large pedunculated submucosal tumors (with videos). *Gastrointest Endosc.* 2008;67:556-560.

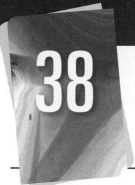

38

Injection Therapy of Esophageal and Gastric Varices

Edward Villa, MD
Uzma D. Siddiqui, MD

Gastrointestinal (GI) variceal bleeding is the most common lethal complication of cirrhosis and accounts for 10% to 30% of all upper GI bleeding. Varices develop at a rate of roughly 8% per year in cirrhotic patients and are present in as many as 50% of cirrhotic patients (5% to 33% in the case of gastric varices).[1] Variceal hemorrhage (VH) occurs at a yearly rate of 5% to 15% (25% in 2 years for gastric varices). Mortality at 6 weeks from first esophageal VH is 20% at 6 weeks, and late rebleeding occurs in about 60% of untreated patients within 1 to 2 years of index hemorrhage.[1]

SCLEROSIS

Sclerosants are tissue irritants that cause vascular thrombosis and endothelial damage, which lead to endofibrosis and vascular obliteration. The sclerosants most commonly used that are available in the United States are fatty acid derivatives (such as ethanolamine oleate, 5% [Ethamolin, QOL Medical, Inc, Woodinville, Sash] and sodium morrhuate, 5% [Scleromate, Glenwood LLC, Englewood, NJ]) or synthetic agents (sodium tetradecyl sulfate, 1% and 3% [Sotradecol, Bioniche Life Sciences, LLC, Belleville, Ontario, Canada; Trombovein, Omega Pharmaceuticals Ltd., Montreal, Quebec, Canada; and Fibro-vein, STD Pharmaceutical, Hereford, England]).[2]

Sclerotherapy has historically been used for bleeding and nonbleeding esophageal varices and for gastric varices extending into the lesser curvature (type 1 gastroesophageal varices [GOV-1] by Sarin Classification) but has largely been supplanted by variceal ligation (VL). Studies have demonstrated that sclerotherapy results in higher mortality compared to sham therapy for primary prophylaxis of esophageal VH.[3,4] There is a 6-month survival of 84% with serial sclerotherapy when combined with vasoactive medications in control esophageal VH, but VL still has been shown to be superior to sclerotherapy with regard to outcomes of rebleeding, variceal eradication, and the rate of complications.[5-7] Adverse events include fever, infections, retrosternal discomfort/pain, dysphagia, injection-induced bleeding, esophageal ulceration with delayed bleeding, esophageal strictures, perforation, mediastinitis, pleural effusion, and bronchoesophageal fistulae.[8]

CYANOACRYLATE INJECTION

Injection with cyanoacrylate variants such as N-butyl-2-cyanoacrylate (cyanoacrylate, enbucrilate, or Histoacryl [B. Braun, Melsungen, Germany]) and 2-octyl cyanoacrylate (Dermabond [Ethicon, Somerville, NJ]) have been utilized in an off-label use in the United States as a successful therapeutic modality for treatment of patients with bleeding type 2 gastroesophageal varices (GOV-2) and isolated fundal varices (IGV-1). Cyanoacrylate (CA) is a monomer in liquid form that upon contact with hydroxyl ions in water or blood rapidly polymerizes into a hard plastic or glue, which results in hemostasis of VH. CA can be injected in combination with a contrast agent (Lipiodol or Ethiodol) for prevention of polymerization within the injection needle and for X-ray visualization.[9]

Injection of CA has resulted in resolution of gastric VH in 87% to 100%; reduction in rebleeding in IGV-1's (85.7%); and eradication of varices in 67.8% to 100%.[10-12] Recurrent bleeding occurred in 23.3% to 35.2% of patients. Among these, 16.7% were successfully retreated with repeat injection, and there was a treatment failure–related mortality rate of 2.2% to 23.7%.[10-12] CA injection is superior to VL with regard to hemostasis and rebleeding rates in GOV-1 and IGV-1 hemorrhage.[11,12]

Most studies quote a 0.5% to 5% adverse event rate.[12-14] Adverse events include fever, rebleeding, ulceration at the injection site, hemothorax, thromboembolic events (pulmonary emboli, stroke, myocardial infarction, other systemic arterial embolizations, portal and mesenteric venous thrombosis, etc.), fistulization, spontaneous bacterial peritonitis, bacteremia, and pneumonia. The use of endoscopic ultrasound (EUS) and audible doppler solely to assess gastric variceal obturation does not appear to significantly affect adverse events or clinical outcomes.[15,16] However, the use of EUS-guided coil deployment performed prior to CA injection into the afferent feeding veins of large fundal gastric varices achieved complete obliteration of the perforating veins in fewer sessions than standard CA injection while resulting in fewer adverse events.[17-20] Preprocedural assessment of the portovenous system should be considered to identify patients with spontaneous portosystemic shunt or patent foramen ovale, and if either is discovered, alternate treatment measures should be considered.[14]

SCLEROTHERAPY OF ESOPHAGEAL AND GASTRIC (GOV-1) VARICES

Indications

1. Acute endoscopic hemostasis and elective obliteration of esophageal VH and GOV-1's.

Contraindications

1. A poorly sedated patient or inability to adequately visualize the field due to risk for perforation or bleeding by tearing the injected varix.

Preparation

1. Insert at least two large-bore intravenous (IV) lines for blood products and IV fluids, as needed. Adequately sedate the patient and perform endotracheal intubation.
2. In the setting of an acute variceal bleed, give a bolus and subsequent continuous infusion of antiportal hypertensive medication (typically, octreotide) as well as an approved antibiotic within 30 minutes of the procedure.
3. A balloon tamponade device (i.e., Sengstaken-Blakemore tube) should be readily available.

Equipment

1. Upper endoscope: A therapeutic upper endoscope is preferred because of its larger working channels but can be performed with a standard upper endoscope.
2. Sclerosant drawn up in nondiluted form in a 10-mL syringe prior to endoscopy. The injection needle should be primed with the sclerosant.

Procedure

1. Perform a complete examination of the upper gastrointestinal tract to exclude other nonvariceal sources of bleeding.
2. Advance the upper endoscope to the hemorrhage site, and advance the catheter. Advance the needle, and inject 0.5 and 2.0 mL of sclerosant immediately distal then proximal to the site of hemorrhage until hemostasis is achieved.

Postprocedure Care

1. Observe for signs of rebleeding, pulmonary complications, fever, and esophageal perforation while keeping the patient NPO for at least 4 to 6 hours postprocedure.
2. Consider using topical medications such as sucralfate and acid-reducing agents.

CYANOACRYLATE OBTURATION OF GASTRIC VARICES

Indications

1. Gastric varices (especially GOV-2's and IGV-1's) with active or stigmata of recent hemorrhage.

Contraindications

1. Increased risk of central nervous system (CNS) embolism. This may occur with hepatopulmonary syndrome or cardiac septal defects with right-to-left shunting. Consider assessment of portovenous circulation and/or echocardiogram prior to the procedure.
2. A poorly sedated patient or inability to adequately visualize the field due to risk for perforation or bleeding by tearing the injected varix.

Preparation

1. Insert at least two large-bore IV lines for blood products and IV fluids, as needed. Adequately sedate the patient and perform endotracheal intubation.
2. In the setting of an acute variceal bleed, give a bolus and subsequent continuous infusion of antiportal hypertensive medication (typically, octreotide) as well as an approved antibiotic within 30 minutes of the procedure.
3. A balloon tamponade device (i.e., Sengstaken-Blakemore tube) should be readily available.

Equipment and Additional Preparation

1. Endoscope: A therapeutic upper endoscope or therapeutic EUS scope are preferred because of their larger working channels. This reduces polymerization within the working channel.
2. Squeeze the refrigerated CA out of the plastic vial into a glass vial and mix in 1:1 ratio with Lipiodol or Ethiodol into a plastic syringe to a final volume of 1 mL of the mixture. Stir the mixture gently with a needle used to dispense the oil, and draw 0.5 mL of the mixture into a 3 mL syringe. With 2-octyl cyanoacrylate (Dermabond), the glue can be directly drawn into a syringe and then injected through the needle, followed by sterile water flush to push the substance through the catheter.
3. Prime the injection catheter or EUS needle with sterile water first. Then follow with injection of the cyanoacrylate agents from step #2. Flush with a 10 mL syringe filled with sterile water.

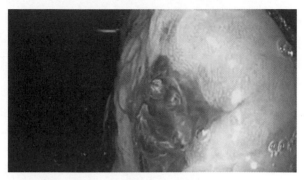

FIG. 38.1 Endoscopic view of an isolated gastric varix.

Procedure

1. Pass the endoscope to bring the fundal varices into view, typically while in the retroflexed position (Fig. 38.1).
2. Irrigate the field, and carefully assess the variceal complex to determine the best site for initial injection (usually to the patient's left as this is the likely "inflow" point).
3. Advance the needle catheter through the working channel, and bring the needle into view. Express a small drop of the mixture to ensure liquidity and absence of premature hardening. Because the cyanoacrylate can polymerize in the cannula, it should not be passed through a pool of blood, as this could cause premature polymerization.
4. Press the needle into the varix at the chosen site (under direct endoscopic or sonographic vision), and rapidly squeeze the water-filled syringe to inject the CA-oil mixture into the variceal lumen in an uninterrupted manner. The varix will swell and turn blue. As the volume reaches 1 to 2 mL (0.5 to 1.0 mL of CA into the varix in every injection), withdraw the needle while there is still flow from the tip, and quickly withdraw the needle cannula. Wait a few minutes for any excess polymer to harden to prevent suctioning hardening glue into the working channel.
5. If performing EUS-guided coil embolization with cyanoacrylate treatment, filling the fundus with water prior to the intervention allows for improved acoustic coupling, which improves endosonographic visualization of the fundal varices and feeder vessels (Fig. 38.2). Measuring the short axis diameter of the varix allows for appropriate selection of coil size. Using a stylet as a pusher, embolization coils can be deployed into the varix through the fine-needle aspiration

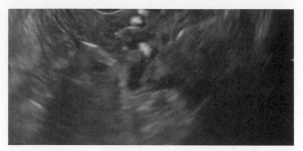

FIG. 38.2 Sonographic view of isolated gastric varix.

(FNA) needle (Fig. 38.3). Typically, one to three embolization coils are injected into the target varix followed by injection of cyanoacrylate until complete obliteration of the varix is noted endosonographically (Fig. 38.4) (Video 38.1).

6. If further hemostasis is necessary, repeat the previous steps with a new injection device.

Postprocedure Care

1. Observe for signs of adverse events, especially rebleeding and embolic events, while keeping the patient NPO for at least 4 to 6 hours postprocedure.

2. Consider using topical medications such as sucralfate and acid-reducing agents.

3. Perform follow-up endoscopy from 24 to 72 hours after the initial session as well as subsequent endoscopies at regular intervals (usually 1 week, 1 month, and then every 3 months for the remaining year), until eradication is confirmed.

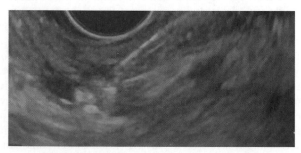

FIG. 38.3 Coil embolization on endoscopic ultrasound.

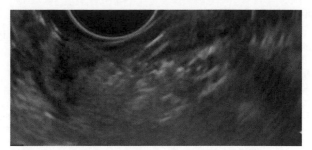

FIG. 38.4 Injection of cyanoacrylate.

Procedural-Related Complications and Adverse Events

1. Premature polymerization: This may occur if precautions are not taken to avoid blood, mucus, or water contact with the CA.
2. Gluing the needle into the varix: This may occur if the needle is not withdrawn as the mixture is flowing. This may require clipping the cannula, removing the scope, and reinserting the scope with endoscopic scissors. Forceful removal of an impacted needle should be avoided, as this may result in severe bleeding.
3. Scope damage: This can result when immediately suctioning the intervention site after injection, as glue can harden within the suction channel. Irrigation of the site with simethicone/water solution and waiting a few minutes prior to suctioning may prevent this problem.
4. Other adverse events: Please refer to the "Cyanoacrylate Injection" section earlier in this chapter for a list of adverse events associated with CA injection.

OTHER USES

1. Bleeding at other sites and enteric fistulae may respond to enbucrilate injection, but these have not been adequately studied.

CPT CODES

43204—Esophagoscopy, flexible, transoral; with injection sclerosis of esophageal varices

43243—Esophagogastroduodenoscopy, flexible, transoral; with injection of esophageal/gastric varices. Upper gastrointestinal endoscopy including esophagus, stomach, and either the duodenum and/or jejunum as appropriate; with injection sclerosis of esophageal and/or gastric varices

Note: Cyanoacrylate injection of gastric varices is not an FDA-approved indication.

ACKNOWLEDGMENT

We thank Dr. Christopher Chapman, MD, for providing the pictures and video used for submission.

References

1. Garcia-Tsao G, Sanyal A, Grace N, Carey W, The Practice Guidelines Committee of the American Association for the Study of Liver Diseases, The Practice Parameters Committee of the American College of Gastroenterology. AASLD Practice Guidelines: prevention and management of the gastroesophageal varices and variceal hemorrhage in cirrhosis. *Hepatology*. 2007;46(3):922-938.

2. Croffie J, Somogyi L, Chuttani R, et al. Sclerosing agents for use in GI endoscopy. *Gastrointest Endosc*. 2007;66(1):1-6.

3. Pagliaro L, D'Amico G, Sorensen T, et al. Prevention of first bleeding in cirrhosis. A meta-analysis of randomized clinical trials of non-surgical treatment. *Ann Intern Med*. 1997;117:59-60.

4. The Veterans Affairs Cooperative Variceal Sclerotherapy Group. Prophylactic sclerotherapy for esophageal varices in men with alcoholic liver disease. A randomized, single-blind, multicenter clinical trial. *N Engl J Med*. 1991;324:1779-1784.

5. Dai C, Liu W, Jiang M, Sun M. Endoscopic variceal ligation compared with endoscopic injection sclerotherapy for treatment of esophageal variceal hemorrhage: a meta-analysis. *World J Gastroenterol*. 2015;21(8):2534-2541.

6. D'Amico G, Pagliaro L, Pietrosi G, Tarantino I. Emergency sclerotherapy versus vasoactive drugs for bleeding oesophageal varices in cirrhotic patients. *Cochrane Database Syst Rev*. 2010;17(3):CD002233. doi:10.1002/14651858. CD002233.pub2.

7. Hwang J, Shergill A, Acosta R, et al. The role of endoscopy in the management of variceal hemorrhage. *Gastrointest Endosc*. 2014;80(2):221-227.

8. Edling J, Bacon B. Pleuropulmonary complications of endoscopic variceal sclerotherapy. *Chest*. 1991;99:1252-1257.

9. Suga T, Akamatsu T, Kawamura Y, et al. Actual behavior of N-butyl-2-cyanoacrylate (Histoacryl) in a blood vessel: a model of the varix. *Endoscopy*. 2002;34(1):73-77.

10. Ríos Castellanos E, Seron P, Gisbert J, Bonfill Cosp X. Endoscopic injection of cyanoacrylate glue versus other endoscopic procedures for acute bleeding gastric varices in people with portal hypertension. *Cochrane Database Syst Rev*. 2015;12(5):CD010180. doi:10.1002/14651858.CD010180.pub2.

11. Qiao W, Ren Y, Bai Y, et al. Cyanoacrylate injection versus band ligation in the endoscopic management of acute gastric variceal bleeding: meta-analysis of randomized, controlled studies based on the PRISMA statement. *Medicine (Baltimore)*. 2015;94(41):e1725.

12. Franco M, Gomes G, Nakao F, et al. Efficacy and safety of endoscopic prophylactic treatment with undiluted cyanoacrylate for gastric varices. *World J Gastrointest Endosc*. 2014;6(6):254-259.

13. Al-Hillawi L, Wong T, Tritto G, Berry P. Pitfalls in histoacryl glue injection therapy for oesophageal, gastric and ectopic varices: a review. *World J Gastrointest Surg*. 2016;8(11):729-734.

14. Tseng Y, Ma L, Luo T, et al. Thromboembolic events secondary to endoscopic cyanoacrylate injection: can we foresee any red flags? *Can J Gastroenterol Hepatol*. 2018;2018:10. Article ID 1940592. https://doi.org/10.1155/2018/1940592.

15. Catron T, Smallfield G, Kang L, Sterling R, Siddiqui M. Endoscopic cyanoacrylate injection with post-injection audible Doppler assessment of gastric varices: a single-institution experience. *Dig Dis Sci*. 2017;62(11):3091-3099.

16. Gubler C, Bauerfeind P. Safe and successful endoscopic initial treatment and long-term eradication of gastric varices by endoscopic ultrasound-guided Histoacryl (*N*-butyl-2-cyanoacrylate) injection. *Scand J Gastroenterol.* 2014;49(9):1136-1142.

17. Romero-Castro R, Ellrichmann M, Ortiz-Moyano C, et al. EUS-guided coil versus cyanoacrylate therapy for the treatment of gastric varices: a multi-center study (with videos). *Gastrointest Endosc.* 2013;78(5):711-721.

18. Romero-Castro R, Pellicer-Bautista F, Giovannini M, et al. Endoscopic ultrasound (EUS)-guided coil embolization therapy in gastric varices. *Endoscopy.* 2010;42(suppl 2):E35-E36. doi:10.1055/s-0029-1215261.Epub 2010 Jan 13.

19. Bhat Y, Weilert F, Fredrick R, et al. EUS-guided treatment of gastric fundal varices with combined injection of coils and cyanoacrylate glue: a large U.S. experience over 6 years (with video). *Gastrointest Endosc.* 2016;83(6):1164-1172.

20. Fujii-Lau L, Law R, Wong Kee Song L, et al. Endoscopic ultrasound (EUS)-guided coil injection therapy of esophagogastric and ectopic varices. *Surg Endosc.* 2016;30(4):1396-1404.

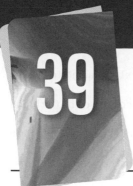

39

Endoscopic Variceal Ligation

Vilas R. Patwardhan, MD
Elliot B. Tapper, MD

Acute variceal hemorrhage (AVH) is a devastating complication of cirrhosis and portal hypertension.[1,2] The expected overall 6-week mortality associated with AVH is 17.7% (95% CI 14.4% to 21.7%), but it should approach 0% in patients with Child A who receives optimal care.[3] A key target for practice improvement is the provision of a high-quality endoscopic procedure. Esophageal band ligation is the first-line therapy for AVH.[4] However, in many (>10%) cases, patients presenting with AVH do not receive any endoscopic therapy.[3] While technical factors and bleeding severity may alter our ability to attain endoscopic hemostasis, operator comfort with endoscopic devices and their indications is essential to improve the outcomes associated with AVH.[5] Band ligation is also an effective therapy for the primary (and secondary) prophylaxis of variceal hemorrhage. This chapter reviews this technique in depth.

INDICATIONS

1. Hemostasis of acutely or recently bleeding esophageal varices
2. Elective obliteration of esophageal varices to prevent recurrent hemorrhage

CONTRAINDICATIONS

1. Esophageal diverticula or suspected esophageal perforation
2. Band ligation is not indicated for gastric or ectopic varices

PREPARATION

Acute bleeding
1. Obtain adequate intravenous (IV) access and start fluid resuscitation if indicated.
2. Bolus IV octreotide 50 mcg followed by infusion at 50 mcg/h.

3. Start intravenous antibiotics (first-line therapy is 1 g of ceftriaxone daily).

4. Consider erythromycin 125 mg IV x1 to facilitate gastric emptying of blood.

5. The patient's blood should be typed and crossed by the blood bank.

6. If hemodynamically stable, the patient should be NPO for 6 hours prior to the examination.

7. Obtain informed, written consent from the patient or a close relative.

8. If hematemesis, delirium, hemodynamic instability, request/arrange endotracheal intubation.

9. If not intubated, administer a topical anesthetic for pharyngeal anesthesia.

10. Obtain medications for sedation (e.g., midazolam and fentanyl). For patients at risk for sedation tolerance, i.e., alcohol consumption, chronic narcotics, or benzodiazepines, consider propofol-based sedation.

11. In the setting of primary or secondary prophylaxis, there is no role for resuscitation, octreotide, antibiotics, type/cross, or routine endotracheal intubation.

EQUIPMENT

1. Upper endoscope. Make sure the ligator device is compatible with the outer diameter and accessory channel length of the endoscope

2. Gloves, safety goggles, or mask with visor, and gown

3. Lubricant

4. 50-mL syringe with Luer-lock tip and sterile saline or water for washing

5. 6- or 7-multiband ligator. Examples include:
   a. Saeed 6 Shooter Multi-Band Ligator (Cook, Bloomington, IN)
   b. (Latex-Free) Speedband Superview Super-7 Band Ligator (Boston Scientific, Natick, MA)
   c. UltraView Multiple Band Ligator (Bard, Covington, GA)

6. As a backup for episodes of band failure: Sodium morrhuate (5%) or sodium tetradecyl (1% or 3%) for injection sclerotherapy

PROCEDURE

1. Perform diagnostic upper endoscopy to document esophageal varices and rule out distal sources of bleeding. Grading schema for varices vary. At a minimum grade varices as small (<5 mm; flatten with insufflation) versus large (>5 mm; do not flatten with insufflation). Document the presence of high-risk

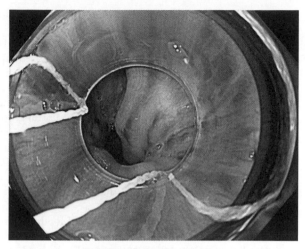

FIG. 39.1 Red wale on a varix.

stigmata such as *red wales* (thinned areas of a variceal column with red discoloration, Fig. 39.1) and *white nipple sign* (localized white fibrin cap on a column indicative of recent bleed). **Note:** Variceal bleeding can be intermittent, and culprit vessels can be smaller if decompressed by prior hemorrhage. Banding must not be deferred if clinical suspicion of bleeding is high but active bleeding is not observed. If technically feasible, band ligation of varices is recommended for all acute upper GI bleed where no other source of bleeding is found.

2. Plan banding strategy. Banding should start at the most caudal/distal extent of the varix but above the gastroesophageal junction (usually 1 to 2 cm). Bands should not be placed in gastric mucosa or on gastric varices. The vast majority of banding should be performed within 5 cm of the gastroesophageal junction. Identify each cord of varices and note the location of the largest protrusions and red markings. Note the distance from the incisors and the location (i.e., 36 cm, 3'o clock).

3. Remove the endoscope, and attach the ligation device. Refer to the specific device instructions for detailed setup instructions.

   a. In general, attachment and operation of the Cook 6 Shooter and Speedband Superview Super-7 are similar and are described below. Both ligator kits come with a ligating unit that is a clear plastic cylinder with preloaded bands and trigger string, a plastic or wire loader, a handle, and an irrigation adapter. Attach the handle to the accessory channel of the endoscope, and push the wire (Super-7) or plastic loader (6 Shooter) into the accessory/

device channel of the endoscope until it exits the distal end of the endoscope insertion tube.

   i. For 6 Shooter: Affix the trigger string to the hook at the end of loader with the knotted end of the string flush with the hook. Pull loader until the cylinder is at the distal end of the endoscope. Insert the endoscope into the cylinder and firmly press. Insert the knotted end of the string, now at the handle, into the central grooved area, it is appropriately attached to the handle. Gently turn the handle to tighten the string, being careful to avoid deploying a band. Confirm that the trigger strings do not obstruct the view of the endoscope, and if they do, rotate the cap so that the strings are in the periphery of the viewing field.

   ii. For the Super-7: Connect the loop of loading wire to the looped wire of cylinder. Remove shrink-wrap from the ligating unit. Affix the wire to the grooved area of the handle perpendicular to the accessory/device port. Gently turn the handle to tighten the string, being careful to avoid deploying a band. Confirm that the trigger strings do not obstruct the view of the endoscope, and if they do, rotate the cap so that the strings are in the periphery of the viewing field.

  b. The UltraView Multiple Band Ligator from Bard is unique, features a retractable ligating unit, and mounts completely to the outside of the endoscope.

4. Lubricate the outside of the ligating unit, and insert it into the esophagus. Note that the ligation device is stiff. Intubation may be more difficult than the diagnostic upper endoscopy due to the added length and size of the ligation device. When possible attempt to intubate in the same orientation as with your diagnostic endoscopy to preserve your original landmarks and positioning of varices.

5. The first varix to be banded should be the most distal cord, ideally also the largest or the one with stigmata of recent hemorrhage. After the appropriate varix site is chosen, the endoscope should be flexed so the varix is perpendicular (as much as possible) with the ligating unit (Fig. 39.2).

6. Suck the varix into the cylinder with constant/maximum suction (Fig. 39.3). If the varix does not enter the ligating unit completely, you may gently torque the scope left or right or gently "push and pull" to coax the varix further into the ligating unit. When the varix is completely sucked into the ligating unit, "redout" will be seen, indicating that the band should be deployed. Misfire, or incomplete deployment of the

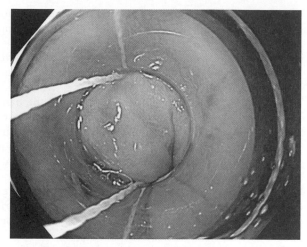

FIG. 39.2 Correct placement of a band ligator on a varix.

band, may occur if the varix is not completely sucked into the ligating unit.

a. If a redout is not achieved, two maneuvers should be considered:

   i. It is possible that the cylinder edge is too tight on the mucosa. Pull off the wall slightly and at a mild angle while applying suction

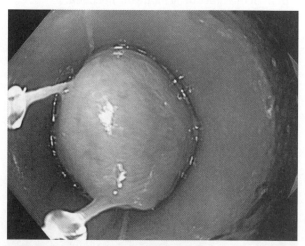

FIG. 39.3 The varix is sucked into the ligating unit but sufficiently for band ligation (need redout).

    ii. A gentle "jiggle" of the insertion tube back-and-forth and torqueing side-to-side may facilitate the fitting of the cylinder over the varix

  b. If the varix does not enter the ligator device more than half-way, consider releasing suction and choosing an alternate location to band.

7. To deploy the band, the knob on the handle of the bander should be rotated approximately 180° clockwise. An increase in tension followed by immediate decrease in tension indicates the band has been deployed. The Super-7 should provide a "click" with more noticeable haptic feedback consistent with band deployment.

8. Following band deployment, apply air insufflation and gently retract the endoscope. Inspect the varix for appropriate placement of the band, hemostasis, and decompression of the varix with photodocumentation (Fig. 39.4).

9. Additional bands should be placed on adjacent cords of varices with high risk features. Multiple bands may be placed on the same varix provided there is adequate distance between them (usually 1- to 2-cm). until varices are completely decompressed.

10. Repeat band ligation of all varices at 14 + 7 day intervals until all varices are obliterated. An average of three to four banding sessions may be necessary to completely obliterate all varices.

11. If high-risk features or stigmata of recent bleeding are found but banding is not technically possible, sclerotherapy may be performed. The clear cap of the banding apparatus can be kept intact in order to facilitate the injection.

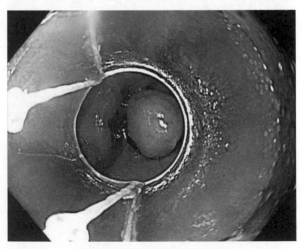

FIG. 39.4 Complete ligation of the varix.

POSTPROCEDURE

1. Monitor vital signs
2. Elevate the head of the bed to reduce aspiration risk
3. Give clear liquids for 6 to 12 hours, soft-solids for the first 12 to 24 hours, then advance the diet as tolerated
4. Avoid nasogastric or feeding tube placement for 24 to 48 hours
5. Continue antibiotic prophylaxis (e.g., 1 g ceftriaxone or oral quinolone for 5 to 7 days after procedure)
6. Patients should be started on therapy to prevent band-ulcer hemorrhage for 10 to 14 days. We prefer using sucralfate slurry (1 g QID). The role of acid suppression (e.g., proton pump inhibitor) is controversial, given its association with infections and hepatic encephalopathy but a short course without refills of proton pump inhibitors is reasonable
7. Patients with a history of AVH without contraindications for nonselective beta-blockage should receive either carvedilol (12.5 mg qHS) or nadolol (20 mg, titrated to a resting heart rate of ~ 55 to 65 beats per minute)
8. The patient should return for severe chest pain, fevers, shortness of breath, hematemesis, or blood per rectum

ADVERSE EVENTS

1. Continued variceal hemorrhage. If endoscopic hemostasis cannot be obtained, consider balloon tamponade (i.e., placement of a Sengstaken-Blakemore or Minnesota tube) and/or emergent transjugular intrahepatic portosystemic shunt or balloon-occluded retrograde transvenous obliteration as well as continued medical management (i.e., IV octreotide, hemodynamic support, and correction of coagulopathy)
2. Superficial esophageal banding ulcers, which may bleed
3. Esophageal strictures
4. Esophageal perforation
5. Aspiration
6. Transient bacteremia
7. Esophageal obstruction
8. Dysphagia and/or odynophagia
9. Chest pain

CPT CODES

43244—Upper gastrointestinal endoscopy including the esophagus, stomach, and either the duodenum and/or jejunum as appropriate; with band ligation of esophageal and/or gastric varices

References

1. Carbonell N, Pauwels A, Serfaty L, Fourdan O, Levy VG, Poupon R. Improved survival after variceal bleeding in patients with cirrhosis over the past two decades. *Hepatology*. 2004;40:652-659.
2. Chojkier M, Conn HO. Esophageal tamponade in the treatment of bleeding varices. *Dig Dis Sci*. 1980;25:267-272.
3. Tapper E, Beste L, Curry M, Bonder A, Waljee A, Saini S. Opportunities for improvement in the contemporary management of acute variceal hemorrhage: a systematic review of observational studies. *Clin Gastroenterol Hepatol*. 2017;15(9):1373-1381.
4. Garcia-Tsao G, Sanyal AJ, Grace ND, Carey W. Prevention and management of gastroesophageal varices and variceal hemorrhage in cirrhosis. *Hepatology*. 2007;46:922-938.
5. Tapper EB, Ezaz G, Patwardhan V, et al. Hospital-level balloon tamponade use is associated with increased mortality for all patients presenting with acute variceal haemorrhage. *Liver Int*. 2018;38:477-483.

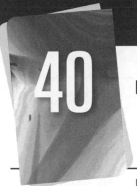

40 Balloon Tamponade

Donovan Inniss, BS
Monica A. Tincopa, MD, MSc

Esophageal varices occur as a consequence of portal hypertension and may develop in up to 50% of patients with cirrhosis, but prevalence varies according to severity of underlying liver disease. Rate of variceal bleeding is dependent on severity of liver disease, size of varices, and presence of high-risk stigmata on endoscopy that is indicative of areas of thinning of the variceal wall. Approximately one-third of patients with varices will experience variceal bleeding with an annual rate of 10% to 15% per year.[1,2] Urgent endoscopic therapy is used as first-line therapy in treating acute variceal bleeding. Endoscopy band ligation is the primary treatment modality. In patients whose bleeding cannot be controlled by endoscopic therapy, emergent therapies via intervention radiology such as transjugular intrahepatic portosystemic shunt (TIPS) should be considered.[1,3] Balloon tamponade plays a role in management of variceal bleeding among patients in whom endoscopic therapy was unsuccessful in controlling bleeding and are in need of a "bridge" therapy in order to acutely stabilize active bleeding until further more definitive intervention can be performed.

The two most commonly used balloon tamponade systems are the Minnesota four-lumen esophagogastric tamponade tube and the three-lumen Sengstaken-Blakemore tube. The Minnesota tube incorporates an internal separate esophageal suction port in addition to the gastric suction port, gastric balloon inflation port, and esophageal balloon inflation port (Fig. 40.1). This esophageal suction port was added in order to help prevent aspiration of esophageal contents. When inflated, the balloons place pressure to decrease blood flow and thus help reduce active bleeding.

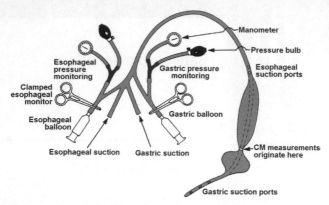

FIG. 40.1 Minnesota four-lumen tube.

INDICATION

1. Acute, life-threatening bleeding from esophageal or gastric varices that is unresponsive to medical and endoscopic therapy.
2. Acute, life-threatening bleeding from esophageal or gastric varices when endoscopic therapy is unavailable.

CONTRAINDICATIONS

Absolute

1. Cessation of variceal bleeding
2. Recent surgery involving the esophagogastric junction
3. Known esophageal stricture

Relative

1. Poorly informed support staff
2. Large hiatal hernia
3. Incomplete lavage
4. Inability to demonstrate a variceal source of bleeding
5. Known severe esophageal ulceration (in these cases, the gastric balloon may be used but not the esophageal balloon)

PREPARATION

1. Ensure appropriate volume resuscitation and pharmacologic therapy with vasoactive medication and antibiotics with a goal to restore and maintain hemodynamic stability.
2. Ensure airway protection. Patients with acute, large volume upper GI bleeds, particularly those who require balloon tamponade for treatment of severe variceal bleeding often require intubation for airway protection given high risk of aspiration in refractory variceal bleeding.

3. Perform endoscopy to confirm the source of bleeding, and attempt band ligation as a primary mode of treating acute variceal bleeding.
4. If endoscopy demonstrates large amounts of blood in the stomach, lavage the stomach with tap water using an adult gastric lavage or other large-bore tube.
5. Initiate evaluation for more definitive therapy via interventional radiology (TIPS or other IR therapy targeted to reduce portal hypertensive bleeding) or surgery.

EQUIPMENT

- Gastroesophageal balloon tamponade tube (Minnesota tube)
- Two three-way stopcocks
- Christmas tree (catheter) adapter
- Two wall-suction setups
- Two padded hemostats to clamp closed the gastric and esophageal balloon ports
- Manometer
- Water-soluble lubricant
- Leur-lock 60 mL syringe
- An over-the-bed traction with a counterweight of 1 lb. or football helmet
- Adhesive tape
- Marking pen
- Scissors
- Bucket of water

PROCEDURE

1. Elevate the head of the bed to 45° and place patient in supine position.
2. Ensure patient is properly sedated and the oropharynx is anesthetized.
3. Remove one plastic peg from the esophageal and one plastic port from the gastric balloon port. Leave the remaining plastic peg in each balloon port.
4. Attach syringe to stopcock and test the balloons by insufflating each with air and examine for leaks under water.
5. Suction all air from the balloons.
6. Lubricate tube and balloons.
7. Clamp hemostats on the two balloon ports.
8. Pass tube through the patient's mouth until the 50-cm mark is located at the gum line. Do not pass the tube through the nares unless orogastric passage is impossible.

9. Remove clamp from gastric balloon port and insufflate 50 mL of air into the gastric balloon port and assess for placement by listening for gastric sounds. Place clamp back on gastric balloon port and confirm placement with an immediate portable radiograph.

10. After x-ray confirmation of tube placement, inflate the gastric balloon with up to additional 200 mL of air. Then replace clamp on gastric balloon port.

11. Gently pull the tube back until resistance is felt against the gastroesophageal junction.

12. With minimum tension on the tube, fix the upper end of the tube to over-the-bed traction with a 1-lb weight or, alternatively, to the crossbar of a football helmet as it exits from the mouth.

13. Mark the tube placement with a marker where the tube exits the mark in order to monitor tube placement.

14. Apply suction to the gastric and esophageal aspiration ports.

15. Observe the nature of the drainage from the gastric and esophageal ports. If bleeding persists from either port, inflate the esophageal balloon. To do this:

    a. Connect the manometer to the esophageal balloon port. Then inflate to a pressure of 30 to 45 mm Hg using the lowest pressure needed to stop bleeding through both the gastric and esophageal ports. Never inflate the esophageal balloon before the gastric balloon.

    b. Clamp the esophageal balloon port.

    c. Check the esophageal balloon pressure with the mercury manometer every 3 hours, or keep the manometer attached for constant monitoring.

POSTPROCEDURE

1. Give nothing by mouth. Institute oral hygiene. If necessary, give medications through the gastric port.

2. Due to the risk of esophageal pressure necrosis, deflation of the esophageal balloon is performed for 5 minutes every 6 hours.

3. Manually check the tube tension at 3-hour intervals. Do not manipulate the tube unnecessarily.

4. Check both the gastric and esophageal return every 2 hours, and flush both lumens if there is any question of clogging. Barium should never be instilled through the tube, since impaction of balloons could occur, requiring removal of the tube.

5. If respiratory distress occurs due to proximal migration of the esophageal balloon with occlusion of the airway, the tube must be removed immediately! *Grasp the tube at the mouth, transect*

with scissors above the grasping hand but below the entrance of the three channel inlets, and pull out the tube.

6. If hemostasis persists for 24 hours and esophageal balloon has been inflated, reduce the pressure in the esophageal balloon 5 mm Hg every 3 hours until 25 mm Hg is reached without bleeding. If bleeding is controlled, deflate the esophageal balloon for 5 minutes every 6 hours to help prevent esophageal necrosis. The esophageal balloon should not be inflated for more than 24 hours.

7. If there is no recurrence of bleeding over the next 6 to 12 hours, deflate the gastric balloon and release tension but leave tube in place.

8. If bleeding recurs, the gastric balloon and, if necessary, the esophageal balloon may be reinflated for an additional 24 hours (Fig. 40.2).

9. If bleeding does not recur by 24 hours after deflation, remove the tube.

ADVERSE EVENTS

Major

1. Aspiration: The most frequent complication. The greatest risk for aspiration occurs during insertion. Airway protection with intubation should be strongly considered.

2. Airway occlusion: Caused by proximal migration of the tube. Preventable by endotracheal intubation. This is usually secondary to deflation of the gastric balloon while the esophageal balloon remains inflated. If tube migration results in airway obstruction, bisecting across all lumens of the tube just distal to bifurcation point enables immediate removal of the entire tube.

3. Esophageal perforation and rupture: Rupture of the esophagus, laceration or ulceration of the stomach, and pressure necrosis of the hypopharynx or alae nasi may occur with prolonged balloon inflation or excessive pressures. Esophageal perforation or rupture can also occur if a gastric balloon is inadvertently placed in the esophagus. Rupture of the esophagus is a particular risk if sclerotherapy has been performed prior to tube placement.

Minor

1. Gastroesophageal and pharyngeal erosions and ulcers caused by local-pressure effects

2. Hiccups

3. Pain

4. Pressure necrosis of nose, lips and tongue, and other facial skin

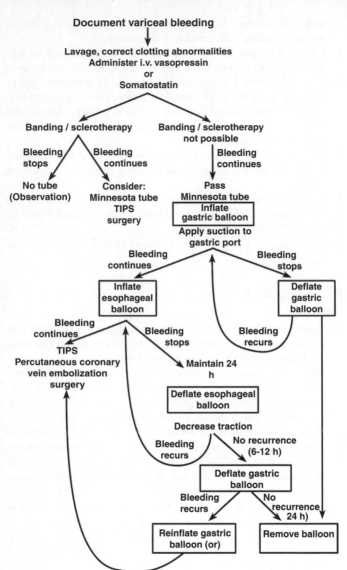

FIG. 40.2 Use of the Minnesota tube in a patient with variceal bleeding. TIPS, transjugular intrahepatic portosystemic shunt.

EFFICACY

With the advent of improved endoscopic techniques and the availability of emergent interventional radiology procedures, balloon tamponade has a limited role in the primary treatment of bleeding varices. Its greatest role may be in temporarily stabilizing the actively bleeding patient in whom initial endoscopic therapy has failed while awaiting emergent TIPS procedure. It is estimated that balloon tamponade can provide effective hemostasis in up to 80% of patients, but efficacy is dependent on overall clinical status of the patient and likely influenced by other factors such as availability of urgent endoscopy and expertise of an endoscopist in variceal band ligation.[4,5] Given the associated severity of underlying liver disease and clinical instability of patients requiring balloon tamponade for control of variceal bleeding, there is significant morbidity and mortality in these patients. Reported mortality in this setting is approximately 20%.[1]

References

1. Garcia-Tsao G, Abraldes JG, Berzigotti A, Bosch J. Portal hypertensive bleeding in cirrhosis: risk stratification, diagnosis, and management: 2016 practice guidance by the American Association for the Study of Liver Diseases. *Hepatology*. 2017;65:310-335.
2. North Italian Endoscopic Club for the Study and Treatment of Esophageal Varices. Prediction of the first variceal hemorrhage in patients with cirrhosis of the liver and esophageal varices. A prospective multicenter study. *N Engl J Med*. 1988;319:983-989.
3. Monescillo A, Martinez-Lagares F, Ruiz-del-Arbol L, et al. Influence of portal hypertension and its early decompression by TIPS placement on the outcome of variceal bleeding. *Hepatology*. 2004;40:793-801.
4. Tapper EB, Ezaz G, Patwardhan V, et al. Hospital-level balloon tamponade use is associated with increased mortality for all patients presenting with acute variceal haemorrhage. *Liver Int*. 2018;38:477-483.
5. Choi JY, Jo YW, Lee SS, et al. Outcomes of patients treated with Sengstaken-Blakemore tube for uncontrolled variceal hemorrhage. *Korean J Int Med*. 2018;33:696-704.

Bariatric Endoscopy

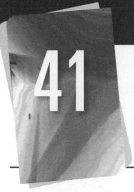

Intragastric Balloon Placement for Weight Loss

Michael C. Bennett, MD
Shelby Sullivan, MD

Intragastric balloons (IGBs) are endoscopically placed devices intended for the management of obesity. They work by occupying space in the stomach and delaying gastric emptying.[1] IGBs have been proven to outperform monitored diet and exercise programs in randomized controlled trials.[2-4]

As of this writing, three IGBs have been approved by the United States Food and Drug Administration (FDA): the ReShape Integrated Dual Balloon System (ReShape Medical, San Clemente, CA), the Orbera Balloon (Fig. 41.1, Apollo Endosurgery, Austin, TX), and the Obalon Balloon System (Fig. 41.2, Obalon Therapeutics, Carlsbad, CA). The ReShape Integrated Dual Balloon System, however, is no longer being manufactured and will not be discussed further. The Orbera balloon is a single, fluid-filled balloon made of medical-grade silicone that can be inflated to between 400 and 700 mL. It is placed endoscopically and removed endoscopically 6 months after placement. The Obalon Balloon System is a swallow-able gas-filled intragastric balloon system comprises three balloons, each filled with 250 mL of a nitrogen-mix gas and removed endoscopically 6 months after administration of the first balloon.

INDICATIONS

Intragastric balloons should be considered for patients with:
- Body mass index (BMI) between 30 and 40 kg/m^2
- Previous unsuccessful weight loss or weight maintenance attempts with lifestyle intervention alone
- BMI outside accepted range above but with medical conditions necessitating weight loss and contraindications to alternate modalities, e.g., surgical therapy[5]

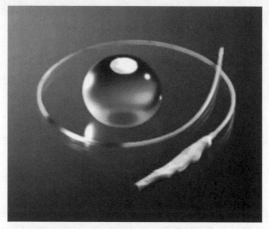

FIG. 41.1 Single fluid-filled balloon (Orbera Balloon). (Reprinted from Abu Dayyeh BK, Edmundowicz SA, Jonnalagadda S, et al. Endoscopic bariatric therapies. *Gastrointest Endosc.* 2015;81(5):1073-1086. Copyright © 2015 American Society for Gastrointestinal Endoscopy. With permission.)

CONTRAINDICATIONS

- Prior foregut or bariatric surgery
- Structural disorder of the gastrointestinal (GI) tract, such as stenosis, neoplasm, hiatal hernia (>2 cm for Obalon and >5 cm for Orbera), or congenital anomaly
- Inflammatory or erosive disorders affecting the GI tract, such as esophagitis, ulcer disease, Crohn disease

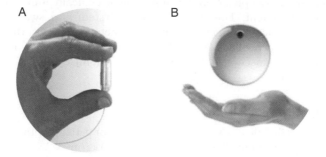

FIG. 41.2 Swallowable gas-filled intragastric balloon system (Obalon Balloon System). Panel A, balloon in capsule attached to catheter. Panel B, balloon fully inflated. (Reprinted from Sullivan S, Swain J, Woodman G, et al. Randomized sham-controlled trial of the 6-month swallowable gas-filled intragastric balloon system for weight loss. *Surg Obes Relat Dis.* 2018;14(12):1876-1889. Copyright © 2018 American Society for Bariatric Surgery. With permission.)

- Motor disorders, such as achalasia or gastroparesis
- Conditions with potential for upper GI bleeding, such as varices or telangectasiasbullet
- Coagulopathy
- Severe comorbid conditions such as cirrhosis
- Use of anticoagulants, antiplatelet medications, nonsteroidal anti-inflammatory drugs (NSAIDs)
- Inability to take proton pump inhibitor (PPI)
- Uncontrolled psychiatric illness, especially addiction or eating disorders
- Pregnancy or breast feeding[6,7]

PREPARATION
Orbera (Single Fluid-Filled Intragastric Balloon) Placement

- Routine preprocedure laboratory evaluation may include complete blood count, comprehensive metabolic panel, coagulation testing, lipid evaluation, hemoglobin A1c, testing for *Helicobacter pylori* infection, and pregnancy testing if applicable.
- Use of a PPI is recommended while the IGB is in place. Begin use of a daily PPI 1 week prior to placement and continue for duration of IGB dwell.
- A suggested regimen of antiemetics and antispasmodics beginning the day of placement and continuing until symptoms resolve: sublingual ondansetron 8 mg every 8 hours and sublingual hyoscyamine 0.125 mg every 4 hours, and aprepitant 40 to 80 mg taken 4 hours prior to placement can be used. Scopolamine patch placed the night before and promethazine can also be considered. Patients may also need pain control for the first few days after placement.
- Prior to balloon placement, patients should have no food or drink for 12 hours.
- Saline-filled balloons can be placed under moderate sedation or with monitored anesthesia care.

Orbera Removal

- 72 hours prior to balloon removal, patients should adhere to a full liquid diet, further restricting to a clear liquid diet 24 hours prior to removal. No food or drink should be consumed for 12 hours prior to the procedure.
- Saline-filled balloon removal can be performed under monitored anesthesia care or general anesthesia.

Obalon (Swallowable Gas-Filled Balloon System) Placement

- Patients considering Obalon IGBs should successfully complete swallows of one placebo Obalon capsule to ensure ability to swallow the encapsulated IGB.

- A contrast esophagram is recommended to rule out structural contraindications such as large hiatal hernia or esophageal stricture.
- Routine preprocedure laboratory evaluation may include complete blood count, comprehensive metabolic panel, coagulation testing, lipid evaluation, hemoglobin A1c, testing for *H. pylori* infection, and pregnancy testing if applicable.
- Use of a PPI is recommended while the IGB is in place. Begin use of a daily PPI 1 week prior to placement and continue for duration of IGB dwell.
- Antiemetics and antispasmodics should be used at the time of placement to reduce the incidence of side effects. A suggested regimen beginning the day before placement and continuing for 4 days includes sublingual ondansetron 8 mg every 8 hours and sublingual hyoscyamine 0.125 mg every 4 hours. This should be repeated for all three balloons, which are administered 2 to 4 weeks apart.
- Prior to balloon placement, patients should have no food or drink for 12 hours.
- Obalon balloon placement does not require sedation.
- Fluoroscopy or digital x-ray is required for visualization of the balloon during placement.

Obalon Removal
- All balloons are removed 6 months after the first balloon was administered.
- Patients should be on liquids 24 hours before removal and should have no food or drink for 12 hours before removal.
- Obalon balloon removal can be performed with monitored anesthesia care or general anesthesia.

EQUIPMENT

Obalon placement requires fluoroscopy, digital x-ray if using the EZ Fill Dispenser or the Obalon Navigation System with Touch Dispenser. Orbera placement and removal, and Obalon removal, require standard equipment for a diagnostic upper endoscopy, in addition to the following for each device:

Orbera Placement
- Orbera balloon placement catheter assembly
- Orbera filling assembly
- 60 mL syringe
- 1000 mL sterile saline bag
- Sterile methylene blue

Orbera Removal

- Two-prong wire grasper (provided in the removal kit) or large endoscopic rat-tooth graspers
- Aspiration catheter (provided in the removal kit)

Obalon Placement

- Dispenser (EZ Fill to use with fluoroscopy or digital x-ray or Touch Dispenser to Use with the Obalon Navigation System)
- If using the EZ Fill Dispenser, fluoroscopy or digital x-ray is needed
- If using the Touch Dispenser, the Obalon Navigation System is needed
- Inflation gas canister
- Encapsulated balloon (in patient's balloon kit, have extra in case of failed swallow)
- Accessory kit including extension tube with three-way stopcock and two 3 mL syringes
- Swallow aids including cups, water, carbonated beverage, applesauce, banana
- Timer or clock

Obalon Removal

- Endoscopic injection/aspiration needle (recommended 6 to 8 mm length, 21 to 23 gauge)
- 15 mm or greater endoscopic rat-tooth alligator forceps

PROCEDURE

Orbera Placement

- Determine inflation volume for the balloon, can be filled from 400 to 700 mL. Once volume of inflation is determined (typically 500 to 600 mL), empty out the excess volume from a 1000 mL saline bag so only the volume to be inflated remains in the bag.
- 2 to 4 mL of methylene can be added to the 1000 mL saline bag, but this is considered off-label use by the FDA.
- Perform a diagnostic esophagogastroduodenoscopy.
- If no contraindications are present, withdraw the endoscope and pass the loaded and lubricated Orbera IGB delivery catheter through the mouth into the esophagus.
- Reinsert the endoscope, and advance the catheter and endoscope together, using direct visualization, into the stomach. Confirm that the entire Orbera balloon is within the stomach using retroflexion.
- Remove the guidewire from the catheter.

- Using the Orbera filling assembly with one-way valve and a 60 mL syringe, inflate the balloon with the predetermined amount of methylene blue–dyed saline, maintaining direct endoscopic visualization.
- Applying even backpressure, withdraw the endoscope and catheter together, which will detach the catheter from the inflated balloon.
- Reinsert the endoscope to confirm that the balloon is inflated within the stomach and without evidence of leak, especially at the filling valve. Inspect the stomach and esophagus for mucosal injury on withdrawal.
- Consider intravenous ondansetron 4 to 8 mg and dexamethasone 4 to 10 mg for control of nausea.
- Consider intravenous administration of 1 to 2 liters of lactated ringers or D5 ½ normal saline to prevent dehydration after the procedure.

Orbera Removal

- Insert the endoscope and identify the balloon within the stomach.
- Advance the aspiration catheter through the endoscope channel into the stomach.
- Advance the needle out of the catheter and puncture the balloon. Advance the catheter 5 cm into the balloon.
- Aspirate the saline from the balloon using a syringe or vacuum suction.
- Grasp the deflated balloon securely with the two prong viper graspers supplied in the removal kit and withdraw the endoscope with the balloon through the mouth.
- Reintroduce the endoscope to assess for mucosal injury, particularly at the esophagogastric junction.

Obalon Placement

Two different systems are available: one for use with fluoroscopy or digital x-ray and one that does not require fluoroscopy or digital x-ray.

Administration With the EZ Fill Dispenser (Fig. 41.3)

- Prepare the EZ fill dispenser by opening the green release valve, attaching the extension tube and inserting the gas can, to prefill the extension tubing. Once the pressure reading is within the predetermined range, the green release valve should be closed.
- The capsule should be submerged in water for no more than 10 seconds and placed in the patient's mouth. The patient should

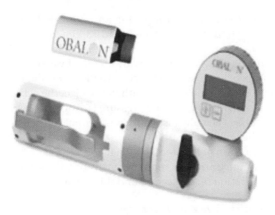

FIG. 41.3 Obalon EZ fill dispenser and gas can. (Reprinted from Sullivan S, Swain J, Woodman G, et al. Randomized sham-controlled trial of the 6-month swallowable gas-filled intragastric balloon system for weight loss. *Surg Obes Relat Dis.* 2018;14(12):1076-1889. Copyright © 2010 American Society for Bariatric Surgery. With permission.)

swallow the encapsulated Obalon balloon, taking care not to bite the catheter. Water should be used to aid swallowing. If this is not successful, carbonated beverage, applesauce, or a soft solid such as a banana can be used to aid passage into the stomach.

- Verify placement of the encapsulated balloon within the stomach using digital x-ray or fluoroscopy to visualize the radiopaque marker in the stomach (below the diaphragm).
- Attach the extension tubing to the end of the catheter coming out of the patient's mouth. Make sure the green release valve is in the closed position. Open the blue valve on the three-way stopcock to allow the gas in the prefilled extension tubing to flow into the deflated balloon. Once the capsule dissolves off of the balloon and the balloon unfolds (which can only occur in the unconstrained space of the stomach), the pressure should drop to below 7 kPa. If pressure remains above 7 kPa, but below 10 kPa reverify position with x-ray prior to inflating.
- Once the balloon is confirmed to be in the stomach by imaging and prepulse pressure measurement, open the green valve to inflate the balloon. Ask the patient to report any pain or pressure in the chest or upper abdomen. Once pressure reading reaches equilibration, ensure stability for 30 seconds with the green valve open. Close the green

valve and confirm stability for an additional 30 seconds. Pressure should be between 9 and 13 kPa, but ideally 12 to 13 kPa.

- Attach a 3 mL syringe filled with 1.5 mL of water to the three-way stopcock. Close the stopcock to the extension tubing and inject 1.5 mL saline into the catheter to eject the catheter from the balloon. Ensure that the pressure is dropping, then pull out the catheter. Visually inspect to ensure that the needle is present at the end of the catheter.
- Verify position of inflated balloon using x-ray.
- The administration is repeated at 2 to 4 week intervals for administration of the second and third balloons.

Administration With the Obalon Navigation System (Fig. 41.4) and Touch Dispenser (Fig. 41.5)

- Prepare the Touch Dispenser by pressing the power button to turn on the system. Once powered up, the system will prompt the user to insert an Obalon inflation gas can. Insert the gas can and close the dispenser lever. The system will automatically perform a system pressure check. The dispenser will display the start new procedure screen when Touch Dispenser is ready for use.
- Prepare the navigation system: enter login and password to access the software and press the new patient administration button and enter the patient's ID.
- Attach the reference sensor to the patient at the midline of the sternum at the xiphoid process. Plug in the reference sensor cable to the sensor interface unit on the Navigation Console.
- The patient should be positioned no further than 12 inches in front of the field generator, with the field generator adjusted to be over the spine at the level of the distal third of the scapula.
- Remove the balloon capsule from the package, hold it at the patient's jugular notch and the navigation system will automatically calibrate denoted by "calibrating" appearing on the Navigation Console screen until calibration is complete.
- The capsule should be submerged in water for no more than 10 seconds and placed in the patient's mouth. The patient should swallow the encapsulated Obalon balloon, taking care not to bite the catheter. Water should be used to aid swallowing. If this is not successful, carbonated beverage, applesauce, or a soft solids such as a banana can be used to aid passage into the stomach.

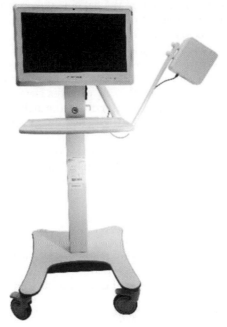

FIG. 41.4 Obalon Navigation System.

- Track the capsule migration into the stomach on the Navigation Console screen. Indications the balloon has reached the stomach include capsule offsets significantly left of the initial midline track, the capsule suddenly accelerates left of lateral, the capsule rotates from vertical to horizontal, and there is vertical movement with respiration.
- Attach the proximal external end of the balloon catheter still outside the patient's mouth to the Touch Dispenser and press the green start button. The system will alert the user when the

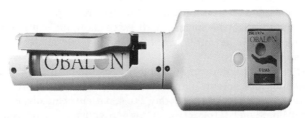

FIG. 41.5 Obalon Touch Dispenser.

capsule has detached from the balloon and conduct an automated pressure check to ensure the balloon is in an unconstrained space (i.e., the stomach).

■ Once the Touch Dispenser has successfully inflated the balloon, the display will show a procedure summary screen. The catheter is then disconnected from the dispenser, and connect the 3 mL syringe filled with 2 mL of water. Depress the syringe rapidly to detach the catheter from the balloon. A second syringe may be needed if the first does not detach the catheter from the balloon.

■ Once detached, pull the catheter out of the patient's mouth and check to ensure the needle at the distal end of the catheter is in the needle sleeve.

Obalon Removal

■ Insert the endoscope and confirm the presence of the Obalon balloons within the stomach.

■ Advance the aspiration needle through the channel. Puncture one of the balloons on the broad surface. Use the adaptor to attach the aspiration catheter directly to suction to deflate the balloon.

■ Remove the catheter and advance a rat-tooth alligator forceps. Grasp the flat edge of the balloon firmly, and withdraw the scope and deflated balloon out through the mouth.

■ Repeat this process with the remaining two balloons.

■ Reinsert the endoscope after all balloons are removed and inspect for mucosal injury.

POSTPROCEDURE

■ Antiemetics and antispasmodics should be continued, as discussed in preparation above. For more severe nausea or pain, brief use of low-dose benzodiazepine or opiate analgesics may be appropriate.

■ For throat or swallowing discomfort following IGB placement or removal, cepacol lozenges and/or a "GI cocktail" solution containing viscous lidocaine may be used.

■ PPI should be continued while the IGB remains in the stomach. Dose can be increased to twice daily for symptoms of reflux or dyspepsia. If symptoms persist, sucralfate solution can be used.

■ Diet should be advanced slowly as tolerated after fluid-filled balloon placement. Initially, a clear liquid diet should be followed for up to 3 days. On day 2 to 4, patients can advance to a full liquid diet. If tolerated, on day 4 to 8 advance to pureed diet with small meals. Around day 7, advance to a soft diet, then to a regular diet without restriction around day 10.

- Diet can typically be advanced more rapidly following Obalon placement, depending on patient tolerance. Diet should be limited to clear liquids on the day of placement, full liquids for 24 hours after and can usually be advanced to a low-calorie diet if symptoms are well controlled.

FOLLOW-UP

- Intragastric balloon therapy is most effective as part of a monitored weight loss program consisting of dietary and behavior counseling at least once a month by trained personnel, typically a registered dietitian with training in adult weight management. Regular contact with patients is recommended.
- Physician follow-up is recommended 1 to 2 weeks after fluid-filled intragastric balloon placement, before balloon removal, and 12 months after the initial placement. Consideration for physician visit at 1 month after placement should also be considered as weight loss at this time point is a predictive factor for weight loss at 12 months.
- Physicians are seeing patients for swallowable gas-filled intragastric balloon placement three times in the first 4 to 8 weeks of therapy. Physician follow-up should occur again before balloon system removal and at 12 months after the initial administration.

ADVERSE EVENTS

Procedure-related adverse events are uncommon. Removal of intragastric balloons can cause trauma at the esophagogastric junction or esophagus, usually superficial and not requiring intervention. Retained food can be seen at removal, so care should be taken to prevent aspiration; use of general anesthesia can be considered for device removal.

Most device-related adverse events are accommodative symptoms including abdominal pain, nausea, vomiting, dyspepsia, gastroesophageal reflux, and eructation. These range from mild to severe, and in some cases may lead to dehydration requiring intravenous fluid administration. Mucosal injury is rare. Comparative adverse event rates in US pivotal trials and postapproval registry studies are shown in Tables 41.1 and 41.2.

CPT CODES

There are no CPT codes specific to placement or removal of intragastric balloons.

TABLE 41.1	Adverse Events in United States Pivotal Trials							
	SAE, n (%)	Pain, n (%)	Nausea, n (%)	Vomiting, n (%)	GERD, n (%)	Early Removal, n (%)	Deflation, n (%)
Orbera[2] n = 160	16 (10.0%)	92 (57.5%)	139 (86.9%)	121 (75.6%)	48 (30%)	30 (18.8%)	0 (0.0%)
Obalon[4] n = 336	1 (0.3%)	244 (72.6%)	188 (56.0%)	58 (17.3%)	Composite dyspepsia and GERD 16.9%	19 (9.6%)	1 (0.1%)

Serious adverse events (SAEs): Orbera: device intolerance (8), dehydration (2), esophageal mucosal injury (2), gastric outlet obstruction (1), gastric perforation (1), aspiration pneumonia (1), cramping and infection (1), laryngospasm (1). Obalon: bleeding gastric ulcer (1).

TABLE 41.2	Adverse Events in United States Registry Series						
	SAE, n (%)	IVFs, n (%)	Pain, n (%)	Nausea, n (%)	Vomiting, n (%)	Early Removal, n (%)	Deflation, n (%)
Orbera[8] n = 321	11 (4%)	26 (8%)	Not reported	Not reported	Not reported	54 (16.6%)	1 (1%)
Obalon[9] N = 1343	2 (0.15%)	1 (0.07%)	71 (5.3%)	63 (4.7%)	31 (2.3%)	135 (10%)	7 (0.18%)

References

1. Gomez V, Woodman G, Abu Dayyeh BK. Delayed gastric emptying as a proposed mechanism of action during intragastric balloon therapy: results of a prospective study. *Obesity (Silver Spring, MD)*. 2016;24:1849-1853.
2. US Food and Drug Administration. Summary of safety and effectiveness data (SSED) ORBERA intragastric balloon system; 2015:1-32. Available at https://www.accessdata.fda.gov/cdrh_docs/pdf14/P140008b.pdf. Accessed May 1, 2018.
3. Ponce J, Woodman G, Swain J, et al. The REDUCE pivotal trial: a prospective, randomized controlled pivotal trial of a dual intragastric balloon for the treatment of obesity. *Surg Obes Relat Dis*. 2015;11:874-881.
4. Sullivan S, Swain J, Woodman G, et al. Randomized sham-controlled trial of the 6-month swallowable gas-filled intragastric balloon system for weight loss. *Surg Obes Relat Dis*. 2018;14:1876-1889.
5. Sullivan S, Kumar N, Edmundowicz SA, et al. ASGE position statement on endoscopic bariatric therapies in clinical practice. *Gastrointest Endosc*. 2015;82:767-772.
6. US Food and Drug Administration. *ORBERA intragastric balloon system directions for use*; 2015:1-35. Available at https://www.accessdata.fda.gov/cdrh_docs/pdf14/P140008c.pdf. Accessed May 1, 2018.
7. US Food and Drug Administration. *Obalon balloon system instructions for use*; 2016:1-24. Available at https://www.accessdata.fda.gov/cdrh_docs/pdf16/p160001d.pdf. Accessed May 1, 2018.
8. Vargas EJ, Pesta CM, Bali A, et al. Single fluid-filled intragastric balloon safe and effective for inducing weight loss in a real-world population. *Clin Gastroenterol Hepatol* 2018;16:1073-1080.e1.
9. Moore RL, Seger MV, Garber SM, et al. Clinical safety and effectiveness of a swallowable gas-filled intragastric balloon system for weight loss: consecutively treated patients in the initial year of U.S. commercialization. *Surg Obes Relat Dis*. 2019;15(3):417-423.

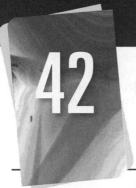

42

Endoscopic Suturing

Qais Dawod, MD
Reem Z. Sharaiha, MD, MSc

BACKGROUND

Endoscopic suturing techniques were firstly introduced by Swain and Mills in 1986.[1]

In 1998, the FDA approved the first flexible endoscopic suturing device, which was primarily used for the management of gastroesophageal reflux disease. Since then, the use of endoscopic sutures in endoscopic procedures has been on the rise. The surgical experience gained from the use of this modality in addition to the rapid new technical and technological advancements in its design has helped physicians expand its use in managing a vast array of gastrointestinal conditions.[2,3]

APPLICATION

Over the past few years, endoscopic suturing utilization in the management of several gastrointestinal conditions has become more prevalent. Endoscopic suturing was particularly helpful in the repair of upper and lower gastrointestinal defects including fistulas, anastomotic leaks, and perforations. In gastrointestinal conditions requiring the placement of esophageal stents to alleviate symptoms, stent migration has been reported in as many as 46% of cases; the recent use of endoscopic suturing for fixation has provided reduced migration rates, as well as better clinical outcomes for patients.[2-5] Endoscopic suturing has also been used to treat ulcer bleeds by oversewing the ulcer bed.[6]

Obesity has been one of the major public health concerns, affecting more than one-third of the adults in the United States. The use of endoscopic suturing for both weight regain following gastric bypass surgery and endoscopic sleeve gastroplasty as a primary procedure, a minimally invasive intervention to counter obesity, has provided effective and sustained results in weight loss.[7] Endoscopic gastric sleeve has been shown to be a safe and effective weigh loss method associated with low adverse event and hospitalization length when compared to laparoscopic sleeve.[8] Using the OverStitch device, for bypass patients, the outlet size is reduced, and in the primary procedure, the stomach is constricted in an accordion-like fashion followed by the use of endoscopic suturing, thus mimicking the surgical technique.

CURRENT DEVICES

Over the past 2 decades, many systems have been developed for endoscopic suturing within the GI tract as listed below. Given that a number of these are not currently utilized in clinical practice, this chapter focuses on the widely used Apollo Endosurgery's Overstitch system.

SUCTION-BASED DEVICE SUTURING SYSTEM

- EndoCinch (Bard, Murray Hill, NJ, USA)
- LSI Solution (Victor, NY, USA)
- Spiderman (Ethicon Endo-Surgery, Cincinnati, OH, USA)
- Sew-Right (Cook Endoscopy, Winston-Salem, NC, USA)
  None of the suction-based suturing system is currently used in clinical practice in humans.[9,10]

WORKING OVERTUBE DELIVERING PRELOADED STITCH SUTURING SYSTEM

- NDO plicator (NDO Surgical, Mansfield, MA, USA)
- EsophyX (EndoGastric Solutions, Redmond, WA, USA)
  EsophyX device is rarely used for endoscopic correction of gastroesophageal reflux disease, while NDO plicator is not commercially available.[11]

FLEXIBLE ENDOSCOPIC STAPLING DEVICE SUTURING SYSTEM

- Power Medical (now Covidien based at New Haven, CT, USA)
  This device is no longer available for clinical use.[12-15]

DELIVERY OF T-TAGS WITH ATTACHED SUTURES THROUGH A HOLLOW NEEDLE SUTURING SYSTEM

- Olympus Optical LTD (Tokyo, Japan)
- Cook Endoscopy (Winston-Salem, NC, USA)
- Ethicon Endo-Surgery Inc (Cincinnati, OH, USA)
  None of these systems is commercially available.[16-19]

CURVED NEEDLE SUTURING SYSTEM

- G-Prox (USGI Medical, San Clemente, CA)
- Eagle Claw (Olympus Optical LTD, Tokyo, Japan)

  G-Prox system is mostly used in bariatric patients for revision of dilated gastrojejunal anastomosis as it requires a special delivery system.[20-27]

- OverStitch (Apollo Endosurgery Inc., Austin, TX, USA) and the Sx (single-channel device). The majority of this article will focus on this system.

  Since 2011, Apollo Endosurgery's OverStitch has been commercially available for human use, considered the most universally used endoscopic suturing device, it allows the creation of endoscopic sutures closely mirroring surgical suturing. This suturing system uses a curved needle which most closely resembles the surgical suturing technique. There are two devices available commercially: the double-channel and the single-channel device (Sx).

PREPARATION

1. Fast the patient for at least 8 hours prior to the procedure.
2. Obtain informed consent from the patient or patient representative, outlining the possible procedural adverse events as well as alternative methods of treatment.
3. Patient would need to be intubated if an upper endoscopy is performed ideally. For lower GI procedures, this would be at the discretion of the endoscopist or the anesthesiologist.
4. Obtain oral suction in the case of retained fluid or inability to clear secretions during the procedure.
5. Start an intravenous line for administration of systemic sedation.
6. For obesity-related procedure, preprocedure medication need to be given for nausea.

EQUIPMENT

1. Double-channel therapeutic Olympus scope for the (Gen 2 OverStitch device) versus a single change if using the Sx device
2. Endoscopic water pump with simethicone in the fluid
3. Overtube device; however, in the hands of experienced endoscopists, the suturing device can be placed safely without the overtube
4. Endoscopic sutures, soaked in water
5. Endoscopic cinches (ensure you have 1 to 2 boxes or >10/case)
6. Helix (depending on the indication for suturing)
7. Lubricant
8. Gloves

PROCEDURE

Apollo OverStitch is a user-friendly device; its use and setup is straightforward. Using a double-channel gastroscope, the device is front loaded prior to inserting the endoscope into the GI tract. The suture is inserted onto the anchor exchange catheter and loaded onto the device. The suture is then transferred to the needle driver. The suture arm is then able to open and close, driving the needle through the first edge of the targeted tissue. The suture then is transferred back to the anchor exchange and thus a full suture loop is completed. The process in then repeated by reloading the suture onto the needle driver again (Fig. 42.1).

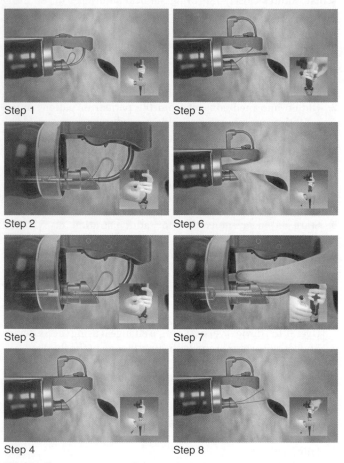

Step 1

Step 2

Step 3

Step 4

Step 5

Step 6

Step 7

Step 8

FIG. 42.1 Tissue suturing guide. (Reprinted with permission from Apollo Endosurgery, Inc.)

The suture pattern is dependent on how many "bites" per suture and the location of each suture bite. The pattern used is based on the procedure indication.

Once the suture pattern is completed, the anchor exchange releases the needle to form a T-bar. This also secures one end of the suture. The other end is secured through a cinching device that guillotines the suture deploying a plastic cinch[23,28] (Fig. 42.2).

Tissue Suturing Guide (Fig. 42.1)

1. After creating suture slack. Close needle body by squeezing the handle.
2. Push anchor exchange forward to engage anchor.
3. Push and hold blue button. Pull back 1 cm.

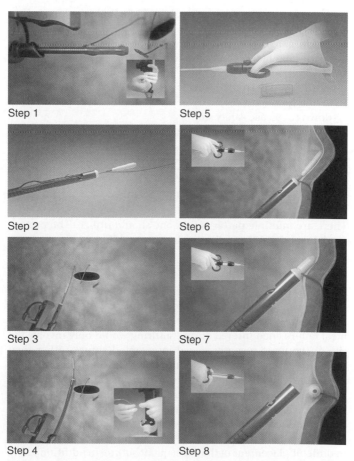

Step 1

Step 5

Step 2

Step 6

Step 3

Step 7

Step 4

Step 8

FIG. 42.2 Cinching guide. (Reprinted with permission from Apollo Endosurgery, Inc.)

4. Squeeze handle open.
5. Advance tissue helix to targeted tissue. Apply forward pressure. Turn blue knob clockwise to engage tissue.
6. Pull tissue helix into needle guard. Close handle to pass anchor and suture.
7. Advance anchor exchange catheter to engage with anchor. Pull anchor exchange without pushing blue button.
8. Turn tissue helix knob counterclockwise to disengage tissue. Open handle. Repeat steps 1 to 8 as needed.

Cinching guide (Fig. 42.2)

1. With the handle open, extend anchor exchange catheter out 3 cm and press blue button to release anchor. Remove anchor exchange.
2. Thread suture through gold tab of cinch. Pull tab along axis of the cinch catheter.
3. Holding slight suture tension, introduce cinch through 3.7 mm scope channel. Extend catheter to first bite location.
4. Holding cinch catheter in place and resting on tissue, pull suture until desired tension is achieved.
5. While holding tension, open cinch handle with palm facing down to release safety stop.
6. Close handle to pull cinch plug into collar.
7. With two hands, continue to squeeze handle.
8. Continue to squeeze until suture is cut and the cinch is deployed. Do not over squeeze handle.

SUTURE PATTERN

There are multiple patterns that one should utilize. The pattern used depends on the indication for suturing (Fig. 42.3).

INTERRUPTED/SIMPLE

This pattern of suturing has been found to exert less drag on tissue during tightening while having no risk of suture entanglement and crossing as compared to running sutures. Any technical failure encountered during suturing would only involve the site of the most recently placed interrupted suture rather than the entire suturing workup. Suture failure after terminating the procedure would not involve the entire closure but rather only a small segment, eliminating risk of dehiscence that is seen in running sutures. One of the drawbacks of this pattern has been the limited visualization and grasping of the edges of the defect encountered after tightening of the first suture which might lead to difficult placement of the subsequent suture. In addition, there is a significant increase in expense proportionate to the number of sutures used.[29]

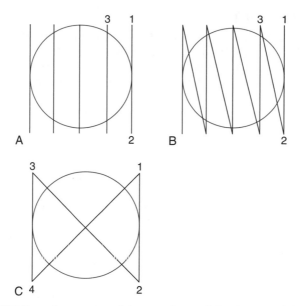

FIG. 42.3 Types of suture pattern. A, Interrupted suture; B, Running suture; C, Figure-of-8 suture.

FIGURE OF 8

This specialized suture pattern is mainly used to repair small circular defects in a circular fashion with equal circumferential tightening toward the center of the defect. Thus, making it ideal suturing pattern for fistula closure and oversewing an ulcer. Inconveniently, this suturing pattern is technically more difficult in contrast to interrupted suturing as well as having a higher risk of suture entanglement. In addition, any failure of the suture due to erosion or breakage would result in loosening of the entire suture and dehiscence of the entire closure.[29]

RUNNING

This suturing pattern allows the endoscopist to have a better visibility of the defect edges until the suturing is completed. While only one stitch and cinch are used, this pattern is considered less expensive than the other suturing patterns. On the other hand, this pattern is associated with tissue drag as the suture goes through multiple bites, requiring careful handling before tightening. Also requires careful technique and experience to avoid entanglement of the long suture. Any encountered failure will result in the loss of the entire workup to that point and would need to start the closure from the beginning. Similarly, any suture failure after terminating the case would result in failure of the entire closure.[29]

ADVERSE EVENTS

Adverse events are minimal and are mainly related to the use of the helix during full-thickness plications. Reported cases in the literature include bleeding, leaking, and gallbladder perforation. Minor adverse events include ulceration or minimal bleeding. In order to minimize these events, one must ensure adequate training of both the endoscopist and the endoscopy staff on the various aspects of the device.

CONCLUSION

The rapid rise of endoscopic suturing is expected to continue. Further innovation and technological advancements are expected to rise. It is anticipated that the indications for suturing as well as its availability will increase over time. The technical difficulties that comes with the handling of the devices will improve in time as will the skills of the endoscopists with continued use and repetition. Various different societies are offering learning opportunities, such as training and simulation labs, that may help shorten the learning curve that is seen with endoscopic suturing, as well as improve technical success while limiting adverse events.

References

1. Swain CP, Mills TN. An endoscopic sewing machine. *Gastrointest Endosc.* 1986;32:36-38.
2. Sharaiha RZ, Kumta NA, DeFilippis EM, et al. A large multicenter experience with endoscopic suturing for management of gastrointestinal defects and stent anchorage in 122 patients: a retrospective review. *J Clin Gastroenterol.* 2016;50:388-392. doi:10.1097/mcg.0000000000000336.
3. Felsher J, Farres H, Chand B, Farver C, Ponsky J. Mucosal apposition in endoscopic suturing. *Gastrointest Endosc.* 2003;58:867-870.
4. Ngamruengphong S, Sharaiha RZ, Sethi A, et al. Endoscopic suturing for the prevention of stent migration in benign upper gastrointestinal conditions: a comparative multicenter study. *Endoscopy.* 2016;48:802-808. doi:10.1055/s-0042-108567.
5. Sharaiha RZ, Kumta NA, Doukides TP, et al. Esophageal stenting with sutures: time to redefine our standards?. *J Clin Gastroenterol.* 2015;49:e57-e60. doi:10.1097/mcg.0000000000000198.
6. Stanley AJ, Laine L. Management of acute upper gastrointestinal bleeding. *Br Med J.* 2019;364:l536. doi:10.1136/bmj.l536.
7. Sharaiha RZ, Kumta NA, Saumoy M, et al. Endoscopic sleeve gastroplasty significantly reduces Body mass index and metabolic complications in obese patients. *Clin Gastroenterol Hepatol.* 2017;15:504-510. doi:10.1016/j.cgh.2016.12.012.
8. Novikov AA, Afaneh C, Saumoy M, et al. Endoscopic sleeve gastroplasty, laparoscopic sleeve gastrectomy, and laparoscopic band for weight loss: how do they compare?. *J Gastrointest Surg.* 2018;22:267-273.
9. Schwartz MP, Schreinemakers JR, Smout AJ. Four-year follow-up of endoscopic gastroplication for the treatment of gastroesophageal reflux disease. *World J Gastrointest Pharmacol Ther.* 2013;4:120-126. doi:10.4292/wjgpt.v4.i4.120.
10. Chen YK. Endoscopic suturing devices for treatment of GERD: too little, too late?. *Gastrointest Endosc.* 2005;62:44-47. doi:10.1016/j.gie.2005.04.013.

11. Yew KC, Chuah SK. Antireflux endoluminal therapies: past and present. *Gastroenterol Res Pract.* 2013;2013:481417. doi:10.1155/2013/481417.
12. Kaehler GF, Langner C, Suchan KL, Freudenberg S, Post S. Endoscopic full-thickness resection of the stomach: an experimental approach. *Surg Endosc.* 2006;20:519-521. doi:10.1007/s00464-005-0147-0.
13. Kaehler G, Grobholz R, Langner C, Suchan K, Post S. A new technique of endoscopic full-thickness resection using a flexible stapler. *Endoscopy.* 2006;38:86-89. doi:10.1055/s-2005-921181.
14. Meireles OR, Kantsevoy SV, Assumpcao LR, et al. Reliable gastric closure after natural orifice translumenal endoscopic surgery (NOTES) using a novel automated flexible stapling device. *Surg Endosc.* 2008;22:1609-1613. doi:10.1007/s00464-008-9750-1.
15. Magno P, Giday SA, Dray X, et al. A new stapler-based full-thickness transgastric access closure: results from an animal pilot trial. *Endoscopy.* 2007;39:876-880. doi:10.1055/s-2007-966896.
16. Raju GS, Shibukawa G, Ahmed I, et al. Endoluminal suturing may overcome the limitations of clip closure of a gaping wide colon perforation (with videos). *Gastrointest Endosc.* 2007;65:906-911. doi:10.1016/j.gie.2006.08.048.
17. Ikeda K, Fritscher-Ravens A, Mosse CA, Mills T, Tajiri H, Swain CP. Endoscopic full-thickness resection with sutured closure in a porcine model. *Gastrointest Endosc.* 2005;62:122-129.
18. Dray X, Krishnamurty DM, Donatelli G, et al. Gastric wall healing after NOTES procedures: closure with endoscopic clips provides superior histological outcome compared with threaded tags closure. *Gastrointest Endosc.* 2010;72:343-350. doi:10.1016/j.gie.2010.02.023.
19. Kantsevoy SV. Endoscopic full-thickness resection: new minimally invasive therapeutic alternative for GI-tract lesions. *Gastrointest Endosc.* 2006;64:90-91. doi:10.1016/j.gie.2006.02.013.
20. Hu B, Chung SC, Sun LC, et al. Endoscopic suturing without extracorporeal knots: a laboratory study. *Gastrointest Endosc.* 2005;62:230-233.
21. Hu B, Chung SC, Sun LC, et al. Eagle Claw II: a novel endosuture device that uses a curved needle for major arterial bleeding: a bench study. *Gastrointest Endosc.* 2005;62:266-270.
22. Kantsevoy SV, Hu B, Jagannath SB, et al. Technical feasibility of endoscopic gastric reduction: a pilot study in a porcine model. *Gastrointest Endosc.* 2007;65:510-513. doi:10.1016/j.gie.2006.07.045.
23. Kantsevoy S. Endoscopic suturing for closure of transmural defects. 2015;17:136-140.
24. Conway NE, Swanström LL. Endoluminal flexible endoscopic suturing for minimally invasive therapies. *Gastrointest Endosc.* 2015;81:262-269.e219. doi:10.1016/j.gie.2014.09.013.
25. Swanstrom LL. Current technology development for natural orifice transluminal endoscopic surgery. *Cir Esp.* 2006;80:283-288.
26. Mullady DK, Lautz DB, Thompson CC. Treatment of weight regain after gastric bypass surgery when using a new endoscopic platform: initial experience and early outcomes (with video). *Gastrointest Endosc.* 2009;70:440-444. doi:10.1016/j.gie.2009.01.042.
27. Ryou M, Mullady DK, Lautz DB, Thompson CC. Pilot study evaluating technical feasibility and early outcomes of second-generation endosurgical platform for treatment of weight regain after gastric bypass surgery. *Surg Obes Relat Dis.* 2009;5:450-454. doi:10.1016/j.soard.2009.03.217.
28. Kantsevoy SV. Endoscopic suturing devices. In: Testoni PA, Arcidiacono PG, Mariani A, eds. *Endoscopic Management of Gastrointestinal Cancer and Precancerous Conditions.* Turin: Edizoni Minerva Medica; 2015:249-255.
29. Stavropoulos SN, Modayil R, Friedel D. Current applications of endoscopic suturing. *World J Gastrointest Endosc.* 2015;7:777-789. doi:10.4253/wjge.v7.i8.777.

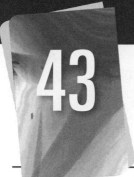

Transoral Outlet Reduction (TORe)

Allison R. Schulman, MD, MPH

Roux-en-Y gastric bypass (RYGB) has traditionally been the most commonly performed bariatric surgical procedure. It involves stapling of the stomach to create a small gastric pouch and connecting it to a portion to the jejunum (known as the Roux limb) to create a gastrojejunal anastomosis (GJA). While diet and lifestyle factors play a role in weight regain after RYGB, studies have demonstrated that a dilated GJA aperture is an independent predictor of weight regain with a linear association.[1] Endoscopic sutured transoral outlet reduction (TORe) is a safe and effective treatment for management of a dilated GJA.

INDICATIONS
1. Dilated GJA (≥15 mm in diameter) (Fig. 43.1)
2. Dumping syndrome

CONTRAINDICATIONS
1. Lack of informed consent
2. Cardiac instability, respiratory insufficiency, or other life-threatening cardiopulmonary conditions
3. Significant bleeding diathesis
4. Warfarin or heparin use
5. Marginal ulceration (i.e., ulceration at the site of the GJA)
6. Lack of patient cooperation
7. Portal hypertension
8. Active tobacco use

PREPARATION
1. Obtain informed consent which includes a detailed discussion with the patient about indications for the procedure, alternative therapy, possible adverse events, and weight loss expectations.

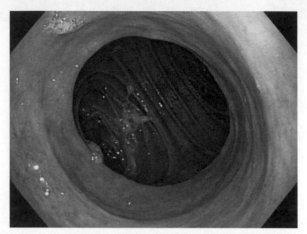

FIG. 43.1 Dilated gastrojejunal anastomosis.

2. An initial upper endoscopy should be performed to assess pouch length and size of the GJA to determine if the RYGB anatomy is amenable to endoscopic-sutured TORe. It is also important to confirm absence of structural abnormalities, marginal ulceration, or severe esophagitis before proceeding. Foreign surgical material such as sutures and staples can also be removed at the time of index endoscopy to prevent interference with eventual reconstruction.[2-6]

3. Bowel preparation: See Chapter 3 on bowel preparation. Bowel preparation is optional and can be considered the night before the procedure to prevent intraprocedure bowel movements and postprocedure abdominal pain, constipation, and/or straining.

4. Preprocedural fast: Liquid diet the day prior to the procedure, and nothing by mouth (NPO) for 12 hours prior to the procedure.

5. Medication: The procedure is performed under general anesthesia with endotracheal intubation, and with CO_2 insufflation. Aggressive antinausea control is essential, including preprocedural administration of a scopolamine patch, dexamethasone, and liberalized use of other antiemetics.

EQUIPMENT

1. Double-channel endoscope (GIF-2T160 or GIF-2T180; Olympus America, Center Valley, PA)

2. Apollo OverStitch Endoscopic Suturing System (Apollo Endosurgery, Austin, TX)

3. Polypropylene nonabsorbable surgical suture (2-0 DemeLENE, DemeTECH, Miami Lakes, FL)
4. An overtube (Guardus; US Endoscopy, Mentor, OH, or OverTube Endoscopic Access System, Apollo Endosurgery)
5. OverStitch Suture Cinch (Apollo Endosurgery)
6. OverStitch Tissue Helix (Apollo Endosurgery)
7. Argon plasma coagulation (APC)
8. Simethicone (60 mL)
9. Through-the-scope (TTS) balloon dilators of various diameters (8 to 12 mm in size)
10. Dilating gun or inflation device to maintain pressure
11. Stopcocks to ensure constant pressure during inflation
12. Monitoring equipment (pulse, blood pressure, with continuous electrocardiogram)
13. Universal precautions with gloves, gowns, masks
14. Protective coverings for universal precautions: gloves, gowns, masks

PROCEDURE

1. Place the patient in left lateral decubitus position.
2. Carbon dioxide should be used exclusively for insufflation throughout the procedure.
3. Perform a complete upper endoscopy with close attention to the posterior jejunal aspect of the GJA to confirm no interval development of a marginal ulceration; the overtube should be preloaded on the upper endoscope.
4. Removal of any foreign material such as surgical staples or sutures that may interfere with the procedure.
5. Insert the overtube carefully, making sure not to push against resistance if encountered at the level of the esophagus; maneuvers such as ensuring the patient's head is parallel to the thorax and performing a jaw thrust can minimize trauma.
6. Instill 60 mL simethicone is instilled down the distal Roux limb to minimize abdominal bloating and distention after the procedure.
7. A 5- to 10-mm area around the margin of the GJA should then be ablated using end-firing forced APC at 30 W and flow rate of 0.8 L/min; this should be performed in a noncontact pattern circumferentially (Fig. 43.2), and all excess argon suctioned prior to removal of the upper endoscope.
8. The endoscopic suturing device (OverStitch, Apollo) should then be attached to a double-channel upper endoscope; the device is composed of a curved suture arm attached to the endoscope tip and an anchor exchange that is deployed through one of the channels and loaded with the first suture.

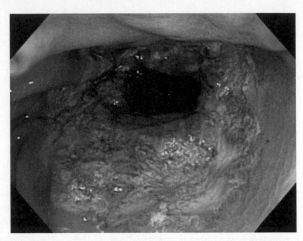

FIG. 43.2 Following argon plasma coagulation in a circumferential pattern around the margin of the gastrojejunal anastomosis to prepare the tissue for endoscopic suturing.

9. With activation of the handle, the suture arm advances the needle through the gastric tissue and passes the needle to the anchor exchange. Opening of the handle then releases the tissue. The anchor then can be passed back to the suture arm in anticipation of additional stitch placement.

10. Sutures can be placed in a variety of different suture patterns (interrupted, purse-string, belts over pants, figure of 8) to reduce the size of the GJA to 8 to 12 mm (Fig. 43.3); the most commonly reported patterns are interrupted and purse-string.[2-6]

    a. In an interrupted pattern, individual sutures are placed sequentially from the lower left to the upper right of the GJA and cinched until the size of the aperture is reduced.

    b. In a purse-string pattern, a single suture is placed around the margin of the GJA in a continuous ring; this stitch pattern is started after a full rotation to the 3 o'clock position and continued in a counter-clockwise fashion, typically requiring 8 to 12 stitches (or bites) with a single suture; a hydrostatic dilation balloon is then passed through the second channel of the endoscope and inflated to a diameter of 8 to 12 mm inside the anastomosis. The single suture is then tightened and cinched over the balloon.

    c. Additional stitches can be placed in the distal gastric pouch just proximal to the anastomosis to reduce gastric volume and reinforce the sutures at the level of the GJA.

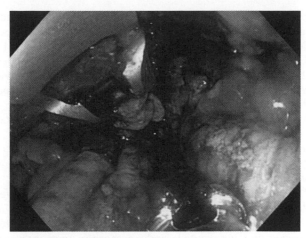

FIG. 43.3 Gastrojejunal anastomosis following transoral outlet reduction (TORe) using endoscopic suturing.

11. After removal of the suturing equipment, a standard upper endoscope was then advanced through the overtube.
12. Close examination of the GJA is performed to confirm suture integrity.
13. Inspection of the esophagus after overtube removal should be performed to ensure no bleeding or laceration; hemostatic clip placement should be considered if either of these adverse events is noted.

POSTPROCEDURE

1. Patients may be discharged the same day or observed for a planned 1-day admission to the hospital following the procedure.
2. Recovery from the sedative/analgesia may take up to several hours, and patients should be informed beforehand that driving is not permitted and that someone should accompany the patient to the procedure in order to safely see him or her home if discharge is desired.
3. Nothing should be administered by mouth the evening of the procedure.
4. Nausea and abdominal pain should be treated at the discretion of the proceduralist and/or the primary inpatient team by intravenous medication.
5. On the first day after the procedure, a clear liquid diet should be instituted for 1 day, followed by full liquids for 4 to 6 weeks.
6. During this time, all medications should be given in a crushed, chewable, or soluble form.

7. For the 2 weeks after the liquid diet, patients should be maintained on a soft-solid diet and then transitioned to solid food.
8. Follow-up clinical examinations should be performed at 4 weeks, 3, and 12 months, with variable follow-up in between; these visits should entail weight recording and interview regarding postprocedure symptoms, dietary and exercise habits, and satiety.

A thorough procedure note in the medical record should contain the following information:
1. Indication for procedure
2. Type of instrument used
3. Medication given and dosages
4. The most distal portion of the intestinal tract intubated (e.g., Roux limb or jejunojejunal anastomosis)
5. Number of sutures used, the pattern of suture placement (e.g., purse-string, interrupted), and whether the aperture is sized (and to what size) using a TTS dilating balloon
6. Detailed description of findings
7. Procedural difficulties (e.g., bleeding, esophageal laceration from overtube placement, other adverse events)
8. Postprocedure condition of the patient
9. Follow-up plan

FOLLOW-UP

The patient should ideally be seen in clinic 1 month, 3 months, 6 months, and 12 months following the procedure. Shorter intervals are required if unexpected symptoms develop. There is no requirement for repeat upper endoscopy or other imaging following the procedure.

ADVERSE EVENTS

1. Cardiopulmonary: Adverse events during TORe procedures can be related to the cardiopulmonary system, with bradycardia, hypotension, and reactions to various sedation medications similar to other endoscopic procedures.
2. Abdominal pain: Abdominal pain following TORe is not uncommon but has only led to emergency evaluation or admission in <4% of patients.[6]
3. Bleeding: Bleeding has been reported in 3% to 4% of patients and can range from intraprocedural oozing at the suture sites (often self-limited) or from the development of marginal ulceration which may require hemoclip placement or epinephrine injection in a small percentage of patients[5,6]).
4. Esophageal trauma: Rarely, patients may develop superficial mucosal proximal esophageal abrasions and tears which may require prophylactic clipping.[5,6]

5. Device-related adverse events: Include suture breakage, needle entrapment in tissue, and accidental needle drop. This is reported to occur in approximately 1% of cases.
6. Gastrojejunal stricture: Very rare and should be treated with serial balloon dilations.

CPT CODES[a]

43999—Unlisted procedure
43850—Revision of gastroduodenal anastomosis (gastrojejunostomy) with reconstruction, with or without vagotomy

References

1. Abu Dayyeh BK, Lautz DB, Thompson CC. Gastrojejunal stoma diameter predicts weight regain after Roux-en-Y gastric bypass. *Clin Gastroenterol Hepatol.* 2011;9(3):228-233.
2. Thompson CC, Chand B, Chen YK, et al. Endoscopic suturing for transoral outlet reduction increases weight loss after Roux-en-Y gastric bypass surgery. *Gastroenterology.* 2013;145:129-137.e3.
3. Kumar N, Thompson CC. Comparison of a superficial suturing device with a full-thickness suturing device for transoral outlet reduction (with videos). *Gastrointest Endosc.* 2014;79:984-989.
4. Kumar N, Thompson CC. Transoral outlet reduction for weight regain after gastric bypass: long-term follow-up. *Gastrointest Endosc.* 2016;83:776-779.
5. Schulman AR, Kumar N, Thompson CC. Transoral outlet reduction: a comparison of purse-string with interrupted stitch technique. *Gastrointest Endosc.* 2018;87(5):1222-1228.
6. Jirapinyo P, Kröner P, Thompson C. Purse-string transoral outlet reduction (TORe) is effective at inducing weight loss and improvement in metabolic comorbidities after Roux-en-Y gastric bypass. *Endoscopy.* 2018;50:371-377.

---

[a]Practice patterns vary based on the location and insurance provider.

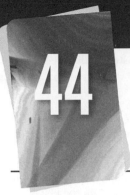

44 Endoscopic Management of Postsurgical Adverse Events

Amar Mandalia, MD
Allison R. Schulman, MD, MPH

Gastrointestinal surgery is commonly performed for a variety of indications in the upper and lower gastrointestinal (GI) tract. There are a number of unique adverse events that can develop in this patient population and are managed endoscopically. This chapter will focus on endoscopic procedural considerations for common adverse events following surgery and will include a brief overview of the epidemiology, pathophysiology, and management of each adverse event.

ANASTOMOTIC ULCERATION

Anastomotic ulceration, also known as marginal ulceration, is reported in up to 8.6% of patients who have undergone partial or total gastrectomy, 5% to 27% of patients with pancreaticoduodenectomy, 0.6% to 16% of patients who have undergone Roux-en-Y gastric bypass (RYGB), and 0.8% of patients following ileocectomy.[1-7] These ulcerations occur at the resection margin of the intestinal wall. The mechanism of development is multifactorial, with a variety of proposed risk factors including but is not limited to ischemia and tension at the anastomosis, tissue irritants such as smoking, various medications, diabetes mellitus, and the presence of foreign material (such as staples or sutures). When symptoms occur, they include pain, obstruction, GI bleeding, perforation, or anemia. Diagnosis is made endoscopically by either upper endoscopy or colonoscopy, depending on location.

DIAGNOSIS AND ENDOSCOPIC MANAGEMENT
Indications
1. High clinical suspicion of the presence of an anastomotic ulcer
2. Overt GI bleeding
3. Unexplained anemia

Contraindications

1. See Chapters 5 and 19 for esophagogastroduodenoscopy and colonoscopy for contraindications

Preparation

1. Obtain informed consent which includes a detailed discussion with the patient about indications for the procedure and possible adverse events.
2. The patient should be nil per os (NPO) for at least 4 to 6 hours prior to endoscopic evaluation; if a colonoscopy is planned, bowel preparation is required (see Chapter 3 for details).
3. Patients with GI bleeding should be appropriately managed and adequately resuscitated prior to pursuing endoscopic evaluation.

Equipment

1. Upper GI tract surgery: use of either a single- or double-channel upper endoscope; if significant bleeding is suspected/encountered, should preferentially use a wide single-channel or a two-channel therapeutic upper endoscope to enhance aspiration.
2. Lower GI tract surgery: use of a colonoscope (see colonoscopy Chapter 19).
3. Use of CO_2 insufflation.
4. Ancillary equipment for hemostasis such as epinephrine 1:10,000, hemostatic clips, bipolar cautery, or argon plasma coagulation.
5. Ancillary equipment for foreign material removal such as forceps, endoscopic scissors, or loop cutters.

Procedure

1. Perform a complete examination of the upper and/or lower GI tract to exclude other causes of pain, anemia, or obstruction; if an anastomotic ulceration is encountered, do not pass beyond it as this can increase the risk of perforation.
2. Identify the location of the anastomotic ulcer and examine the ulcer for bleeding or stigmata of recent bleeding such as a visible vessel or pigmented red spot; if present, treat accordingly with injection and/or hemostatic clipping and/or cautery (see Chapters 35 to 37 on management of upper GI bleeding).
3. If no active bleeding or high-risk stigmata or recent bleeding, examine the area for foreign bodies such as staples or sutures. If present, use forceps to remove staples and sutures, and consider use of endoscopic scissors or loop cutters for refractory material.

Postprocedure Care

1. Observe the patient for signs of bleeding, fever, and/or perforation. Pain medication may be indicated.
2. Use acid-suppressing medication in open capsule or soluble form for upper GI anastomotic ulcers; consider use of liquid sucralfate.[8]
3. Repeat the procedure in 8 to 12 weeks to evaluate for healing of the ulcer.

Adverse Events

1. Cardiopulmonary: The most common adverse events during colonoscopic examinations are related to the cardiopulmonary system, with bradycardia, hypotension, and reactions to various sedation medications.
2. Perforation: More serious adverse events such as perforation occur in <1% of examinations, but the risk is increased in the setting of a deep-cratered anastomotic ulceration and during therapeutic intervention. See Chapters 5 and 19 on upper endoscopy and colonoscopy for management.
3. Rebleeding: See Chapters 35 to 37 on management of upper GI bleeding.
4. Infection: Rare, see Chapters 5 and 19 on upper endoscopy and colonoscopy for more information.

ANASTOMOTIC STENOSIS/STRICTURE

Anastomotic luminal stenosis may form after esophagectomy (9.1% to 65.8%), partial or total gastrectomy (1.1% to 8.0%), pancreaticoduodenectomy, RYGB (2% to 23%), sleeve gastrectomy (0.1% to 3.9%), and colorectal surgery (0% to 30%).[9-18] Anastomotic biliary strictures can occur after liver transplantation (14.2%) and are covered in detail in the Chapter 28.[19] Etiologies of stricture formation include ischemia, anastomotic tension, inflammation, surgical technique, and recurrence of malignancy. Luminal strictures can present as obstructive symptoms and inability to tolerate meals. The strictures are typically benign but can also be due to a recurrence of malignancy at the anastomoses. Endoscopic management varies by location and by complexity of stricture. This subsection will outline the various endoscopic tools that can be used to treat anastomotic strictures and stenoses.

Indications

1. Esophageal stricture
2. Gastroenteral anastomotic (gastrojejunal [Fig. 44.1] or gastroduodenal) stricture
3. Gastric stenosis following sleeve gastrectomy (Fig. 44.2)
4. Ileocolonic, colo-colonic, or colorectal anastomotic stricture

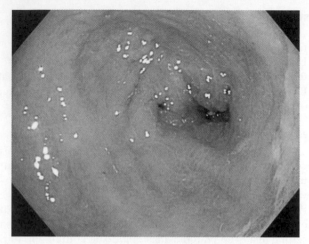

FIG. 44.1 Gastrojejunal anastomotic stricture following Roux-en-Y Gastric Bypass.

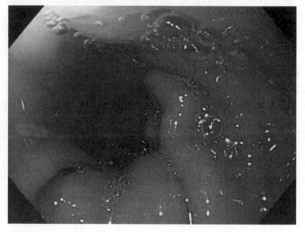

FIG. 44.2 Bilious fluid proximal to gastric sleeve stenosis following sleeve gastrectomy.

Contraindications

1. Inflammation or ulceration at the site of stenosis
2. Active bleeding at the site of the stenosis
3. Long stricture (>5 cm)
4. Evidence of acute abdomen
5. Evidence of abdominal perforation
6. Bleeding diathesis
7. Recent anticoagulation use

Preparation

1. The patient should be NPO for 4 to 6 hours
2. Could consider decompression by nasogastric tube to low intermittent suction depending on the clinical situation
3. Obtain written consent. Be sure to include an associated increased risk of perforation and blood-borne infection with dilation
4. Anesthesia assistance should be considered for these cases

Equipment

1. Upper endoscope or pediatric/adult colonoscope depending on location of stricture; consider ultraslim scope for cases with severe narrowing
2. hrough-the-scope (TTS) balloon dilators of various sizes
3. Pneumatic dilators and fluoroscopy for gastric sleeve stenosis

Procedure

1. Perform a complete examination of the upper gastrointestinal tract or the lower gastrointestinal tract to evaluate for causes of obstruction
2. Identify the location of the stricture
3. If the stricture appears malignant, then it would be important to biopsy it and avoid dilation
4. If the stricture is benign, note whether the stricture is circumferential and traversable
5. If it is not traversable and precludes you from completing a full examination, consider switching to a small caliber scope (≤6 mm) to complete your examination. Note that a small caliber scope will not allow for TTS balloon dilation
6. If the stricture is traversable, note for resistance
7. For simple anastomotic strictures or gastric sleeve stenosis, a TTS balloon can be used for dilation
   a. Choose the appropriate TTS balloon size for dilation: options include 6-7-8 mm, 8-9-10 mm, 10-11-12 mm, 12-13.5-15 mm, 15-16.5-18 mm, and 18-19-20 mm. Deliver the TTS balloon through the biopsy channel; for stenosis of the gastrojejunal anastomosis following RYGB, dilation past 15 mm should generally be avoided given risk of weight regain
8. Note for gastric sleeve stenosis, the TTS balloon should be used to dilate the incisura and the pylorus; if the patient does not respond to a TTS dilation of 20 mm then it would be advisable to step up to pneumatic dilation (Fig. 44.3)[20]
   a. Start with the 30 mm pneumatic balloon and grade the resistance. Note that maximal PSI may not be reached at the first session. Ensure that the pneumatic balloon does not span the gastroesophageal junction or the pylorus

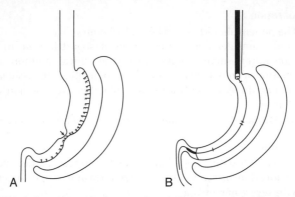

FIG. 44.3 A, Arrow demonstrating stenosis at the incisura angularis following sleeve gastrectomy. B, Pneumatic balloon dilation of gastric sleeve stenosis.

    b. Repeat the procedure in 2 weeks if symptomatic improvement is not achieved. Use the same size balloon until maximum PSI is reached or use a pneumatic balloon that is 5 mm greater in size than the previous balloon

9. Carefully align the balloon with narrowest point of the stricture and ask your technician to inflate the balloon to the indicated size. Wrap your left pinky finger over the balloon catheter for stabilization and control

    a. Technician should evaluate degree of resistance

    b. There is no standardization regarding number of seconds for which dilation should be performed with an inflated balloon. Typically, dilation can be performed for 1 minute and redilation can be performed with another size; however, for pneumatic dilation, the dilation is often performed for several minutes

    c. The number of dilations performed during one endoscopy is also not standardized, but generally it is recommended to not dilate more than three consecutive sizes (i.e., "the rules of three")

    d. After completion of the dilation, examine the area for mucosal tears and ensure that perforation is not present

    e. Remove your balloon dilator from your scope and withdraw the scope

    f. Several subsequent sessions may be required for dilation

Postprocedure

1. Observe the patient for signs of fever, bleeding, and/or perforation

2. Advise the patient to seek emergent care if obstructive symptoms reoccur, if he/she develops worsening pain, or if there is concern for overt gastrointestinal bleeding

3. Schedule a follow-up endoscopy/colonoscopy as needed for further dilations

Adverse Events

1. Cardiopulmonary: The most common adverse events during endoscopic examinations are related to the cardiopulmonary system, with bradycardia, hypotension, and reactions to various sedation medications.

2. Perforation: This adverse event can occur in approximately 2% of patients undergoing dilation with TTS. The perforation risk using pneumatic balloons is also increased, but it is considered to be <1% for dilation of gastric sleeve stenosis.[21,22]

3. Restenosis: Restenosis can occur at any point after the initial dilation. If it does occur, it may require a repeat procedure to treat the stenosis.

4. Infection: Bacteremia is increased to approximately 5% in patients who undergo a dilation technique.

5. Pain: Common adverse event after dilation procedures. It would be important to rule out perforation and restenosis/obstruction as pain medication could mask this symptom.

POSTSURGICAL LEAKS

Postsurgical leaks occur along a suture or staple line, with an incidence of 10.6% following esophagectomy, 1.5% to 1.8% following gastrectomy, 0.5% to 8.3% following RYGB, and 0.3% to 7.0% following laparoscopic sleeve gastrectomy.[23-26] Before any intervention is undertaken, it is crucial to identify the location of the leak using cross-sectional imaging or combined endoscopic and fluoroscopic interrogation of possible sites, as that will dictate the appropriate management.

The location and chronicity of the leak dictates potential management strategies, and endoscopic practice varies among proceduralists. As a general principle, it is important to treat downstream obstruction and remove foreign material from the leak site including staples, sutures, and drains that may be in close proximity. In this chapter, we will cover stent placement for acute/early leaks (≤6 weeks). We will not review treatment of late/chronic leaks (>6 weeks), as management is dependent on location of leak, expertise of proceduralist, and regional variability; closure techniques (including cap-mounted clip placement, endoscopic suturing, and injectable biomaterials/compounds), septotomy, and double pigtail catheter drainage are all variably performed and will not be described here.

SELF-EXPANDABLE METAL STENT PLACEMENT

Indication
1. Esophageal leaks or acute/early postsurgical gastric leaks (≤6 weeks)

Contraindication
1. Extensive esophageal luminal dehiscence (>70%)
2. Hemodynamic instability
3. Bleeding diathesis
4. Undrained periesophageal or perigastric collection or abscess

Equipment
1. Wide-channel or dual-channel upper endoscope
2. Fluoroscopy if desired
3. Fully covered or partially covered self-expandable metal stent (SEMS); the longest/widest stents are generally selected in the setting of a leak, following sleeve gastrectomy and ideally bridge the distal esophagus and pylorus
4. Guidewire
5. Dilators (hydrostatic and/or pneumatic); see chapter xxx.
6. Consider Apollo OverStitch Endoscopic Suturing System (Apollo Endosurgery, Austin, TX), Polypropylene nonab-sorbable surgical suture (2-0 DemeLENE, DemeTECH, Miami Lakes, FL), and OverStitch Suture Cinch (Apollo Endosurgery)

Preparation
1. Obtain written consent from the patient
2. Patient should be NPO 4 to 6 hours prior to the procedure
3. Antibiotics if source control has not been obtained
4. Perform this procedure with an anesthesiologist present
5. Ensure that your endoscopic technician is familiar with the deployment of the esophageal stent

Procedure
1. Perform a diagnostic upper endoscopy and identify the location of the leak by combined endoscopic and fluoroscopic interrogation of possible sites if necessary
2. Treat down-stream obstruction with endoscopic dilation (discuss with referring surgeon and exercise caution in early period following surgery)
3. Remove foreign material from the leak site including staples, sutures, and drains that may be in close proximity (discuss with referring surgeon and exercise caution in early period following surgery)

4. Consider marking the leak site with contrast injection, endoscopic clips, or use of external fluoroscopic markers, such as coins, paper clips, or other metallic objects to delineate the desired location of stenting

5. Obtain guidewire access and advance the stent over the guidewire

6. Stents can be deployed under fluoroscopic guidance, endoscopic guidance, or a combination of the two; either the physician can directly operate the deployment catheter to control the stepwise release of the stent or the deployment can be controlled by an assistant/technician while the physician holds the delivery catheter itself and makes necessary adjustments prior to deployment

7. In leaks following sleeve gastrectomy, the longest/widest stents are generally selected with the goal of bridging the distal esophagus and pylorus; could consider placement of overlapping stents

8. If a fully covered SEMS is selected, consider endoscopic suturing of the proximal end to prevent migration

Postprocedure

1. Provide information to the patient on the esophageal stent diet; generally patients are instructed to take clear liquids for 24 hours following placement, then advance diet over the following days. They should be instructed to eat small bites of food and always chew food well, avoiding raw/leafy vegetables indefinitely.

2. Stay in a sitting position for at least 2 hours after each meal. Sleep with the head of your bed raised to 30 to 45 degrees.

3. High-dose proton pump inhibitors (PPIs).

Adverse Events

1. Pain—can be absent to severe, and tends to abate over the first week following stent placement. If pain is protracted and/or severe, endoscopic removal of the stent is often possible.

2. Bleeding—often mild, subclinical; overt gastrointestinal bleeding is rare.

3. Perforation—very rare in acute setting, can occur in delayed fashion.

4. Gastroesophageal reflux disease (GERD)—often develops if the stent is placed across the gastroesophageal junction.

5. Stent migration—delayed adverse event and more often occurs with fully covered stents that are not anchored in place.

6. Aspiration.

BILIARY/PANCREATIC PATHOLOGY REQUIRING ERCP IN POSTSURGICAL ANATOMY

Certain types of surgical procedures are compatible with conventional endoscopic retrograde cholangiopancreatography (ERCP) techniques, given accessibility of the duodenum and major papilla. These include but are not limited to esophagectomy with gastric pull-up, Billroth I, choledochoduodenostomy, and bariatric surgery that does not alter the conformation of the small bowel (including laparoscopic sleeve gastrectomy, vertical-banded gastroplasty, and laparoscopic-adjustable gastric banding). On the other hand, Billroth II gastrectomy, pancreaticoduodenectomy, Roux-en-Y hepaticojejunostomy, RYGB, and biliopancreatic diversion with or without a duodenal switch oftentimes require nonstandard ERCP technique. The selection of an appropriate endoscope and accessory devices depends on the surgical anatomy.

Indication
1. *See Chapter 25 for all indications

Contraindications
1. Marginal ulceration—this should be excluded prior to advancing the endoscope
2. Uncorrected coagulation abnormalities
3. Concern for visceral perforation

Preparation
1. Obtain written consent
2. NPO for at least 4 to 6 hours
3. Review all relevant operative reports to understand the type of surgical reconstruction including the length of surgically created limbs and the type of anastomosis
4. Ensure that your endoscopic nurse and technician are familiar with the procedure
5. Consider a multidisciplinary approach with close collaboration with the surgeon and/or interventional radiologist when needed
6. Anesthesia support
7. Fluoroscopy
8. CO_2 insufflation
9. Consider use of a clear cap to aid in visualization and cannulation as above

Equipment/Procedure
The equipment and procedure vary considerably based on the postoperative surgical anatomy and the approach to obtain ampullary access. A variety of factors must be considered:
1. Positioning of the patient; supine or left lateral approach may be preferred over prone positioning in altered surgical anatomy.

2. Distance between anastomosis and ampulla; if short (30 to 50 cm) ,consider duodenoscope or wide-channel gastroscope; otherwise consider pediatric colonoscope, enteroscope, or device-assisted enteroscope; furthermore, use of fluoroscopy may help identify the pancreaticobiliary limb, and tattooing may be considered to aid in future identification.

3. Potential direction or biliary or pancreatic orifice; for example, in Billroth II anatomy, the biliary orifice will be toward the 5 o'clock position as compared to 11 o'clock in normal anatomy; consider use of devices that improve orientation for cannulation including rotatable or specially designed sphincterotomes or bendable cannulas. Additionally, use of a clear cap to aid in visualization and cannulation.

4. Compatibility of diagnostic and therapeutic devices with the chosen endoscope.

5. In RYGB anatomy, endoscopic options for management include laparoscopic-assisted gastrostomy with transgastric ERCP, percutaneous gastrostomy with transgastric ERCP, or endoscopic ultrasound-directed transgastric ERCP procedure, where a lumen-apposing metal stent is placed through the gastric pouch and into the remnant stomach to allow access. These procedures are specific to RYGB anatomy and will not be discussed in detail.

Postprocedure

1. *See Chapter 25 for postprocedure care.

Adverse Events

1. *See Chapter 25 for adverse events associated with conventional ERCP such as bleeding, pancreatitis, and perforation.

2. Perforation at the gastrojejunal anastomosis, jejunojejunal anastomoses, and Roux-en-Y reconstruction must also be considered during ERCP in the postsurgical setting.

3. If endoscopic ultrasound-directed transgastric ERCP is performed, stent dislodgement/migration and nonhealing gastrogastric fistula must be considered.

References

1. Azagury DE, Abu Dayyeh BK, Greenwalt IT, Thompson CC. Marginal ulceration after Roux-en-Y gastric bypass surgery: characteristics, risk factors, treatment, and outcomes. *Endoscopy.* 2011;43(11):950-954.

2. Chari ST, Keate RF. Ileocolonic anastomotic ulcers: a case series and review of the literature. *Am J Gastroenterol.* 2000;95(5):1239-1243.

3. Chung WC, Jeon EJ, Lee K-M, et al. Incidence and clinical features of endoscopic ulcers developing after gastrectomy. *World J Gastroenterol.* 2012;18(25):3260-3266.

4. Csendes A, Burgos AM, Altuve J, Bonacic S. Incidence of marginal ulcer 1 month and 1 to 2 years after gastric bypass: a prospective consecutive endoscopic evaluation of 442 patients with morbid obesity. *Obes Surg.* 2009;19(2):135-138.

5. Rasmussen JJ, Fuller W, Ali MR. Marginal ulceration after laparoscopic gastric bypass: an analysis of predisposing factors in 260 patients. *Surg Endosc.* 2007;21(7):1090-1094.

6. Sacks BC, Mattar SG, Qureshi FG, et al. Incidence of marginal ulcers and the use of absorbable anastomotic sutures in laparoscopic Roux-en-Y gastric bypass. *Surg Obes Relat Dis.* 2006;2(1):11-16.

7. Wu JM, Tsai MK, Hu RH, Chang KJ, Lee PH, Tien YW. Reflux esophagitis and marginal ulcer after pancreaticoduodenectomy. *J Gastrointest Surg.* 2011;15(5):824-828.

8. Schulman AR, Chan WW, Devery A, Ryan MB, Thompson CC. Opened proton pump inhibitor capsules reduce time to healing compared with intact capsules for marginal ulceration following Roux-en-Y gastric bypass. *Clin Gastroenterol Hepatol.* 2017;15(4):494-500.e1.

9. Briel JW, Tamhankar AP, Hagen JA, et al. Prevalence and risk factors for ischemia, leak, and stricture of esophageal anastomosis: gastric pull-up versus colon interposition. *J Am Coll Surg.* 2004;198(4):536-541; discussion 41-2.

10. Burgos AM, Csendes A, Braghetto I. Gastric stenosis after laparoscopic sleeve gastrectomy in morbidly obese patients. *Obes Surg.* 2013;23(9):1481-1486.

11. Gagner M, Deitel M, Erickson AL, Crosby RD. Survey on laparoscopic sleeve gastrectomy (LSG) at the fourth international consensus summit on sleeve gastrectomy. *Obes Surg.* 2013;23(12):2013-2017.

12. Gagner M, Deitel M, Kalberer TL, Erickson AL, Crosby RD. The second international consensus summit for sleeve gastrectomy, March 19-21, 2009. *Surg Obes Relat Dis.* 2009;5(4):476-485.

13. Helmiö M, Victorzon M, Ovaska J, et al. SLEEVEPASS: a randomized prospective multicenter study comparing laparoscopic sleeve gastrectomy and gastric bypass in the treatment of morbid obesity: preliminary results. *Surg Endosc.* 2012;26(9):2521-2526.

14. Khalayleh H, Pines G, Imam A, Sapojnikov S, Buyeviz V, Mavor E. Anastomotic stricture rates following Roux-en-Y gastric bypass for morbid obesity: a comparison between linear and circular-stapled anastomosis. *J Laparoendosc Adv Surg Tech A.* 2018;28(6):631-636.

15. Mendelson AH, Small AJ, Agarwalla A, Scott FI, Kochman ML. Esophageal anastomotic strictures: outcomes of endoscopic dilation, risk of recurrence and refractory stenosis, and effect of foreign body removal. *Clin Gastroenterol Hepatol.* 2015;13(2):263-271.e1.

16. Park JY, Song HY, Kim JH, et al. Benign anastomotic strictures after esophagectomy: long-term effectiveness of balloon dilation and factors affecting recurrence in 155 patients. *Am J Roentgenol.* 2012;198(5):1208-1213.

17. Ribeiro-Parenti L, Arapis K, Chosidow D, Dumont JL, Demetriou M, Marmuse JP. Gastrojejunostomy stricture rate: comparison between antecolic and retrocolic laparoscopic Roux-en-Y gastric bypass. *Surg Obes Relat Dis.* 2015;11(5):1076-1084.

18. Xiong JJ, Altaf K, Javed MA, et al. Roux-en-Y versus Billroth I reconstruction after distal gastrectomy for gastric cancer: a meta-analysis. *World J Gastroenterol.* 2013;19(7):1124-1134.

19. Landi F, de'Angelis N, Sepulveda A, et al. Endoscopic treatment of anastomotic biliary stricture after adult deceased donor liver transplantation with multiple plastic stents versus self-expandable metal stents: a systematic review and meta-analysis. *Transpl Int.* 2018;31(2):131-151.

20. Schulman AR, Thompson CC. Complications of bariatric surgery: what you can expect to see in your GI practice. *Am J Gastroenterol.* 2017;112:1640.

21. Caro L, Sanchez C, Rodriguez P, Bosch J. Endoscopic balloon dilation of anastomotic strictures occurring after laparoscopic gastric bypass for morbid obesity. *Dig Dis (Basel, Switzerland)*. 2008;26(4):314-317.

22. Ukleja A, Afonso BB, Pimentel R, Szomstein S, Rosenthal R. Outcome of endoscopic balloon dilation of strictures after laparoscopic gastric bypass. *Surg Endosc*. 2008;22(8):1746-1750.

23. Alizadeh RF, Li S, Inaba C, et al. Risk factors for gastrointestinal leak after bariatric surgery: MBSAQIP analysis. *J Am Coll Surg*. 2018;227(1):135-141.

24. Aurora AR, Khaitan L, Saber AA. Sleeve gastrectomy and the risk of leak: a systematic analysis of 4,888 patients. *Surg Endosc*. 2012;26(6):1509-1515.

25. Jiang L, Yang K-H, Guan Q-L, et al. Laparoscopy-assisted gastrectomy versus open gastrectomy for resectable gastric cancer: an update meta-analysis based on randomized controlled trials. *Surg Endosc*. 2013;27(7):2466-2480.

26. Kim J, Azagury D, Eisenberg D, DeMaria E, Campos GM. ASMBS position statement on prevention, detection, and treatment of gastrointestinal leak after gastric bypass and sleeve gastrectomy, including the roles of imaging, surgical exploration, and nonoperative management. *Surg Obes Relat Dis*. 2015;11(4):739-748.

Endoscopic Submucosal Dissection and Peroral Endoscopic Myotomy

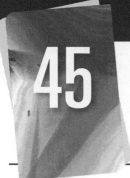

45 Esophageal Endoscopic Submucosal Dissection

Daniel S. Strand, MD
Andrew Y. Wang, MD

Endoscopic submucosal dissection (ESD) is a therapeutic endo-scopic technique that enables the en bloc resection of superficial epithelial neoplasia within the alimentary track. Developed by Japanese endoscopists following the observation that piecemeal endoscopic mucosal resection (EMR) of large lesions resulted in appreciable rates of recurrence, the goal of ESD is the en bloc removal of superficial luminal neoplasms, including in the esoph-agus.[1-3] Although adoption of ESD among Western endoscopists has been slowed by a lack of formalized training and the slow release of specialized endoscopic tools, there is significant enthu-siasm for this procedure as it offers the ability to provide a cura-tive R0 resection for large dysplastic lesions and early esophageal cancers.[4,5]

INDICATIONS

ESD can be used to treat large dysplastic lesions or superficial carcinomas in the esophagus that are well or moderately differ-entiated and ideally confined to the mucosa (m1-m2 for squa-mous carcinoma and m1-m3 for Barrett adenocarcinoma).[6] Such lesions confer a low risk for lymph node metastasis (LNM) and may be amenable to endoscopic cure. ESD may play a role in the cure of esophageal cancers that invade into the superfi-cial submucosa, but the increased risk of LNM must be consid-ered and discussed with the patient. ESD has been reported for both esophageal squamous cell carcinomas (SCCs) and Barrett adenocarcinomas.

Squamous Cell Carcinoma

Because squamous cell carcinoma develops via a field effect, mar-gins can be difficult to discern and ESD—not EMR—should be the first option for treating superficial esophageal squamous dys-plasia. Localized SCC that invades no further than the muscularis mucosae (i.e., T1a lesions, specifically those confined to the m1 and m2 layers) is the ideal target for esophageal ESD, given a low risk for LNM.[7] M3 (deep mucosal) and early T1b (submucosal involvement of <200 μm) SCCs with no evidence of LNM by endoscopic ultrasound (EUS) or cross-sectional imaging can be considered for ESD. These lesions may have an increased risk of LNM up to 15%, depending on size. Lesions with deeper submucosal invasion have an unacceptably high rate of LNM, and ESD should be avoided in patients fit for surgery.[8]

Esophageal Adenocarcinoma

Similar to SCC, the principal indication for ESD in esophageal adenocarcinoma (EAC) arising from Barrett esophagus is a T1a lesion limited to the mucosa or lamina propria, as the risk of LNM is predicted to be less than 2%.[9] This level of LNM is rational, because surgical esophagectomy has a similar risk of overall mortality (2%) and significant additional morbidity. Extension of this indication to include patients with superficial submucosal (sm1/early T1b, <200 μm) involvement may be acceptable in some settings, particularly for those patients who are unsuitable candidates for surgery.[8]

CONTRAINDICATIONS

1. Invasive esophageal carcinoma with extension beyond the superficial submucosa.
2. Radiographic or EUS evidence of locoregional or distant spread (N1 or M1 or greater disease).
3. EAC with known high-risk features: lymphovascular invasion or poor differentiation.[8]
4. Patient is medically unfit for therapeutic endoscopy, procedural sedation, or general anesthesia.
5. Patient has an uncorrectable coagulopathy.
6. Very small lesions (<10 mm) that may be reliably resected *en bloc* via EMR techniques[10] (relative contraindication).

PRE-ESD LESION ASSESSMENT

Establishing the depth and local extent of neoplasia is the major determinant of whether or not to perform ESD for superficial esophageal cancers, provided that the means and experience required to remove the lesion by ESD is present. Therefore, careful preprocedure assessment of any lesion considered for ESD is critical.

1. ***Endoscopic visual assessment***: High-definition white-light inspection and advanced endoscopic imaging are important for detection and assessment of prospective lesions prior

to ESD. Advanced imaging techniques include dye-based chromoendoscopy, optical enhancement technologies (e.g., narrow-band imaging), and methods such as optical coherence tomography or confocal endomicroscopy. While review of these approaches is beyond the scope of this chapter, advanced endoscopists performing ESD should be well versed in use of dye-based and electronic chromoendoscopy. Use of endoscopes capable of optical zoom magnification can offer a diagnostic advantage, in particular when evaluating intrapapillary capillary loops (IPCLs) as a means of diagnosing and staging SCCs. Careful mucosal endoscopic examination of esophageal lesions is essential for delineation of margins, as well as identification of highly dysplastic or malignant foci, which must be removed.[11] For squamous lesions, we found the topical application of a dilute 0.5% Lugol iodine solution (Safecor Health, Woburn, MA) to the esophageal mucosa prior to lesion marking very useful. This will delineate the extent of SCC, as dysplastic or malignant cells will not uptake the dilute iodine, whereas normal squamous cells will. Barrett esophagus can be surveyed after the application of acetic acid, which may facilitate the endoscopic diagnosis of high-grade intraepithelial neoplasia or cancer with a sensitivity of up to 96%.[11]

2. *Endoscopic ultrasound*: EUS can be considered prior to esophageal ESD but is not mandatory. The ability of EUS to accurately discriminate endoscopic resectability (T1 vs T2) is imperfect, even when high-frequency EUS miniprobes are used. Up to 25% of lesions may be understaged by EUS, while up to 12% may be overstaged when compared to pathology.[12] Despite tempered enthusiasm for EUS in T-staging, EUS using a dedicated radial or linear echoendoscope is valuable for nodal staging, and linear EUS and fine-needle aspiration should be performed if suspicious lymph nodes are identified.

EQUIPMENT

1. *General*: All basic equipment required for diagnostic or therapeutic upper endoscopy, including carbon dioxide insufflation and endoscopes with dedicated water jet capability, should be available and used during esophageal ESD cases. See the previous chapter on upper endoscopy for additional information.

2. *Endoscopic knives*: ESD "knives" can broadly be categorized as needle-type, insulated-tip-type, and scissors-type. Commercially available needle-type knives for esophageal ESD include HookKnife (Olympus America, Center Valley, PA), DualKnife (Olympus), Triangle Tip knife (Olympus), and Flush Knife (Fujifilm Endoscopy, Wayne, NJ). The I- and T-type

HybridKnife are needle-type knives that can be used with the ERBEJet2 (ERBE USA, Marietta, GA) to lift lesions typically using 20 to 25 psi of force. The ITknife nano (Olympus) is an insulated-tip ESD knife suited for esophageal ESD. Scissors-type ESD devices include the Clutch Cutter (Fujifilm) and the SB Knife (Olympus). Selection of an appropriate instrument varies based upon lesion location and expertise.

3. *Injection solutions*: A variety of options for submucosal injection are available including: normal saline (with or without epinephrine, 1:100,000 to 1:250,000 final dilution), 50% dextrose in water, hyaluronic acid, 0.83% hydroxypropyl methylcellulose, 6% hydroxyethyl starch in normal saline, and a commercially available premixed combination of a viscous agent with methylene blue (Eleview, Aries Pharmaceutical, San Diego, CA).

4. *Electrosurgical generators and settings*: A modern, programmable, adaptive electrosurgical unit (ESU) with the capacity to provide various cut and coagulation currents, and measure tissue resistance, is required for successful ESD. Typical current types used during ESD include blended cutting current (e.g., EndoCut) and forced/swift/spray/soft-coagulation modes (specifically when using a VIO 300D ESU, ERBE, although ESUs from other vendors offer similar modes).

5. *Hemostatic equipment*: Through-the scope endoscopic clips and hemostatic forceps (e.g., Coagrasper, Olympus), must be available when performing ESD, in particularly for preemptive coagulation of large vessels and for bleeding control. Other devices such as over-the-scope clips, covered esophageal stents, and endoscopic suturing platforms can also be desirable in case of severe bleeding or perforation during ESD.

6. *Distal attachment caps*: An array of clear, distal attachment caps are available and are necessary to aid visualization and allow some tissue traction during ESD. Both soft straight caps (available from Olympus and from US Endoscopy, Mentor, OH) and tapered-end caps (short ST Hood, Fujifilm) are commercially available.

PROCEDURE

Anesthesia and Airway Protection

General endotracheal anesthesia is recommended for all esophageal ESDs as procedures will likely be extended in duration and also for airway protection in the event of bleeding, which will necessitate irrigation with water. Early in the learning curve or for complex ESDs, procedures may last longer than 2 to 3 hours. In such cases, sequential compression devices and a warming blanket are also recommended for patients under general anesthesia.

Inspection and Marking

Once the endoscope is introduced and advanced to the lesion selected for ESD, careful visual inspection is necessary. The lateral margins should be examined, and optical or dye-based chromoendoscopy should be employed. Endoscopes with an optical magnification feature can be helpful. The lesion margins are then marked circumferentially approximately 5 mm outside the lateral edge using short bursts of low-power soft-coagulation current (Effect 4, 20W, using an ERBE ESU). The tip of the DualKnife with the blade retracted is often used for this purpose, as can APC (precise mode, ERBE). Care should be taken to avoid overt penetration of the mucosa by electrocautery, both to avoid injuring underlying tissue and to prevent leakage of submucosal fluid that is later injected.

Submucosal Injection

Dynamic submucosal injection should be performed to lift the esophageal lesion off the muscularis propria. For large lesions, portions of the lesion can be lifted sequentially as the ESD progresses. Inadequate lifting may increase the risk of perforation, whereas too much submucosal injection can prevent successful ESD as the esophageal lumen can become pseudo-obstructed.

Choosing Among ESD Techniques

For endoscopists early in their learning curve for esophageal ESD, it is recommended that smaller lesions (probably limited to 2 to 3 cm in size), encompassing no greater than one-third of the esophageal lumen be attempted. Such lesions are typically amenable to traditional ESD, which involves circumferential mucosal incision followed by submucosal dissection. For lesions with superficial ulceration or if fibrosis is expected, a pocket method has been advocated, which can be facilitated by using a tapered cap (short ST Hood, Fujifilm). The pocket method begins with a one-third proximal circumferential incision, followed by dissection underneath the lesion, with gradual extension of the circumferential incision. For longer and wider lesions, a tunnel method has been described, which involves mucosal incision at the proximal and distal aspect of the lesion.[13] A submucosal tunnel connecting both incisions is then made, and finally the lateral portions of the mucosa are incised. Endoscopists experienced in per oral endoscopic myotomy (POEM) will find the tunnel method familiar.

Tips for Mucosal Incision

After completion of marking, mucosal incision is the next step, be it a traditional circumferential incision or partial incision as part of a pocket or a tunnel method. While esophageal ESD can be done with needle-type knives, insulated-tip knifes, and scissors-type knives, usually the version with a shorter blade or smaller tip is used as the esophagus is a thin-walled luminal structure (in contradistinction to the stomach). Similarly, a variety of submucosal injection fluids have been used, which may vary by country and referral center. We typically utilize 6% hydroxyethyl starch in normal saline tinted with methylene blue. While not routine, a small amount of epinephrine can be added (1:100,000 to 1:250,000 final dilution) if increased lesion vascularity or elevated risk of bleeding is expected.

If a needle-type knife is used, incision is performed in a pushing fashion. If an insulated-tip knife is used, incision is performed in a pulling motion. A needle-type knife is needed to make a 1-cm long mucosal entry incision typically at the side of the lesion farthest away from the scope to allow use of the insulated-tip knives. Conversely, a needle-type knife can help the speed of ESD using scissors-type knives by starting the mucosal incision at the side of the lesion closest to the scope.

Many modern adaptive electrosurgical generators can be used for ESD, and most endoscopists use an EndoCut mode (VIO 300 D, ERBE) or a similar PulseCut mode (ESG-100, Olympus) for mucosal incision. These similar proprietary waveforms begin their duty cycles with a pure cut phase. A common pattern for mucosal incision is a tap-tap-tap, which employs only the cutting phase of the duty cycle. The result is then inspected before continuing the incision in the desired direction. This cut-cut-cut then inspect rhythm is a classic way of performing ESD safely and allows for more precise knife control.

Many novices also do not cut through the entire mucosal layer, which will make the ESD much more difficult. To facilitate easier ESD, an adequate lift followed by incision through the entire mucosa to expose the blue-tinted submucosa is essential before further extending the mucosal incision.

Submucosal Dissection

After partial or circumferential incision is completed, the submucosal injection is then performed. An adequate submucosal lift is critical and repeated injections can be required. If possible, use of the cap to get underneath the opened mucosal layer will stabilize the scope and aid in submucosal dissection. It is advisable for those early in their learning phase to consider performing submucosal dissection at a halfway point in the expanded blue-tinted submucosal layer. However, for lesions with deep invasion, dissection of the submucosa right atop the muscularis propria may be required. As vessels branch in the submucosal space closer to the mucosa, dissection at a deeper layer can mean dealing with fewer vessels, though these may be larger in caliber.

Submucosal dissection is typically performed using coagulation current, although different waveforms are employed by different ESD experts. Typical waveforms might include forced coag (ERBE and Olympus), swift coag (ERBE) or spray coag (ERBE). While Spray Coag is advantageous during POEM procedures, it can be less precise than other waveforms. We prefer using Swift Coag 40 to 50W for submucosal dissection.

During submucosal dissection, careful attention must be paid to visible submucosal vessels before they are incised. For vessels smaller in width than the ESD knife, (typically <1 mm) changing the coagulation setting or altering the submucosal dissection is typically unnecessary, and these vessels can be coagulated (and sometimes cut) without bleeding. For larger vessels (1 to 2 mm in size), it is useful to dissect the submucosa to skeletonize the vessel, as if severed cut arteries can contract. Vessels of this size can then be coagulated using the ESD knife without changing the coagulation current. For very large vessels, hemostatic forceps (Coagrasper, Olympus) should be used in combination with soft coagulation current at 50 to 80W, (ERBE and Olympus). Typically, the larger red vessels seen in the submucosa are thinner-walled veins, and the smaller white accompanying vessels are arteries. In cases where bleeding produces visual impairment, we have found that using the cap to provide mechanical tamponade to the area while irrigating is very useful, which allows time to switch to hemostatic forceps if needed. Precise localization of a bleeding source is critical for hemostasis and to reduce inadvertent tissue damage during bleeding control.

Gravity and Traction

Depending upon a lesion's anatomical location, pooling of fluid and blood during submucosal dissection can obscure visibility in esophageal ESD. For easier ESD, if the patient can be positioned so the lesion is in an antigravity position. However, manipulating the position of a patient while under general endotracheal anesthesia may be difficult. To further minimize interference by gravity, dissection should be initiated near the dependent portion of the lesion.

Traction methods are available that can improve submucosal exposure by retracting pliable mucosal tissue. To provide traction, a hemostatic clip is opened after to introduction through the endoscope and silk surgical line or dental floss is tied around one arm of the clip. The clip is then used to grasp the partially dissected mucosal flap of the lesion's edge.[14] Gentle traction is applied by hand to retract the mucosal flap and to better expose the submucosa. This technique can be helpful for more proximal gastric lesions. For small esophageal lesions, clip traction is not usually required. However, when circumferential ESD is performed, clip traction can be a valuable adjunctive technique to increase speed of submucosal dissection. A suture-pulley method has also been described, whereby a second clip can be deployed anchoring the suture against the opposite luminal wall. This can help with dissection of the oral side of an esophageal lesion.

IMMEDIATE ADVERSE EVENTS

1. **Bleeding**: Bleeding can occur at any stage during ESD and should be addressed immediately. Lavage using a water jet for lesion localization and to prevent clotting is essential. Sometimes additional submucosal dissection may be required to expose the bleeding vessel. Hemostasis can then be performed using the ESD knife and/or hemostatic forceps.

2. **Perforation**: Limited, linear perforations may occur in up to 6% of esophageal ESD procedures.[15] Esophageal perforation can lead to significant mediastinitis, mediastinal emphysema, pneumothorax, or midline shift. Perforations at the gastroesophageal junction can result in peritoneal free air and peritonitis. Immediate recognition of a full-thickness perforation is critical in performing ESD to afford treatment and to mitigate delayed adverse outcomes. Such perforations, when small, may be repaired effectively using endoscopic clips and a course of antibiotics would be recommended. Again, additional submucosal dissection is often needed to expose the muscularis propria prior to closing a perforation for precise clip closure and so that clip closure does not prevent completion of the ESD. Esophageal stenting is an adjunctive technique in case of a large perforation that cannot be closed by using endoclips or endoscopic suturing. Surgery is rarely necessary following endoscopic closure.

POSTPROCEDURAL CARE

1. **General recovery and diet**: Following esophageal ESD, we typically recommend that patients follow a clear liquid diet for 24 to 48 hours, then full liquids to complete 1 week, followed by soft foods for the following week (days 7 to 14). For cases of suspected perforation and clip closure or in patients who report symptoms following their procedure, we recommend

inpatient observation and obtaining a postprocedural esopha-gram. We recommend an 8-week course of proton-pump inhibitor therapy to reduce acid secretion so as to promote healing of the post-ESD esophageal ulcer.

2. ***Esophageal stricture***: Esophageal stricture formation is a long-term complication of ESD in patients who undergo extensive near-circumferential or circumferential resection[16] and is not often a problem for ESD of <1/2 the esophageal circumference. For patients at risk for stricturing, a follow-up esophagogastroduodenoscopy(EGD) in 2 weeks is advised, at which time stricture dilation can be performed if necessary and repeated dilations may be required.[17] Injection of triam-cinolone immediately following ESD has been described as potentially beneficial in the prevention of strictures in patients thought to be at increased risk.[18]

3. ***Surveillance after ESD***: Pathological specimens should be fixed to cork or Styrofoam, oriented, and then submitted for formalin fixation and pathological analysis. While R0 resection of lesions with good prognostic features and a low risk for LN metastasis might be surveyed up to 1 year later (as has been done in Asian countries), we would recommend follow-up EGD in 3 to 6 months for surveillance in the United States. For patients with submucosally invasive cancers removed by ESD that are at increased risk for LNM (i.e., >5% to 10% risk), but who refuse surgery or are not good surgical candidates, more frequent endoscopic surveillance will be required in addition to periodic cross-sectional imaging.

PROCEDURAL REIMBURSEMENT

There are no specific Current Procedural Terminology (CPT) billing codes for esophageal ESD. As such, these procedures are typically submitted under code 43499 (unlisted procedure, esoph-agus). Despite the lack of a dedicated CPT code, some insurance carriers will reimburse for ESD procedures if sufficient documen-tation is submitted and prior authorization is obtained.

References

1. Makuuchi H. Endoscopic mucosal resection for mucosal cancer in the esophagus. *Gastrointest Endosc Clin N Am.* 2001;11(3):445-458.

2. Pech O, Gossner L, May A, Vieth M, Stolte M, Ell C. Endoscopic resection of superficial esophageal squamous-cell carcinomas: Western experience. *Am J Gastroenterol.* 2004;99(7):1226-1232.

3. Yang D, Coman RM, Kahaleh M, et al. Endoscopic submucosal dissec-tion for Barrett's early neoplasia: a multicenter study in the United States. *Gastrointest Endosc.* 2017;86(4):600-607.

4. Coman RM, Gotoda T, Draganov PV. Training in endoscopic submucosal dis-section. *World J Gastrointest Endosc.* 2013;5(8):369-378.

5. Kotzev AI, Yang D, Draganov PV. How to master endoscopic submucosal dissection in the USA. *Dig Endosc.* 2019;31(1):94-100.

6. Draganov PV, Wang AY, Othman MO, Fukami N. Clinical practice of endoscopic submucosal dissection in the United States. *Clin Gastroenterol Hepatol.* 2019;17(1):16-25.

7. Stein HJ, Feith M, Bruecher BL, Naehrig J, Sarbia M, Siewert JR. Early esophageal cancer: pattern of lymphatic spread and prognostic factors for long-term survival after surgical resection. *Ann Surg.* 2005;242(4):566-573; discussion 73-5.

8. Pimentel-Nunes P, Dinis-Ribeiro M, Ponchon T, et al. Endoscopic submucosal dissection: European Society of Gastrointestinal Endoscopy (ESGE) guideline. *Endoscopy.* 2015;47(9):829-854.

9. Dunbar KB, Spechler SJ. The risk of lymph-node metastases in patients with high-grade dysplasia or intramucosal carcinoma in Barrett's esophagus: a systematic review. *Am J Gastroenterol.* 2012;107(6):850-862; quiz 63.

10. Ishihara R, Iishi H, Takeuchi Y, et al. Local recurrence of large squamous-cell carcinoma of the esophagus after endoscopic resection. *Gastrointest Endosc.* 2008;67(6):799-804.

11. Kaltenbach T, Sano Y, Friedland S, Soetikno R, American Gastroenterological Association. American Gastroenterological Association (AGA) Institute technology assessment on image-enhanced endoscopy. *Gastroenterology.* 2008;134(1):327-340.

12. Larghi A, Lightdale CJ, Memeo L, Bhagat G, Okpara N, Rotterdam H. EUS followed by EMR for staging of high-grade dysplasia and early cancer in Barrett's esophagus. *Gastrointest Endosc.* 2005;62(1):16-23.

13. Arantes V, Albuquerque W, Freitas Dias CA, Demas Alvares Cabral MM, Yamamoto H. Standardized endoscopic submucosal tunnel dissection for management of early esophageal tumors (with video). *Gastrointest Endosc.* 2013;78(6):946-952.

14. Oyama T. Counter traction makes endoscopic submucosal dissection easier. *Clin Endosc.* 2012;45(4):375-378.

15. Fujishiro M, Yahagi N, Kakushima N, et al. Endoscopic submucosal dissection of esophageal squamous cell neoplasms. *Clin Gastroenterol Hepatol.* 2006;4(6):688-694.

16. Ono S, Fujishiro M, Niimi K, et al. Predictors of postoperative stricture after esophageal endoscopic submucosal dissection for superficial squamous cell neoplasms. *Endoscopy.* 2009;41(8):661-665.

17. Takahashi H, Arimura Y, Okahara S, et al. Risk of perforation during dilation for esophageal strictures after endoscopic resection in patients with early squamous cell carcinoma. *Endoscopy.* 2011;43(3):184-189.

18. Hanaoka N, Ishihara R, Takeuchi Y, et al. Intralesional steroid injection to prevent stricture after endoscopic submucosal dissection for esophageal cancer: a controlled prospective study. *Endoscopy.* 2012;44(11):1007-1011.

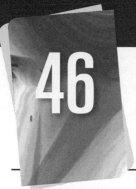

46

Gastric Endoscopic Submucosal Dissection

Makoto Nishimura, MD
Norio Fukami, MD

Gastric endoscopic submucosal dissection (ESD) is a technique of endoscopic resection that removes lesions by a free-hand dissection at the level of submucosal layer with injection solution, knives, and electrosurgical unit most suitable for larger gastric dysplastic lesions including early gastric cancer. This procedure was developed in Japan and currently prevailed because of the high curatively from cancer and low recurrence rate of dysplasia and cancer than conventional endoscopic mucosal resection (EMR). Since the stomach has its unique anatomical shape of sac, removal strategies are required for smooth and successful ESD tailored to a location of the lesion utilizing the benefit of gravity. Nowadays, wide variety of devices specific to the ESD procedure are available in the United States and setting of electrosurgical unit needs to be well understood to accomplish successful gastric ESD. Precise hemostasis or rather a prevention of active bleeding is also important because the anatomy of the gastric wall is proven to be rich in large blood vessels compared to other organs such as the esophagus and the colorectum. It is noted that ESD at the upper stomach has higher chance of experiencing arterial bleeding because of the rich arterial supply from the left gastric artery.

In this section, the indication, preparation, equipment, and procedural steps are described.

INDICATIONS

Indications of gastric ESD were established by the Japanese Gastric Cancer Association[1] and has been recently revised to expand the criteria.[2,3] In the United States, no established indications have officially been endorsed; however, recent publication from American Gastroenterology Association suggested to adopt those indications. In essence, gastric ESD should be applied to the lesions without ulceration and are highly suggested to be limited to mucosa or not to invade deeper than the shallow submucosal layer.[2] Another indication would be a large area of dysplasia (i.e., adenoma), which is unable to be removed en bloc by conventional techniques. Prior to ESD, the lesion should be assessed endoscopically for its extension and a depth of invasion to assess for possible submucosal invasion and also to rule out deeper invasion by endoscopic ultrasonography as needed. In cases when extension of the lesion is subtle and difficult to be determined, four-quadrant biopsies can be performed a few weeks prior to ESD to confirm its extent and to determine a lateral margin (i.e., a mapping biopsy). If the lesion is considered to fulfill the criteria described below, ESD may be chosen as a primary endoscopic treatment for gastric cancer and assess whether curative resection was achieved upon reviewing resected specimen. Patient's performance status, comorbidity, and medications, especially an anticoagulant agent, are to be taken into an account when choosing the best treatment modality.

Absolute Indication

- Intramucosal gastric cancer (cT1a), <2 cm, well-differentiated adenocarcinoma, without ulceration (EMR/ESD)
- Intramucosal gastric cancer (cT1a), >2 cm, well-differentiated adenocarcinoma, without ulceration (ESD)
- Intramucosal gastric cancer (cT1a), <3 cm, well-differentiated adenocarcinoma, with ulceration (ESD)

Expanded Indication

- Intramucosal gastric cancer (cT1a), ≤2 cm, undifferentiated adenocarcinoma, without ulceration

Relative Indication

- Early gastric cancer, other than the listed lesion as above absolute indication and expanded indication, without surgical indication because of age or comorbidity, might be considered under fully informed consent of risks and benefits.

Contraindications

- Gastric cancer with deep submucosal invasion
- Gastric cancer with deep ulceration
- Intramucosal gastric cancer, >2 cm, undifferentiated adenocarcinoma

PREPARATION

Gastric ESD should be performed with informed consent from the patient explaining the specific concept of removal of mucosal and submucosal layer away from the muscle layer, ESD as an alternative to EMR or surgery with certain benefits for a certain group of patients, and possible complications with slightly higher rates compared to EMR, possible incomplete attempt and termination of ESD due to a variety of factors complicating ESD procedure, and possible requirement of additional treatment such as surgery or multimodal therapy depending on the pathological stage after ESD. Patient is required to discontinue anticoagulation agents before gastric ESD according to the guideline. The patient required to be NPO after midnight as for regular upper endoscopic procedures. Patient and family member should be informed about the importance of follow-ups (i.e., postresection surveillance esophagogastroduodenoscopy (EGD) and cross-sectional imaging as indicated) and a possibility of additional surgical treatment as shown in the algorithm (Fig. 46.1). Prior to ESD, blood test (CBC, chemistry, and prothrombin time–international normalized ratio [PT-INR]), and EKG are preferable but not mandatory to assess patient's condition prior to the procedure based on patient's comorbidity.

ANESTHESIA AND PATIENT POSITION

Monitored anesthesia care or general anesthesia administered by anesthesia service is commonly used for gastric ESD. General anesthesia is recommended for a procedure that is expected to take long hours or for a patient with a risk of aspiration.[4] General anesthesia is also to be considered for patients with large hiatal hernia or with a lesion at the gastroesophageal junction. Patient is positioned to the left lateral decubitus or may be on supine position. If the lesion is difficult to be accessed because it is located at incisura or lesser curvature of the body, then right lateral decubitus may be useful.

EQUIPMENT

Equipment of ESD includes injectable solution, dedicated ESD knives, and other devices (Fig. 46.2A-D).

Endoscope

Endoscopes with waterjet function are highly recommended for gastric ESD (Fig. 46.2A).

Solutions

For gastric ESD, 0.4% sodium hyaluronate (MucoUp, Boston Scientific, Japan) with a small amount of epinephrine and indigo carmine dye is widely used into submucosal injection in Japan.[5] In the United States, hydroxyethyl starch in sodium chloride (Voluven, Fresenius Kabi, USA), hydroxypropyl methylcellulose (HPMC),

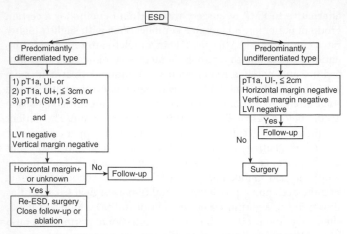

FIG. 46.1 Algorithm for post–endoscopic submucosal dissection (ESD) treatment of gastric cancer. (Reprinted from Japanese Gastric Cancer Association. Japanese Gastric Cancer Treatment Guidelines 2018 (version 5). With permission.)

or SIC-8000 (Eleview, Aries Pharmaceuticals, Inc.) are commonly used for ESD mixed with dye and with or without epinephrine, all of which are more effective alternatives to saline solution.[6,7]

Distal Attachments

Various transparent hood or distal attachment caps are available to facilitate the dissection of submucosal tissue creating a clear view and traction within submucosal space during ESD (Olympus, USA, US Endoscopy, USA, and Fujifilm USA; Fig. 46.2B).

Injection needles; larger gauge than 23G is recommended for injection needle.

Some injection fluid does not flow well with certain needle (i.e., Carr-Locke needle), and pretesting is recommended to ensure smooth flow of fluid.

Knives

Various ESD knives are available with unique features.
- IT2 knife (KD-611L, Olympus)
- IT-nano knife (KD-612 L/U, Olympus)
- Dualknife J (KD-655L, Olympus)
- SB knife (MD-47703 W/L, Sumitomo Bakelite)
- HybridKnife (T/O/I-type, ERBE, Germany)
- FlushKnife (DK2618 J/DK2623 J, Fujifilm)
- ClutchCutter (DP2618DT-35/30, Fujifilm, USA) (some are shown in Fig. 46.2D)

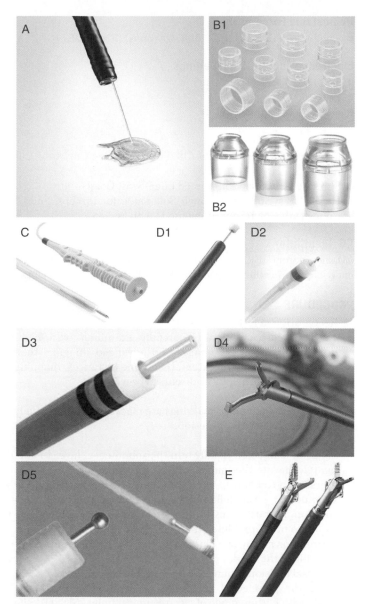

FIG. 46.2 A and B1, B2, Endoscope with waterjet function. C, Injected needle. D, Knives—1) IT-nano knife, 2) Dual-J knife, 3) HybridKnife, 4) SB knife, 5) FlushKnife. E, hemostasis forceps. (Parts A, C, E reprinted with permission from Olympus America, Inc; Part B, reprinted with permission from (a) Olympus America, Inc. and (b) © Fujifilm Medical Systems, U.S.A.; Part D, reprinted with permission from (a) and (b) Olympus America, Inc., (c) ERBE, U.S.A, © Erbe Elektromedizin GmbH, (d) and (e) © Fujifilm Medical Systems, U.S.A.)

Hemostasis Forceps

■ Coagrasper (FD-411UR/410LR, Olympus) (Fig. 46.2E)

Electrosurgical Unit and Settings

■ VIO (300D, ERBE, Germany)
■ ESG-100 (Olympus, USA)
■ Gi4000 (US Endoscopy) etc.

Settings

■ Circumferential cut; Endo Cut/Pulse Cut/Dry Cut/Auto Cut mode
■ Submucosal dissection; Forced Coag/Swift Coag mode
■ Hemostasis; Soft Coag/Touch Soft mode for forceps, Forced Coag/Swift Coag/Spray Coag mode with knives

CO_2 Insufflator

CO_2 insufflator (UCR, Olympus) is mandatory for any interventional endoscopic procedures especially ESD and submucosal tunneling.

PROCEDURE

1. Recognition of lesion and its extension
   Targeted gastric lesion is carefully examined with high-definition endoscopic images and advanced imaging, then determined the lateral extent. (For some instances, mapping biopsy would be helpful as discussed previously.)
2. Marking
   Using tip of the knives, markings are placed circumferentially 3 to 5 mm outside of the lesion.
3. Injection of solution
   Solution is injected rapidly into the submucosal layer to adequately elevate the mucosa. Saline injection may be used as a first step to confirm appropriate injection of fluid into the submucosal layer, followed by injection of dedicated ESD solution. In most of institution, small amount of epinephrine (equal to or more diluted than 1: 100,000 dilution) and indigo carmine or methylene blue dye are mixed to the solution for coloring of the fluid.
4. Mucosal incision around the targeted lesion
   Using the preselected ESD knife, circumferential incision is made with cutting mode of electrosurgical unit (ESU). IT knife requires initial incision by other needle knife, which is usually made at three sites (triangle configuration) or at four quadrants. IT knives work best by pulling motion, compared to the tip-style knife with which pushing motion works better. This can be completed at once or by stepwise depending on the technique used.

5. Submucosal dissection

   Immediately after a circumferential incision, a submucosa layer is exposed. Additional submucosal injection facilitates further exposure of and access to the submucosal layer. Steady tension is applied to the tissue with cap and a knife contacted with the target tissue; short bursts of activation on ESU are applied repeatedly to perform dissection of submucosal tissue. Hemostatic forceps are used when large vessels are seen to preemptively coagulate or to achieve hemostasis. To control bleeding, it is important to identify a bleeding spot by a water irrigation using waterjet function for an effective hemostasis completed by precisely grasping the vessel at the bleeding spot with hemostasis forceps.

6. Completing ESD

   Dissection should be started first from the lowest point of gravity so that the gravity can be used to our advantage. Pocket creation method or additional traction method can be used to facilitate procedure or if there is substantial submucosal fibrosis. En bloc resection is the goal of ESD (e.g., removal of the lesion in one piece with adequate margin), and steps 3, 4, and 5 are repeated until the resection is completed.

7. Retrieval of lesion and preparation for pathological assessment

   Roth net or forceps grasper is used to facilitate the retrieval of the resected specimen. Scope should be reinserted and additional hemostasis or clipping should be applied as necessary to prevent delayed bleeding or perforation. The resected specimen should be carefully pinned at the edge onto rubber or cork board for a proper orientation and pathological assessment (Figs. 46.3 and 46.4).

ADDITIONAL TREATMENT

Final pathology result would dictate a need for further therapy. Additional surgery is recommended in cases judged to be non-curative resection and observation with proper surveillance in cases fulfilling criteria for curative resection.[8,9]

ADVERSE EVENTS

1. Cardiopulmonary adverse events: Despite proper preprocedural assessment and preparation, cardiopulmonary adverse events may occur during the procedure. Careful planning and monitoring during anesthesia are of utmost importance, and endotracheal intubation under general anesthesia might reduce the risk of aspiration pneumonia.[10,11]

2. Perforation—intraprocedural and delayed perforation: Reported perforation risk of ESD is 0.3% to 5.8% in gastric

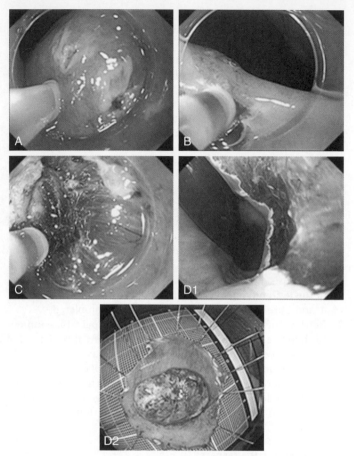

FIG. 46.3 A, Injection solution into the submucosal layer. B, Circumferential cut. C, Submucosal dissection. D1, En bloc resection of cardiac lesion (retroflexion view) and D2, pinned resected specimen.

ESD.[11] To avoid perforation, the endoscopist needs to recognize different anatomical features of gastric muscle depends on the location. The risk of perforation increases at lesser curvature and fundus of the stomach because muscularis propria becomes thinner. Also, excessive hemostasis by hemostatic forceps should be avoided to reduce a risk for delayed perforation from deeper thermal injury. Almost all perforations caused by the ESD knife are small in size and are recognized early. Timely endoscopic clip application or postresection suturing is effective to seal the perforation in nearly all cases.

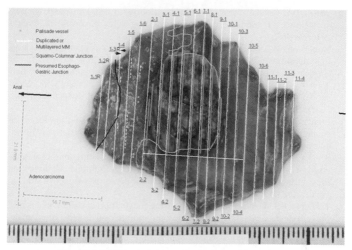

FIG. 46.4 Pathological assessment of resected specimen.

3. Bleeding—intraprocedural and delayed bleeding: Good visualization of submucosal tissue is very important for an identification of large vessels to prevent premature cutting and a resultant significant bleeding. Preemptive coagulation on large vessel or artery prevents intraprocedural bleeding and reduces delayed bleeding after a completion of gastric ESD.[9]

SUMMARY

Gastric ESD is a new treatment option for early gastric cancer and large gastric dysplasia. It extended the capability of endoscopic treatment way beyond EMR, and many more patients are cured by endoscopic resection using ESD technique. Proper patient selection is very important to achieve maximal benefits for patients. ESD steps are simple but they require intensive training to be competent. Detailed analysis on the outcomes of ESD procedure and pathological report is mandatory to properly counsel patients with the final result and to guide on future surveillance or adjuvant therapy.

References

1. Japanese Gastric Cancer Association. Japanese gastric cancer treatment guidelines 2014 (ver. 4). *Gastric Cancer.* 2017;20:1-19.
2. Draganov PV, Wang AY, Othman MO, Fukami N. AGA Institute Clinical Practice update: endoscopic submucosal dissection in the United States. *Clin Gastroenterol Hepatol.* 2019;17(1):16-25.e1.
3. Japanese Gastric Cancer Association. Japanese gastric cancer treatment guidelines 2018 (ver. 5). 2018.

4. Yurtlu DA, Aslan F, Ayvat P, et al. Propofol-based sedation versus general anesthesia for endoscopic submucosal dissection. *Medicine (Baltimore)*. 2016;95:e3680.

5. Yamamoto H. Endoscopic submucosal dissection of early cancers and large flat adenomas. *Clin Gastroenterol Hepatol*. 2005;3:S74-S76.

6. Girotra M, Triadafilopoulos G, Friedland S. Utility and performance characteristics of a novel submucosal injection agent (Eleview˜) for endoscopic mucosal resection and endoscopic submucosal dissection. *Transl Gastroenterol Hepatol*. 2018;3:32.

7. Mehta N, Strong AT, Franco M, et al. Optimal injection solution for endoscopic submucosal dissection: a randomized controlled trial of Western solutions in a porcine model. *Dig Endosc*. 2018;30:347-353.

8. Ito H, Gotoda T, Oyama T, et al. Long-term oncological outcomes of submucosal manipulation during non-curative endoscopic submucosal dissection for submucosal invasive gastric cancer: a multicenter retrospective study in Japan. *Surg Endosc*. 2018;32:196-203.

9. Takizawa K, Oda I, Gotoda T, et al. Routine coagulation of visible vessels may prevent delayed bleeding after endoscopic submucosal dissection–an analysis of risk factors. *Endoscopy*. 2008;40:179-183.

10. Wadhwa V, Issa D, Garg S, et al. Similar risk of cardiopulmonary adverse events between propofol and traditional anesthesia for gastrointestinal endoscopy: a systematic review and meta-analysis. *Clin Gastroenterol Hepatol*. 2017;15:194-206.

11. Yamashita K, Shiwaku H, Ohmiya T, et al. Efficacy and safety of endoscopic submucosal dissection under general anesthesia. *World J Gastrointest Endosc*. 2016;8:466-471.

47

Colon Endoscopic Submucosal Dissection

Sergey V. Kantsevoy, MD, PhD

Endoscopic submucosal dissection (ESD) was developed in Japan for *en bloc* removal of gastric cancer and precancerous lesions located in the upper gastrointestinal (GI) tract.[1,2] ESD is now also used for removal of lesions located in esophagus, colon, and small bowel.[3,4]

In United States, a well-established screening for colorectal cancer has led to increased detection of precancerous colonic lesions (polyps) and early colon cancer.[5] Traditionally these lesions were removed with endoscopic mucosal resection (EMR) utilizing various endoscopic snares. However, *en bloc* resection rate during EMR is relatively low and only possible for relatively small lesions fitting the size of endoscopic snare.[6] Removal of large colonic lesions with EMR requires a piecemeal resection with a high rate (16%) of residual polyps on follow-up colonoscopy.[7]

Compared to EMR, ESD allows *en bloc* resection even for large and flat colonic lesions.[6]

INDICATIONS

1. Nongranular-type polyps over 20 mm in size (Fig. 47.1).
2. Granular-type polyps above 30 mm in size and laterally spreading tumors.
3. Well-differentiated early (T1) colorectal cancer not involving deep submucosal layer.
4. Submucosal colorectal lesions not involving muscularis layer of colonic wall.

CONTRAINDICATIONS

1. Noncorrectable blood coagulation disorders
2. Ulcerated lesions
3. Poorly differentiated, aggressive malignant lesions

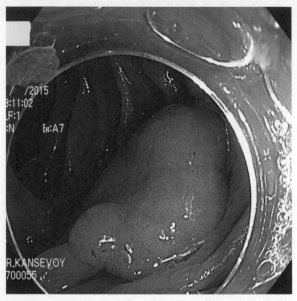

FIG. 47.1 Large colonic polyp. Large, nongranular-type, sessile (Is) polyp located in transverse colon.

4. Malignant lesion infiltrating deep submucosal and muscularis layer of colonic wall
5. Enlarged lymph nodes suspicious for malignant involvement near colonic lesion

Extensive submucosal fibrosis under a colonic lesion could be a relative contraindication to ESD due to higher risk of full-thickness colonic perforation.

EQUIPMENT

Traditional devices and accessories for colonic ESD include:
1. Colonoscope with a water jet.

   Bleeding of various degrees (from capillary to arterial) is relatively common during ESD.[8] When the bleeding is encountered, a special accessory for thermal (Coagrasper, ESD knives—see details below) or mechanical (endoscopic clips) hemostasis is inserted through the biopsy channel of the colonoscope. Because the biopsy channel is now occupied with hemostatic device, flushing the blood away from the view field can only be achieved through a dedicated water jet build into the colonoscope.
2. Equipment for carbon dioxide insufflation.

   ESD usually requires prolonged period of time. Carbon dioxide is absorbed from GI tract much faster than room air.[9] To

decrease abdominal distention during long endoscopic procedures, carbon dioxide insufflation should be used during ESD.
In addition, if colonic perforation happens during ESD, carbon
dioxide is absorbed from peritoneal cavity more rapidly than
room air decreasing the chance of abdominal compartment
syndrome and postprocedural prolonged subcostal pain due
to pneumoperitoneum.

3. Distal attachments (Olympus America, Center Valley, PA or
Fujifilm, Saitama, Japan).

   Distal attachment is a small transparent hood preloaded on
the distal tip of the endoscope. Distal attachment pushes the
tissue away from the endoscope's lens facilitating entrance of
the endoscope's tip into submucosal space and dissection of
the submucosal fibers.

4. Injection needles.

   Multiple injection needles are currently available. We pre-
fer 25 or 26 gauge injection needles (Injector Force Max and
NeedleMaster, Olympus America, Center Valley, PA) although
other injection needles (Interject injection needle made by
Boston Scientific, Carr-Locke injection needle made by US
Endoscopy, etc) can also be used during colonic ESD.

5. Dedicated ESD knives:

   a. DualKnife and DualKnife J (Olympus America, Center
   Valley, PA)

      DualKnife is a very versatile device, which can be used for
   all steps of ESD: marking, circumferential incision around
   the lesion, hemostasis, and dissection of submucosal fibers.
   DualKnife and DualKnife J have fixed length of its protruding portion (2 mm for gastric length device and 1.5 mm
   for colonic length device) and small rounded ball at its tip.
   DualKnife can be used in two positions: (1) Fully open position—is used to make a circumferential incision and dissection of submucosal fibers. (2) Fully closed position—is
   used for marking and endoscopic hemostasis.

      DualKnife J also allows injection of fluid into the submu-
   cosal space eliminating the need to exchange the knife for
   injection needle and significantly speeding up submucosal
   dissection.

   b. ITknife nano (Olympus America, Center Valley, PA)
      ITknife nano has isolated tip (with ceramic ball) to decrease
   the chance of inadvertent colonic perforation.

   c. HookKnife (Olympus America, Center Valley, PA)
      HookKnife is a very effective device especially in case of
   extensive submucosal fibrosis. However, control of hook's
   tip and rotation of the hook require special training of the
   assistant, which should be done prior to the start of ESD.

d. HybridKnife (ERBE USA, Marietta, GA)

HybridKnife is a combination knife allowing performance of all steps of ESD: marking, submucosal injection of fluid, circumferential incision around the lesion, hemostasis, and dissection of submucosal fibers.

Injection of fluid is performed through the channel inside the HybridKnife. The operator can control the length of the protruding portion of the knife. Use of HybridKnife eliminates the need for exchange to a needle for submucosal fluid injection and significantly speeds up ESD in the colon and upper GI tract.

HybridKnife in the United States is currently available in two configurations: straight (I-type) and T-shape (T-type). A third configuration (O-type with isolated tip) will soon be available in United States.

e. FlushKnife (Fujifilm, Saitama, Japan)

FlushKnife resembles in appearance DualKnife J: it also has two positions (fully open and fully closed) of a fixed-length protruding tip with a metal ball at its end and ability to inject fluid into the submucosal space through the knife. Similarly to DualKnife J and HybridKnife, FlushKnife eliminates the need for exchange to an injection needle and significantly speeds up ESD.

6. Endoscopic hemostatic forceps—Coagrasper (Olympus Corporation, Center Valley, PA).

Coagrasper resembles hot biopsy forceps. However, the branches of Coagrasper are blunt (not sharp). Grasping a blood vessel with sharp branches of a hot biopsy forceps can damage the blood vessel's wall causing significant bleeding. To the contrary, endoscopists can grasp the blood vessel with a Coagrasper without causing any damage to the vessel, and then application of electric current will seal the lumen of the vessel preventing or stopping the bleeding.

7. Endoscopic clips.

Traditional endoscopic clips (Resolution and Resolution 360 [Boston Scientific, Natick, MA], QuickClip2 and QuickClip Pro [Olympus America, Center Valley, PA], Instinct [Cook Medical, Winston-Salem, NC]) are sometimes used for endoscopic hemostasis and closure of accidental perforations during ESD.

8. Endoscopic suturing device—Overstitch (Apollo Endosurgery, Austin, TX).

Previous study demonstrated superior results of endoscopic suturing closure of colonic perforations with Overstitch endoscopic suturing system compared to closure with traditional endoscopic clips.[10] Overstitch also allows suturing closure of large mucosal defects post ESD, decreasing the chance of delayed bleeding and delayed perforations and eliminating the need for hospital admission for observation post colonic ESD.

PROCEDURAL STEPS

Colonic ESD is performed in several consecutive steps:
1. Submucosal injection (Fig. 47.2).

Submucosal injection is used to expand the submucosal space. Expansion of the submucosal space lifts the mucosal lesion and separates it from the underlying muscularis layer.

During ESD in the stomach and esophagus, injection of the submucosal solution makes it difficult to see the outer margins of the gastric/esophageal mucosal lesion. For that reason, outer margins of esophageal/gastric lesions are identified with cautery marks ("marking" step) prior to submucosal injection. However, during colonic ESD "marking" is not necessary because, in the colon, injection of a submucosal solution makes difference between the polyp and surrounding normal mucosa more pronounced, clearly identifying the outer borders of the lesion.

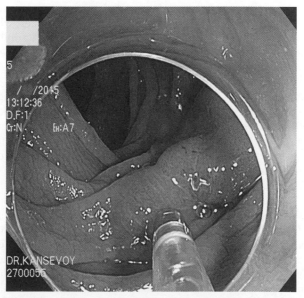

FIG. 47.2 Submucosal injection. The needle is inserted into the submucosal space approximately 4 to 5 mm away from the lateral border of the polyp. Submucosal injection of fluid colored with indigo carmine is performed to raise the mucosal lesion.

It is a common practice to add a blue dye (indigo carmine or methylene blue) to the injection solution. Submucosal space contains relatively loose fibers, accepting the dye and turning into a blue color. Muscularis layer contains dense fibers and is not changing its color after submucosal injection (stays white). This difference between blue color of the submucosal space and white color of the muscularis layer allows determining the dissection plane for ESD.

Various solutions are currently used for submucosal injection during ESD in the United States. Normal saline is readily available, but it rapidly migrates from the site of injection not leaving enough time to perform endoscopic dissection. However, several commercially available ESD knives (ERBE knife, DualKnife J, Flushknife) allow repeat injection through the knife, and normal saline can be successfully used through these devices for colonic ESD.

Volume expanders such as Hespan (6% hetastarch in 0.9% sodium chloride injection, B. Braun Medical) and Voluven (6% hydroxyethyl starch 130/0.4 in 0.9% sodium chloride, Fresenius Kabi Norge A.S., Halden Norway) are easy to inject and provide submucosal cushion, which lasts longer than normal saline.

Eleview (Aries Pharmaceutical Inc, San Diego, CA) is the first dedicated solution for submucosal injection cleared by Food and Drug Administration and currently commercially available in United States. Eleview is preloaded in 10 mL ampules, which can be stored at room temperature away from direct sunlight. Injection of Eleview can be done through any 23, 25, or 26 gauge endoscopic injection needles.

2. Circumferencial incision around the lesion (Fig. 47.3).

After adequate submucosal cushion is created by submucosal injection, the injection needle is removed and ESD knife is inserted through the biopsy channel of the endoscope. A circumferential cut around the lesion is performed to establish lateral margins of dissection separating the polyp from surrounding normal mucosa.

3. Dissection of the submucosal fibers (Fig. 47.4).

Dissection of submucosal fibers above the muscularis layer establishes the deep margin of resection separating the mucosal lesion from the underlying muscularis layer of the colonic wall. The plane of dissection usually leaves approximately one-third of the depth of the submucosal space above the muscularis layer and two-thirds of the depth of the submucosal layer below the mucosa. Multiple blood vessels of various calibers could be seen in the submucosal space. Smaller vessels could be cauterized with the tip of the ESD knife. Larger vessels should be preemptively cauterized with Coagrasper to prevent massive bleeding.

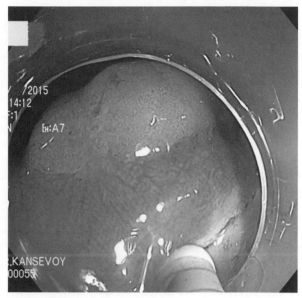

FIG. 47.3 Circumferential incision. Circumferential incision around the lesion is started using the DualKnife. Please note safety terminal plate (white) and gray color line of the DualKnife are above the mucosa—to prevent deep injury of the muscle by the tip of the DualKnife.

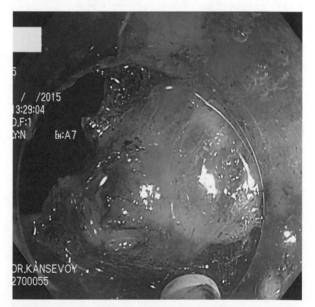

FIG. 47.4 Dissection of submucosal fibers. Under precise visual control, black-colored submucosal fibers are dissected with the DualKnife.

During ESD, only intensely blue-colored submucosal tissue should be cut. If the color fades (becomes less blue or even white), risk of damage of muscularis layer and full-thickness perforation increases. Additional injection of submucosal solution should be made to restore intensely blue color of the submucosal space to continue dissection.

Some endoscopists recommend only partial (sectoral) cut instead of full-circumferential incision. Partial cut slows dissipation of injected fluid from the submucosal space allowing more time for dissection of the submucosal fibers. After sectoral dissection is completed, next submucosal injection is made to expand the adjacent sector to continue ESD.

4. Closure of the large mucosal defects post colonic ESD.

Completion of ESD creates large mucosal defect exposing submucosal and muscular layers (Fig. 47.5). Previous studies demonstrated increased risk of delayed bleeding from large mucosal defects post EMR and ESD.[11] Closure of the defects larger than 2 cm in size significantly decreased the rate of delayed adverse events post removal of large colonic lesions.[11,12]

We use Overstitch endoscopic suturing device for closure of all large mucosal defects post colonic ESD. Suturing closure

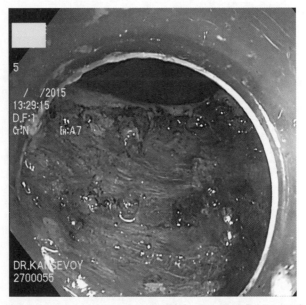

FIG. 47.5 Endoscopic submucosal dissection (ESD) is completed. *En bloc* resection of the colonic lesion is completed. Large mucosal defect post ESD demonstrates intact muscularis layer.

significantly decreased the risk of delayed bleeding and delayed perforation post ESD, eliminated the need for hospital admission, and resulted in significant cost saving—over $5000 per patient.[12]

ADVERSE EVENTS

Intraprocedural bleeding is frequently encountered during colonic ESD. It is usually amenable to endoscopic hemostasis using electrocautery with the tip of DualKnife in closed position (to prevent perforation) or Coagrasper.

Perforation is the most fearsome adverse event during colonic ESD. As soon as endoscopic perforation is diagnosed, intravenous antibiotics with broad coverage (against gram-negative and anaerobic bacteria) should be administered (we usually use 400 mg of Ciprofloxacin and 500 mg of Metronidazole). Frequent palpation of the patient's abdomen and monitoring of the vital signs are necessary to check for abdominal distension and prevention of abdominal compartment syndrome.

Endoscopic suturing device allows full-thickness closure of colonic perforations eliminating the need for surgery.[10,13] However, if colonic defect cannot be reliably closed endoscopically, immediate surgery is needed to prevent peritonitis.

References

1. Fujishiro M, Yahagi N, Nakamura M, et al. Successful outcomes of a novel endoscopic treatment for GI tumors: endoscopic submucosal dissection with a mixture of high-molecular-weight hyaluronic acid, glycerin, and sugar. *Gastrointest Endosc.* 2006;63:243-249.
2. Larghi A, Waxman I. State of the art on endoscopic mucosal resection and endoscopic submucosal dissection. *Gastrointest Endosc Clin N Am.* 2007;17:441-469, v.
3. Nakajima T, Saito Y, Tanaka S, et al. Current status of endoscopic resection strategy for large, early colorectal neoplasia in Japan. *Surg Endosc.* 2013;27:3262-3270.
4. Kantsevoy SV, Adler DG, Conway JD, et al. Endoscopic mucosal resection and endoscopic submucosal dissection. *Gastrointest Endosc.* 2008;68:11-18.
5. Rex DK, Schoenfeld PS, Cohen J, et al. Quality indicators for colonoscopy. *Gastrointest Endosc.* 2014;81:31-53.
6. Fujiya M, Tanaka K, Dokoshi T, et al. Efficacy and adverse events of EMR and endoscopic submucosal dissection for the treatment of colon neoplasms: a meta-analysis of studies comparing EMR and endoscopic submucosal dissection. *Gastrointest Endosc.* 2015;81:583-595.
7. Moss A, Williams SJ, Hourigan LF, et al. Long-term adenoma recurrence following wide-field endoscopic mucosal resection (WF-EMR) for advanced colonic mucosal neoplasia is infrequent: results and risk factors in 1000 cases from the Australian Colonic EMR (ACE) study. *Gut.* 2015;64:57-65.
8. Draganov PV, Gotoda T, Chavalitdhamrong D, et al. Techniques of endoscopic submucosal dissection: application for the Western endoscopist?. *Gastrointest Endosc.* 2013;78:677-688.
9. Saltzman HA, Sieker HO. Intestinal response to changing gaseous environments: normobaric and hyperbaric observations. *Ann N Y Acad Sci.* 1968;150:31-39.

10. Kantsevoy SV, Bitner M, Hajiyeva G, et al. Endoscopic management of colonic perforations: clips versus suturing closure (with videos). *Gastrointest Endosc*. 2016;84:487-493.

11. Liaquat H, Rohn E, Rex DK. Prophylactic clip closure reduced the risk of delayed postpolypectomy hemorrhage: experience in 277 clipped large sessile or flat colorectal lesions and 247 control lesions. *Gastrointest Endosc*. 2013;77:401-407.

12. Kantsevoy SV, Bitner M, Mitrakov AA, et al. Endoscopic suturing closure of large mucosal defects after endoscopic submucosal dissection is technically feasible, fast, and eliminates the need for hospitalization (with videos). *Gastrointest Endosc*. 2014;79:503-507.

13. Kantsevoy SV, Bitner M, Davis JM, et al. Endoscopic suturing closure of large iatrogenic colonic perforation. *Gastrointest Endosc*. 2015;82:754-755.

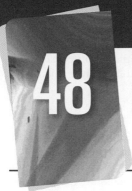

48

Esophageal Peroral Endoscopic Myotomy

Amy Hosmer, MD
Ryan Law, DO

Prior to 2008, the standard of care for the treatment of achalasia was Heller myotomy. Since that time, the development of per-oral endoscopic myotomy (POEM) has largely supplanted surgical intervention.[1] POEM is an endoscopic procedure that allows division of the muscular fibers of the esophagus, including the lower esophageal sphincter to mimic the surgical gold standard. Available data suggest a high rate of procedural and clinical success with a low adverse event rate. Long-term studies will be necessary to determine the durability of this intervention.

INDICATIONS

Absolute Indications
- Classic achalasia (type I, II, III)

Extended Indications
- Hypertensive lower esophageal sphincter
- Jackhammer esophagus
- Diffuse esophageal spasm
- Repeat esophageal myotomy after prior laparoscopic Heller myotomy (LHM) or POEM

CONTRAINDICATIONS[a]
- Advanced or end-stage achalasia
- Large epiphrenic diverticula in the surgical field
- Prior irradiation to the mediastinum or esophagus
- Severe pulmonary disease
- Coagulopathy, INR >1.5
- Baseline platelet count <50,000/mm^3

---

[a]Current contraindications for POEM are based only on expert consensus.[2]

- Prior esophageal endoscopic mucosal resection or other mucosal ablative therapy (i.e., endoscopic submucosal dissection [ESD], photodynamic therapy, radiofrequency ablation)
- Cirrhosis with portal hypertension

PREPARATION

1. Initiate a full liquid diet 3 days prior to the procedure and begin a "clear-liquids-only" diet 24 hours prior to the procedure
2. Patients on anticoagulants and antiplatelet agents should stop or alter their medication after discussion with the prescribing physician
3. Obtain standard preoperative consent by the surgeon/endoscopist and anesthesiologist including risks/benefits/alternatives
4. Place patient in supine position
5. Expose abdomen during procedure to monitor pneumoperitoneum
6. Procedure performed under general anesthesia with endotracheal intubation using a paralytic
7. Give a single dose of prophylactic heparin (10,000 units subcutaneous)
8. Consider a single dose of antibiotic prophylaxis
9. Ensure air insufflation is turned off on the processor

EQUIPMENT

- Standard gastroscope and accompanying tower/processor/monitor
- CO_2 insufflator with full canister or wall attachment
- Electrosurgical generator
- Spray catheter
- Injection needle
- Clear cap for the gastroscope
- ESD knife
- Hemostatic forceps
- Endoscopic clips
- Normal saline + indigo carmine/methylene blue
- Veress needle

PROCEDURE (ESOPHAGEAL POEM, VIDEO 48.1)

1. *Pre-POEM EGD.* Prior to POEM, a routine esophagoduodenoscopy (EGD) is performed to clean and lavage contents within the esophagus and stomach. Precise measurements should be obtained to determine the location of the gastroesophageal (GE) junction. The starting point of the circular myotomy and location of the submucosal incision will be based on this measurement. Finally, the esophagus is irrigated with antibiotic solution (i.e., gentamicin 180 mg mixed into 240 mL of sterile saline).

2. *Mucosal incision.* The submucosal injection/incision will be performed on the anterior esophageal wall ~2 cm proximal to where the myotomy will begin at the 2 o'clock position (alternative: 5 o'clock position [posterior myotomy]). Once identified, 10 mL of saline + indigo carmine/methylene blue will be injected into the submucosal space using a standard sclerotherapy needle. An ESD knife will then be used to create a 1.5 to 2 cm longitudinal incision using a blended current (i.e., EndoCut mode 2, 50 W) to gain full access to the submucosal space (Fig. 48.1).

3. *Submucosal tunneling/dissection.* The distal attachment (clear cap) is instrumental in early tunnel creation and aids access to the submucosal space. Once the tunnel is begun, subsequent injection of saline + indigo carmine/methylene blue (10 mL/injection) into the distal submucosal space using a spray catheter is necessary every few centimeters to identify the submucosal plane. Dissection of the submucosal plane closest to the circular muscle using either blended current (Endocut mode 2, 50 W) or coagulation current (Spray coagulation, effect 2, 50 W) is carried out with avoidance of the mucosa (Fig. 48.2). Small vessels or bleeding encountered in the esophagus can be treated with the ESD knife (spray coagulation); larger vessels (>2 mm) should be treated with hemostatic forceps (soft coagulation mode, 80 W, effect 5). The GE junction is identified by the spindle vein and/or palisading vessels. Additionally, the submucosal tunnel narrows at this point making scope passage more challenging. These findings,

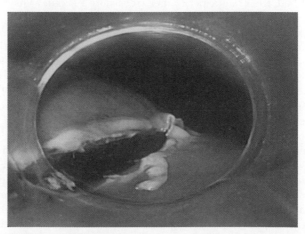

FIG. 48.1 A 2 cm longitudinal mucosal incision to gain access to the submucosal space to initiate tunneling.

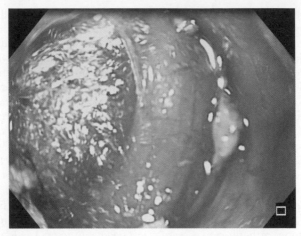

FIG. 48.2 Creation of the submucosal tunnel involves dissecting along the plane between the submucosa (gray) and circular esophageal muscle (white). In this image, the dissection plane runs from 12 o'clock to 6 o'clock.

as well as measurement, signify the GE junction. After passing the GE junction, the tunnel opens widely in the gastric cardia. Following dissection into the gastric cardia (≥3 cm beyond GE junction), the gastroscope should then be withdrawn from the tunnel and passed into the esophageal lumen then retroflexed in the stomach to verify adequate tunnel length. The gastroscope is then returned to the tunnel for close inspection for bleeding or vessels that may bleed subsequently. If identified, the Coagrasper (larger vessels) or TT knife is used for coagulation/coaptation.

4. *Myotomy.* We perform a selective circular myotomy, not a full-thickness myotomy (Fig. 48.3). We aim to preserve the longitudinal muscle; however, the longitudinal muscle may split/separate during the myotomy. This is unavoidable and should not generate concern. The myotomy is initiated ~2 cm below the mucosotomy. Entry through the circular muscle is achieved using spray coagulation mode to identify the circular-longitudinal muscle plane. Once identified, the circular muscle tissue is grabbed with the ESD knife and divided while retracting the knife tip into the distal attachment cap to prevent both mucosal and longitudinal muscle injuries. Spray coagulation can be used to divide the circular muscle; however, a blended current may be necessary for thicker muscle fibers (i.e., lower esophageal sphincter). The myotomy should be continued for 2 to 3 cm into the gastric cardia. Bleeding vessels should be treated promptly using either the ESD knife (spray

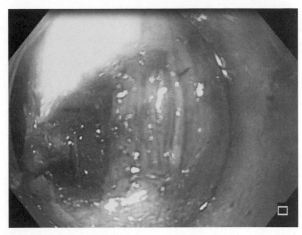

FIG. 48.3 The selective circular myotomy is carried out by dividing the circular muscle and preserving the longitudinal muscle.

coagulation) for smaller vessels or the Coagrasper (soft coagulation) for larger vessels. Prophylactic coagulation/coaptation of blood vessels should be performed to prevent bleeding.

5. *Tunnel closure.* The tunnel is copiously irrigated with sterile saline. Antibiotic solution (i.e., gentamycin 80 g in 20 mL normal saline) is sprayed into the tunnel and suctioned. The submucosal tunnel is then completely closed with endoclips or endoscopic suturing (Fig. 48.4).

POSTPROCEDURE

Following POEM patients should be admitted for overnight observation. Patients will be kept NPO. Oral proton-pump inhibitors will be initiated and continued for 6 months. Acetaminophen can be administered as needed for pain control. Antiemetics, broad-spectrum antibiotics, and narcotic analgesics may be required in select cases. Contrast esophagram (or CT esophagram) and chest x-ray should be obtained the following morning. If no esophageal leak is identified and contrast passes smoothly through the GE junction on esophagram, a clear liquid diet will be initiated and the patient will be discharged.

The patient should continue a clear liquid diet for 3 days then can advance to a full liquid diet until postprocedure clinic follow-up (generally 1 to 2 weeks after discharge). Anticoagulants and antiplatelet agents will be resumed on a case-by-case basis with the assistance of the prescribing provider. Generally, these agents can be resumed within 24 to 72 hours. Patients will be scheduled for a standard postoperative visit 7 days after discharge.

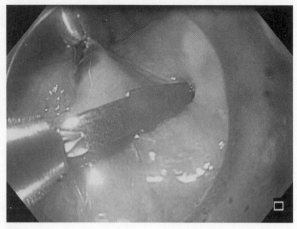

FIG. 48.4 Following completion of the circular myotomy and irrigation of the tunnel, the mucosotomy is closed with a series of endoclips.

Patients should follow-up in clinic no less frequent than once yearly thereafter for repeat symptom assessment and additional evaluation if necessary which may include a timed barium esophagram, EndoFLIP, esophageal manometry, upper endoscopy, or pH monitoring.

ADVERSE EVENTS[3]

Intraprocedural

Bleeding: Bleeding from the submucosal tunnel is not uncommon and easily treated in most cases. Bleeding which occurs during creation of the submucosal tunnel can routinely be managed with the ESD knife (spray coagulation for smaller vessels) or hemostatic forceps (soft coagulation for larger vessels). Instillation of normal saline into the tunnel via the gastroscope irrigation jet can localize the bleeding vessel.

Inadvertent mucosotomy: Inadvertent mucosal tears can occur during tunnel creation or during the myotomy. This occurs secondary to inadvertent energy application to the mucosal flap, most commonly at or near the GE junction due to the tight working space in that area. These defects should be closed with standard endoclips or endoscopic suturing at the end of the procedure to prevent leakage of luminal contents into the tunnel.

Tension pneumoperitoneum/pneumothorax: Subcutaneous emphysema and mild pneumoperitoneum are not uncommon and generally require no intervention. In rare cases, patients may develop tension pneumothorax (less common; requires intraoperative chest tube placement) or tension pneumoperitoneum (more common; requires intraoperative Veress needle placement).

Delayed

Delayed bleeding: Patients with delayed bleeding may have dysphagia, hematemesis, or chest pain related to the blood clot within the submucosal tunnel. Upper endoscopy should be performed emergently with removal of endoclips/endoscopic sutures to access the submucosal tunnel. Hematoma within the submucosal tunnel can lead to pressure necrosis of the mucosal flap, thus clotted blood should be carefully evacuated from the tunnel. The bleeding site should be treated using the hemostatic forceps (soft coagulation, 80 W, effect 5). Following hemostasis, the entry mucosotomy should be closed with endoclips/endoscopic sutures.

Mediastinitis/peritonitis: While extremely uncommon, this occurs secondary to an esophageal leak with an increased risk when inadvertent mucosotomy occurs during tunnel creation or myotomy. In most scenarios, treatment will require initiation of broad-spectrum intravenous antibiotic therapy and surgical drainage.

Late

Gastroesophageal reflux disease (GERD): The incidence of GERD following POEM may be up to 40%.[4] Patients with symptoms (i.e., heartburn, reflux, etc.) may need to undergo upper endoscopy and/or pH testing. Continuation of proton-pump inhibitor therapy may be necessary.

Failed myotomy: Inadequate symptom relief following POEM may be related to an insufficient myotomy. Repeat intervention may be required either with posterior POEM or with LHM.[5]

References

1. Inoue H, Minami H, Kobayashi Y, et al. Peroral endoscopic myotomy (POEM) for esophageal achalasia. *Endoscopy*. 2010;42:265-271.
2. Stavropoulos SN, Modayil RJ, Friedel D, Savides T. The International per oral endoscopic myotomy Survey (IPOEMS): a snapshot of the global POEM experience. *Surg Endosc*. 2013;27:3322-3338.
3. Haito-Chavez Y, Inoue H, Beard KW, et al. Comprehensive analysis of adverse events associated with per oral endoscopic myotomy in 1826 patients: an International Multicenter Study. *Am J Gastroenterol*. 2017;112:1267-1276.
4. Repici A, Fuccio L, Maselli R, et al. GERD after per-oral endoscopic myotomy as compared with Heller's myotomy with fundoplication: a systematic review with meta-analysis. *Gastrointest Endosc*. 2018;87:934-943 e18.
5. Ngamruengphong S, Inoue H, Ujiki MB, et al. Efficacy and safety of peroral endoscopic myotomy for treatment of achalasia after failed Heller myotomy. *Clin Gastroenterol Hepatol*. 2017;15:1531-1537 e3.

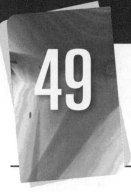

49

Gastric Per-Oral Endoscopic Myotomy

Maen Masadeh, MD
Rami El Abiad, MD
Mouen A. Khashab, MD

Gastroparetic patients present with a wide variety of symptoms that include nausea, vomiting, early satiety, and weight loss. Gastroparesis inflicts a significant burden on the patient and the healthcare system.[1-3] Hospitalizations related to gastroparesis as the primary diagnosis has increased by 158% between 1995 and 2004.[1] The pathogenesis of the disease is heterogeneous and not fully understood, which renders treatment challenging. The loss of myenteric interstitial cells of Cajal, myopathy, and neuropathy with secondary derangement in gastric motility and accommodation are thought to be part of the pathophysiology. Pylorospasm and loss of synchrony between the antrum and the duodenum further aggravate the problem.[4]

Treatment of gastroparesis can be challenging for both patients and physicians. Conservative management with dietary modification is recommended. Low-residue diet can alleviate the key symptoms of gastroparesis in patients with diabetes. [5]Medical therapy is limited by considerable side effects, such as cardiac arrhythmias, extrapyramidal symptoms, and tachyphylaxis. Pylorus-directed therapies aim to decrease pyloric spasms. Botulinum toxin injection may be effective in certain subset of patients (females, younger ages, idiopathic gastroparesis)[6] but lacks effectiveness in randomized controlled trials.[7,8] Pylorus stenting, which is usually used as a palliative treatment for malignant gastric outlet obstruction, has been studied retrospectively in gastroparesis. Seventy-five percent of gastroparesis patients with pylorus stenting had positive clinical response, which is not long lived, as the stents are prone to migration.[9] Surgical pyloroplasty aims at decreasing pylorospasm. It has been shown to be effective in reducing gastric emptying time in 86% of patients in a large study of 177 patients.[10]

Pylorus-directed therapies are promising and have been increasingly used for the treatment of refractory gastroparesis. In this chapter, we describe clinical indications, contraindications, complications, and technical aspects of gastric per-oral endoscopic myotomy (G-POEM), which was first described in 2013 by Khashab et al.[11]

INDICATIONS AND PATIENT SELECTION

Patients with retention of >10% at 4 hours on gastric emptying scintigraphy (GES) regardless of the etiology are considered to have gastroparesis. Those who fail conservative treatment with dietary modification and/or medications including prokinetic agents are considered for G-POEM. Endoscopic functional luminal imaging probe (endoFLIP) may be used to measure the pressure, diameter, and distensibility of the pylorus[12] and is a promising modality which could help identify patients who would benefit from pyloric intervention such as G-POEM. Gastroparesis symptoms like postprandial fullness and early satiety have been shown to be inversely related to diameter and cross-sectional area of the pylorus.[13] Also, pyloric pressure was found to be high in about 50% of patients with nausea and vomiting in the setting of delayed gastric emptying.[14] However, the use of endoFLIP in triaging optimal candidates for G-POEM is still investigational.

CONTRAINDICATIONS

Absolute

- Patients who are deemed unfit to undergo an elective endoscopy with general anesthesia due to cardiovascular or pulmonary morbid conditions
- Pregnancy
- Diabetic patients with diabetic ketoacidosis

Relative

- Patients with pain predominant symptoms on high-dose narcotics
- Patients with hemoglobin A1c > 10

PROCEDURE TEAM

G-POEM team involves an advanced endoscopist with experience in submucosal endoscopy, a trained endoscopy technician, and an anesthesia team. The procedure can be performed in the operating room or the endoscopy suite.

PREPARATION

Patients are placed on liquid diet for 1 to 2 days prior to the procedure. This ensures clear endoscopic views and reduces the risk of aspiration.

Antiplatelet and/or anticoagulant medications should be stopped prior to the procedure after consultation with the treating physician whenever needed.[15] Patients with prior gastric surgery involving the pylorus or antrum and those on anticoagulation that cannot be stopped/held are contraindicated.

Periprocedural prophylactic intravenous antibiotics are used, usually a second-generation cephalosporin.

EQUIPMENT

A high-definition gastroscope with water jet is used. Disposable distal attachment is secured at the tip of the gastroscope using zinc oxide-based tape (HyTape). Carbon dioxide is used for insufflation to reduce the risk of pneumoperitoneum and gas-related adverse events. Either a triangle tip knife (Olympus, Tokyo, Japan) or HybridKnife (Erbe, Tubingen, Germany) can be used to create the tunnel and perform the myotomy. Some experts prefer using the insulated tip knife (Olympus) for pyloromyotomy as the ceramic tip protects against injury of the duodenal wall, which runs close and perpendicular to the pyloric ring.

TECHNIQUE

The procedure is divided into four steps: Mucosal incision and entry into the tunnel, creation of the submucosal tunnel, pyloromyotomy, and closure of mucosal entry site.

Step 1: Mucosal Incision and Entry into the Tunnel

There is no default site to approach the pylorus. Anterior and lesser curvature approaches have been described,[16] but this could make entering the channel difficult. We prefer the greater curvature approach at 5 o'clock. A submucosal lift is made using blue-dyed saline, then a 2-cm longitudinal mucosal cut is performed about 3 to 4 cm proximal to the pylorus (Erbe EndoCut Q 3:1:1 or Dry Cut 50 W Effect 2) (Fig. 49.1). Distal attachment is used to separate the edges and expose the submucosal space. Dissection of the submucosal fibers is then performed using the same current as above, and the endoscope is gently maneuvered into the submucosal space.

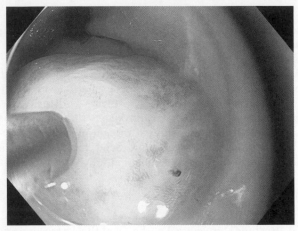

FIG. 49.1 Submucosal injection with blue-dyed saline and bleb formation; a mucosal longitudinal incision is performed 3 to 4 cm proximal to the pylorus.

Step 2: Creation of the Submucosal Tunnel

During this step, avoidance of mucosal injury is crucial and the operator should maintain the muscularis propria at 6 o'clock and the mucosa at 12 o'clock. Repetitive methylene blue/saline mix injection (using spray catheter, injection needle, knife, or endoscope jet) helps providing a submucosal cushion and separating the muscularis propria during tunneling. Tunneling or submucosal fiber dissection is then performed using Endocut Q, Dry Cut, or Spray coagulation currents (Fig. 49.2). Submucosal penetrating vessels are frequently encountered; those should be prophylactically coagulated using a coagulation grasping forceps (soft coagulation, 80 W and effect 5). The end point of the tunnel is when the posterior aspect of the pyloric ring (half-moon) is exposed (Fig. 49.3). Further dissection into the duodenum is not recommended, as risk of perforation is high.

Step 3: Pyloromyotomy

After exposing the pylorus, myotomy can be performed preferably by using an insulated tip knife (IT-2 or IT-nano, Olympus) to avoid duodenal mucosal injury. A full-thickness myotomy is achieved using Endocut Q current, with close attention to the serosa and intra-abdominal organs (Fig. 49.4). The direction of myotomy is usually retrograde, starting at the pylorus and ending 1 to 2 cm proximally before the antral circular muscles. Cutting antral circular muscles could theoretically worsen gastroparesis symptoms, by abating the antral phase of digestion and propelling food into the pylorus.

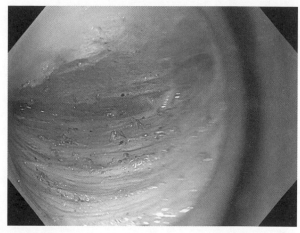

FIG. 49.2 Tunneling is achieved by dissecting submucosal fibers with careful attention to the mucosal layer.

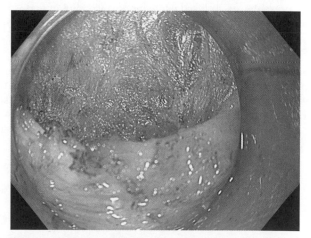

FIG. 49.3 The muscular layer with the distinct "half-moon" shape identifies the pylorus.

Step 4: Closure of Mucosal Entry

After completing the myotomy, the submucosal tunnel is examined for any signs of bleeding and/or any blood vessels that have the potential to bleed. If present, those are coagulated to ensure hemostasis and avoid future bleeding. The edges of the mucosectomy site are approximated and closed using hemostasis clips or endoscopic suturing (Overstitch; Apollo Endosurgery, Austin, TX) (Fig. 49.5). The mucosa is then examined from the gastric

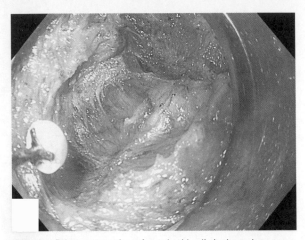

FIG. 49.4 Pyloromyotomy is performed, with a limited antral myotomy.

lumen for any signs of thermal injury and/or mucosal rupture, and if present, this is closed using hemostasis clips or endoscopic suturing as well.

POSTPROCEDURAL CARE AND FOLLOW-UP

Although there is no standard postprocedural care, patients are admitted for 1 day after the procedure. Patients are initiated/kept on high-dose proton-pump inhibitors for 1 month, as gastric antral ulcers could develop. Soft diet is started on postoperative day 1. After 1 week, the diet is advanced to a thicker consistency

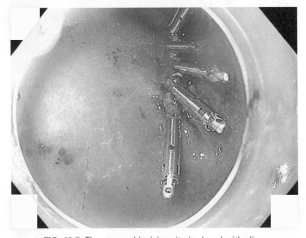

FIG. 49.5 The mucosal incision site is closed with clips.

and gauged to patient's tolerance. Obtaining upper gastrointestinal series postoperatively is controversial and should be judged based on the endoscopist confidence of a reliable mucosectomy closure. Outpatient follow-up is usually arranged in 4 to 6 weeks (or earlier if needed). On follow-up, symptom assessment and gastric emptying study should be obtained, although they do not always correlate, as symptom improvement could occur without a significant change in gastric emptying. Partial responders are encouraged to adhere to gastroparesis diet, and if needed, take their prokinetic/antiemetic agents.

ADVERSE EVENTS
Early Complications
- Capnoperitoneum
- Bleeding
- Peritoneal abscess/peritonitis
- Mucosal perforation
- Leakage

Late Complications
Although long-term follow-up data are limited to date, studies reported the following long-term complications.[17,18]
- Ulcer (pyloric or prepyloric)
- Stricture formation

  Importantly, dumping syndrome has not been reported after G-POEM.

PROCEDURAL OUTCOMES
The procedure was first performed by Khashab et al[11] in 2013 and showed successful results. Since then, multiple case reports and case series have been reported. They all confirmed the efficacy and safety of this procedure in the treatment of gastroparesis. Shlomovitz et al[19] reported a retrospective analysis of seven patients with gastroparesis who underwent G-POEM. All procedures were technically successful. Clinical success was achieved in 85% of cases, with statistically significant improvement in nausea and epigastric burning ($P < .05$). There was one late complication in which a patient presented with a bleeding ulcer at the pyloric channel, treated with blood transfusion and placement of clips. A multicenter study by Khashab et al[20] included 30 patients with refractory gastroparesis who underwent G-POEM. Procedure was technically successful in all patients. Complications were encountered in 2 (6.7%), one with capnoperitoneum and one with prepyloric ulcer. Clinical success rate was 86% at a median follow-up of 5.5 months. To date,

the largest study included 47 patients by Rodriguez et al[16,17] This group favored the lesser curvature approach, and technical success rate was 100%. Although there was a statistically significant improvement in every component of Gastroparesis Cardinal Symptom Index and improvement in gastric emptying, normalization of gastric emptying was not reported. This is in contrary to other studies, where normalization of gastric emptying was described in up to 70% of patients. Gonzalez et al[17] reported the only prospective study to date. It included 29 patients with a median follow-up of 10 months. Clinical success was 79% and 69% at 3 and 6 months, respectively, with normalization of GES in 70% of patients.

HELPFUL TIPS

Novel technologies are used to better understand the physiologic changes of the pylorus in patients with gastroparesis and perhaps identify patient subsets who would benefit the most from G-POEM. As mentioned in *Indications and patient selection* section, the use of endoFLIP is an emerging tool to assess pyloric compliance,[12] diameter,[13] and distensibility[14] in correlation with patients' symptoms. Despite the need for more data, endoFLIP seems to be the most promising modality that could assist in identifying patients with pylorospasm-predominant gastroparesis who could benefit the most from the procedure.

References

1. Wang YR, Fisher RS, Parkman HP. Gastroparesis-related hospitalizations in the United States: trends, characteristics, and outcomes, 1995-2004. *Am J Gastroenterol*. 2008;103:313-322.

2. Wadhwa V, Mehta D, Jobanputra Y, Lopez R, Thota PN,Sanaka MR. Healthcare utilization and costs associated with gastroparesis.*World J Gastroenterol*. 2017;23:4428-4436.

3. Lacy BE, Crowell MD, Mathis C, Bauer D, Heinberg LJ. Gastroparesis: quality of life and health care utilization. *J Clin Gastroenterol*. 2018;52:20-24.

4. Parkman HP, McCallum RW, *Gastroparesis*: Pathophysiology, Presentation, and Treatment. Clinical Gastroenterology. New York: Humana Press; 2012: xvi, 422.

5. Olausson EA, Störsrud S, Grundin H, Isaksson M, Attvall S, Simrén M. A small particle size diet reduces upper gastrointestinal symptoms in patients with diabetic gastroparesis: a randomized controlled trial. *Am J Gastroenterol*. 2014;109:375-385.

6. Coleski R, Anderson MA, Hasler WL. Factors associated with symptom response to pyloric injection of botulinum toxin in a large series of gastroparesis patients. *Dig Dis Sci*. 2009;54:2634-2642.

7. Arts J, Holvoet L, Caenepeel P, et al. Clinical trial: a randomized-controlled crossover study of intrapyloric injection of botulinum toxin in gastroparesis. *Aliment Pharmacol Ther*. 2007;26:1251-1258.

8. Friedenberg FK, Palit A, Parkman HP, Hanlon A, Nelson DB. Botulinum toxin A for the treatment of delayed gastric emptying. *Am J Gastroenterol*. 2008;103:416-423.

9. Khashab MA, Besharati S, Ngamruengphong S, et al. Refractory gastropare-sis can be successfully managed with endoscopic transpyloric stent place-ment and fixation (with video). *Gastrointest Endosc.* 2015;82:1106-1109.

10. Shada AL, Dunst CM, Pescarus R, et al. Laparoscopic pyloroplasty is a safe and effective first-line surgical therapy for refractory gastroparesis. *Surg Endosc.* 2016;30:1326-1332.

11. Khashab MA, Stein E, Clarke JO, et al. Gastric peroral endoscopic myotomy for refractory gastroparesis: first human endoscopic pyloromyotomy (with video). *Gastrointest Endosc.* 2013;78:764-768.

12. Gourcerol G, Tissier F, Melchior C, et al. Impaired fasting pyloric compliance in gastroparesis and the therapeutic response to pyloric dilatation. *Aliment Pharmacol Ther.* 2015;41:360-367.

13. Malik Z, Sankineni A, Parkman HP. Assessing pyloric sphincter pathophys-iology using EndoFLIP in patients with gastroparesis. *Neurogastroenterol Motil.* 2015;27:524-531.

14. Snape WJ, Lin MS, Agarwal N, Shaw RE. Evaluation of the pylorus with con-current intraluminal pressure and EndoFLIP in patients with nausea and vomiting. *Neurogastroenterol Motil.* 2016;28:758-764.

15. Acosta RD, Abraham NS, Chandrasekhara V, et al. The management of antithrombotic agents for patients undergoing GI endoscopy. *Gastrointest Endosc.* 2016;83:3-16.

16. Rodriguez JH, Haskins IN, Strong AT, et al. Per oral endoscopic pyloromyot-omy for refractory gastroparesis: initial results from a single institution. *Surg Endosc.* 2017;31:5381-5388.

17. Gonzalez JM, Benezech A, Vitton V, Barthet M. G-POEM with antro-pyloromyotomy for the treatment of refractory gastroparesis: mid-term follow-up and factors predicting outcome. *Aliment Pharmacol Ther.* 2017;46:364-370.

18. Ngamruengphong S, Inoue H, Ujiki MB, et al. Efficacy and safety of peroral endoscopic myotomy for treatment of achalasia after failed Heller myotomy. *Clin Gastroenterol Hepatol.* 2017;15:1531-1537.e1533.

19. Shlomovitz E, Pescarus R, Cassera MA, et al. Early human experience with per-oral endoscopic pyloromyotomy (POP). *Surg Endosc.* 2015;29:543-551.

20. Khashab MA, Ngamruengphong S, Carr-Locke D, et al. Gastric per-oral endoscopic myotomy for refractory gastroparesis: results from the first multicenter study on endoscopic pyloromyotomy (with video). *Gastrointest Endosc.* 2017;85:123-128.

PART TEN

Percutaneous Gastrointestinal-Related Procedures

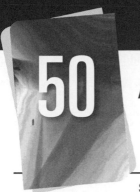

Abdominal Paracentesis

Shreya Sengupta, MD

Abdominal paracentesis with appropriate ascitic fluid analysis is one of the most rapid and cost-effective methods of diagnosing the cause of ascites.[1] Paracentesis is safely and routinely performed in both the inpatient and outpatient settings.

INDICATIONS

1. Evaluation of new-onset ascites
2. Evaluation for spontaneous bacterial peritonitis in all patients with ascites and abdominal pain, fever, unexplained encephalopathy, leukocytosis, worsening renal function, or gastrointestinal bleeding
3. Evaluation for subclinical infection in all patients with ascites requiring hospitalization
4. Treatment of symptomatic ascites[2]

CONTRAINDICATIONS

Coagulopathy should preclude paracentesis only when there is clinically evident fibrinolysis or clinically evident disseminated intravascular coagulation.[1] There is no data to suggest coagulation parameter cutoffs beyond which paracentesis should be avoided as the incidence of clinically significant bleeding in patients with underlying liver disease is low.[1,2] Paracentesis should be performed with caution in pregnant patients or in patients with organomegaly, bowel obstruction, intra-abdominal adhesions, or a distended urinary bladder. The paracentesis catheter should avoid sites of cutaneous infection, visibly engorged cutaneous vessels, surgical scars, or abdominal wall hematomas.[2]

PREPARATION OF PATIENT

1. Explain the risks, benefits, and details of the procedure to the patient.

2. Obtain written informed consent.
3. Ask the patient to empty his or her bladder.

EQUIPMENT

1. Sterile gloves and face shield
2. Skin preparation solution (i.e., chlorhexidine, iodine solution; sterile gauze)
3. Draping towels
4. Local anesthetic (lidocaine, 1%) and needles
5. Syringes: 10 mL, 50 mL
6. Paracentesis needles:
   a. No. 16, 18, 20, or 22 gauge
   b. Spinal needle (No. 18, 20 gauge) for obese patients
   c. Caldwell needle, long angiocath
7. Sterile specimen tubes
8. Blood culture bottles for bedside inoculation, if infection suspected
9. Vacutainer or wall suction setup for large-volume paracentesis

PROCEDURE

Diagnostic Paracentesis

1. Position the patient supine with the head slightly elevated to allow fluid to accumulate in the lower abdomen.
2. Identify the point of aspiration on either flank, usually two finger breadths cephalad and two finger breadths medial to the anterior superior iliac spine. An alternative location is in the midline midway between the umbilicus and pubic bone. Although the midline is relatively avascular, the abdominal wall in the left lower quadrant is thinner with a larger pool of fluid than in the midline.[3] Be careful to avoid abdominal wall scars, as bowel may be fixed to the wall, and visible collaterals. The rectus muscles should also be avoided because the epigastric arteries travel within the rectus sheath (Fig. 50.1).
3. Confirm dullness to percussion in the site selected for needle entry. If available, use bedside ultrasonography to find an appropriate pocket of ascites fluid that does not contain loops of bowel or solid organs. Mark the chosen entry site with a skin-marking pen. At many institutions, radiology can be consulted to mark the site with largest fluid pocket.
4. Put on sterile gloves.
5. Sterilize the site with an iodine solution or with chlorhexidine using small to large circles to clean the area.
6. Arrange sterile draping towels or a sterile drape.
7. Infiltrate the skin and subcutaneous tissue with a local anesthetic. Using a 22- or 25-gauge, 1.5 in. or longer needle, place a wheal of anesthetic (e.g., 1% to 2% lidocaine) in the epidermis

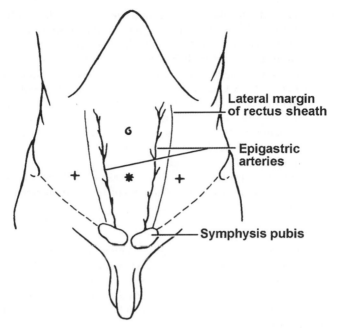

FIG. 50.1 Various sites of paracentesis. (+) preferred; (*) secondary.

at the entry site. Advance the needle along the anticipated trajectory of the paracentesis needle to anesthetize deeper structures, alternatively injecting anesthetic and pulling back on the plunger to ensure the needle has not penetrated a vascular structure. Stop advancing once peritoneal fluid begins to fill the syringe and inject additional anesthetic to numb the sensitive parietal peritoneum. In total, 5 to 10 mL of lidocaine is generally used.[2,4]

8. Attach a 20- or 22-gauge needle to a 10-mL syringe. Spinal needles (3.5-in. needles) are needed only in the setting of a large panniculus.

9. Insert the needle into the peritoneal cavity using a "Z-tract" to minimize leakage of ascites after the procedure. To create a Z-tract, use one gloved hand to move the skin approximately 2 cm in any direction in relation to the deep abdominal wall and then insert the paracentesis needle. The skin is not released until the needle has penetrated the peritoneum and fluid flows. When the needle is removed, the skin slips back into its original position and seals the leak. Although not backed by data, the theory behind the Z-tract maneuver is that if the needle is inserted directly into the fluid without a Z-tract, the straight line of flow allows fluid to leak out more easily.

10. Advance the needle in 2 to 3 mm increments, with gentle aspiration of the syringe between needle advancements while the needle is stationary. If no fluid returns after several attempts, ultrasonography can be used to identify a site.

11. When fluid is flowing, stabilize the needle to ensure a steady flow and attach a larger 30 to 60 mL syringe to the needle. It is not unusual for flow to stop as bowel or omentum are suctioned over the bevel of the needle.

12. For a diagnostic paracentesis, as little as 1 to 5 mL of fluid can be sufficient for fluid analysis, but the recommendation is to obtain 25 mL of ascites fluid.

13. Remove the needle, and place an adhesive bandage or pressure dressing over the site. The patient may resume normal activities.

Therapeutic Paracentesis

A therapeutic paracentesis is similar to diagnostic paracentesis except that a larger bore needle (14 to 18 gauge) is used and much greater amounts of fluid are removed. A large-volume paracentesis has been defined as the removal of greater than 5 L of fluid. The removal of more than 8 to 10 L of ascites fluid is not recommended.

1. Obtain the necessary equipment including a paracentesis tray with paracentesis catheter (7 in. long, with no. 14-gauge × 2-in. needle) and multiple 1-L vacuum bottles.

2. Prepare the patient as for diagnostic paracentesis. Select the paracentesis site as described above. Clean and drape the selected site. Infiltrate the skin and subcutaneous tissue with a local anesthetic.

3. Place an intravenous heparin lock if an albumin infusion of 5 g for each liter removed has been planned. Albumin has been recommended for removal of greater than 5 L to minimize increases in renin and aldosterone and, therefore, to minimize volume depletion.[5] However, no study has demonstrated a survival advantage for patients who have received albumin.

4. Using the paracentesis catheter attached to a 10-mL syringe, slowly advance the needle and catheter into the peritoneal cavity using the Z-tract technique. Intermittently aspirate fluid until a steady flow is achieved.

5. Attach tubing to the catheter and insert it into a 1-L vacuum bottle, or attach to a wall suction with a large canister.

6. Aspirate 4 to 6 L of ascitic fluid using this apparatus over 30 to 60 minutes.

7. Remove the catheter, and place a bandage or absorbable suture at the puncture site. A pressure bandage may be applied.

8. Send a sample of fluid from each paracentesis for cell count and differential and culture to detect the onset of unsuspected bacterial peritonitis.

9. For every liter of fluid removed, please give 6 to 8 g (per liter of ascites removed) of 25% albumin. This postparacentesis volume expansion should be given if >5 L is removed. We use 25% albumin due to the lower sodium load as compared to 5% albumin.

ANALYSIS OF FLUID

The analysis of the aspirated fluid will be determined by the individual patient and his or her presentation. If uncomplicated cirrhotic ascites is suspected, the initial laboratory investigation should include at least an ascitic fluid cell count and differential, total protein, and albumin (Table 50.1).[4] If the results of these tests are unexpectedly abnormal, further testing can be performed. For new-onset ascites, an accompanying serum liver function or comprehensive metabolic panel should be sent to allow calculation of the SAAG (serum ascites albumin gradient).

If spontaneous or secondary bacterial peritonitis is suspected, bacterial culture in blood culture bottles should be performed at the bedside. Gram stain and cell counts with differential should be obtained. If there is concern for secondary bacterial peritonitis, total protein, lactate dehydrogenase, and glucose are obtained. Other studies, such as acid-fast bacilli (AFB) smear and culture, cytology, triglycerides, and bilirubin, can be ordered based on pretest probability of disease. Ascitic fluid profiles for various disease states appear in Table 50.2.[5]

 Testing of Ascitic Fluid

Recommended
Cell count and differential
Albumin
Culture
Gram stain
Glucose
Lactate dehydrogenase (LDH)
Optional (Depending on Clinical Setting and Ascites Appearance)
Amylase
Triglycerides
Bilirubin
Tuberculosis staining
Cytology

TABLE 50.2	Ascitic Fluid Profiles
Type of Ascites	**Typical Paracentesis Findings**
Portal hypertensive ascites	Clear, straw-colored fluid, with ascitic fluid neutrophil count of <250 cells/mm³; high serum-ascites albumin gradient (SAAG), i.e., serum albumin minus ascitic fluid albumin >1.1 g/dL.
Spontaneous bacterial peritonitis	Ascitic fluid neutrophil count of >250 cells/mm³ (need to subtract 1 polymorphonuclear neutrophil (PMN) for every 250 red blood cells [RBCs] in hemorrhagic ascites); some variants may have as few as 100 cells/mm³. Usually a single offending microbe. Glucose usually >50 mg/dL.
Secondary bacterial peritonitis	Ascitic fluid neutrophil count of >250 cells/mm³ (need to subtract 1 PMN for every 250 RBCs in hemorrhagic ascites); surgically treatable intra-abdominal source of infection; often polymicro bial. Glucose usually <50 mg/dL.
Chylous ascites	Milky colored fluid, ascites triglycerides >200 mg/dL, often accompanied by malignant cells, usually low SAAG.
Pancreatic ascites	Clear or straw-colored fluid, ascites amylase generally >200 IU/L. Usually low SAAG.
Choleperitoneum (bile leak into ascites)	Brown-tinged fluid, ascites bilirubin > serum bilirubin and greater than 6 mg/dL.
Malignant	Often blood-tinged or chylous, may be clear. Usually low SAAG; malignant cells on cytology.
Tuberculous	May be clear, chylous, or blood-tinged. Low SAAG; positive smear for AFB.
Congestive heart failure	Clear, PMNs <250 cells/mm³. Usually high SAAG.

ADVERSE EVENTS

The incidence of serious adverse events from paracentesis is rare.[2] Adverse events were reported in only about 1% of patients (abdominal wall hematomas), despite the fact that 71% of the patients had an abnormal prothrombin time. Other adverse events, like persistent leakage of ascites fluid, localized infection, injury to intra-abdominal organs, and puncture of the inferior epigastric artery, are rare with an estimated incidence of less than 0.2%.[2,6] Large-volume paracentesis can be complicated by circulatory dysfunction with severe cases leading to hepatorenal syndrome and death. Though the use of albumin as a plasma expander remains controversial, many experts recommend giving 6 to 8 g of 25% albumin for every liter of ascites fluid removed in patients who have had more than 5 L of ascites fluid removed.[7]

References

1. Runyon BA. Management of adult patients with ascites due to cirrhosis: an update. *Hepatology.* 2009;49(6):2087-2107.

2. Thomsen T, Shaffer R, White B, Setnik G. Paracentesis. *N Engl J Med.* 2006;355:19.

3. Sakai H, Mendler MH, Runyon BA. Choosing the location for non-image guided abdominal paracentesis. *Liver Int.* 2005;25:984-986.

4. McGibbon A, Chen G. An evidence-based manual for abdominal paracentesis. *Dig Dis Sci.* 2007;52:3307-3315.

5. Moore KP, Arroyo V. The management of ascites in cirrhosis: report on the consensus conference of the International Ascites Club. *Hepatology.* 2003;38(1):258-266.

6. De Gottardi A, Hadengue A. Risk of complications after abdominal paracentesis in cirrhotic patients: a prospective study. *Clin Gastroenterol Hepatol.* 2009;7(8):906-909.

7. Gines P, Cardenas A, Arroyo V, Rodes J. Management of cirrhosis and ascites. *N Engl J Med.* 2004;350:1646-1654.

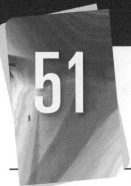

51 Percutaneous Liver Biopsy

Shreya Sengupta, MD

Liver biopsy has a central role in the evaluation of patients with suspected liver disease and can assess the nature and severity of disease. It can also be useful in monitoring the efficacy of various treatments. There are several methods for performing liver biopsy, which include percutaneous, transjugular, or laparoscopic biopsy; endoscopic ultrasound or computer tomography (CT)-guided approach is also being used. Although percutaneous liver biopsy is safe and routinely performed, a transjugular approach should be considered when standard liver biopsy is contraindicated.[1] New noninvasive tests have reduced the need for liver biopsy, but this procedure continues to have a role in the diagnosis of some liver disease, resolving questions regarding stages of fibrosis, and for addressing research questions.[2]

INDICATIONS

1. Diagnosis
   a. Multiple parenchymal liver diseases
   b. Abnormal liver tests of unknown etiology
   c. Fever of unknown origin
   d. Focal or diffuse abnormalities on imaging studies
   e. Hepatic mass—imaging can be diagnostic for HCC and certain types of cholangiocarcinoma (hilar) should not be biopsied; however, biopsy can be considered in certain situations
2. Prognosis—staging of known parenchymal liver disease
3. Management—developing treatment plans based on histologic analysis[3]
   a. Rejection in the transplanted liver

CONTRAINDICATIONS

Specifying contraindications to liver biopsy is difficult given the scarcity of data. Contraindications will vary depending on the physician and local expertise, and most of the contraindications listed below are considered to be relative. In clinical practice, patients who are uncooperative, are morbidly obese, or have an increased risk of bleeding are of greatest concern.[1,3]

Absolute Contraindications

1. Uncooperative patient
2. Severe coagulopathy (no set cutoff for INR (international normalized ratio) but may consider INR > 2 as severe coagulopathy)
3. Infection of the hepatic bed
4. Extrahepatic biliary obstruction
5. Inability to identify an adequate biopsy site by percussion and/or ultrasound

Relative Contraindications

1. Ascites
2. Morbid obesity
3. Possible vascular lesions
4. Amyloidosis
5. Hydatid disease

PREPARATION

1. Complete a history and physical examination, assessing for personal or family history of excessive bleeding.
2. Review medications, particularly those known to affect bleeding parameters.
3. Evaluate coagulation status with prothrombin time, platelet count, and a complete blood count prior to the biopsy. Bleeding time may be considered, particularly in patients with renal failure or a history of excessive bleeding.
4. Obtain written informed consent.
5. There is no clear evidence in the literature regarding fasting status. Some centers recommend NPO (nil per os) status prior to the procedure, while other centers advocate for a preprocedural light snack to avoid a vasovagal response and to ensure that the gallbladder is contracted.
6. Conscious sedation is not routinely required. However, the use of light sedation is safe and does not increase the risk of the procedure.

7. Review computed tomography (CT) or magnetic resonance imaging (MRI) scans of the liver; this may aid in selection of a biopsy site.

8. Instruct the patient on what to expect and on the need to follow commands regarding respiration.[1,4]

EQUIPMENT

There are three different categories of liver biopsy needles.

1. Aspiration needles (Jamshidi, Klatskin, Menghini). The Jamshidi needle is the preferred needle at many centers.

2. Cutting needles (Tru-cut, Vim-Silverman)

3. Spring-loaded cutting needles that have triggering mechanisms

If cirrhosis is suspected, a cutting needle is preferred over an aspiration-type needle to minimize fragmentation of fibrotic tissue. The intrahepatic phase of the biopsy is shorter when using aspiration needles, potentially decreasing the risks of the procedure.[4]

The following supplies will be needed at the bedside for the biopsy:

1. Liver biopsy tray including biopsy needle, scalpel, gauze, saline, 10-mL syringe, 25- to 27-gauge needle (for anesthetic infiltration) and Betadine (or chlorhexidine)

2. Sterile towels

3. Gloves

4. Lidocaine (5 to 10 mL of a 1% solution)

5. Sterile containers for serology and culture specimens

6. Adhesive bandage

PROCEDURE

1. Position the patient supine near the edge of the bed, with his or her right hand under the head and left arm by the left side.

2. Percuss the area of maximum liver dullness in both inspiratory and expiratory phases over the right hemithorax in the midaxillary line (usually between the eighth or ninth intercostal spaces), and mark the spot (Fig. 51.1).

3. Confirm the selected biopsy site with bedside ultrasound.

4. Disinfect the biopsy site using povidone-iodine (Betadine)-soaked gauze pads or a chlorhexidine swab (Chloraprep).

5. Infiltrate the site with local anesthetic, inserting the needle along the superior margin of the rib in order to avoid the intercostal artery. Once the superficial skin is anesthetized, inject lidocaine into the deeper structures.

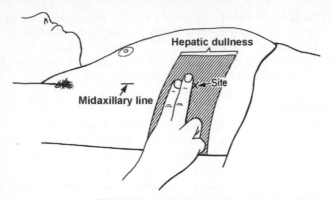

FIG. 51.1 Percutaneous liver biopsy.

6. Prepare the biopsy needle. If a suction needle is used, attach it to a 10-mL syringe filled with sterile saline.

7. Make a small skin incision so the needle can be passed easily through the skin.

8. Insert the biopsy needle through the incision with the tip directed toward the xiphoid process, creating a tract that is parallel to the floor. Guide the needle with the left hand.

9. Continue to apply negative pressure (suction) on the syringe while the needle passes through the subcutaneous tissue and the intercostal muscles. Place the left hand on the biopsy needle 3 cm from the skin.

10. While the patient holds his or her breath in expiration phase, continue to apply negative pressure on the syringe plunger and quickly advance the biopsy needle 3 cm within the liver, and come out quickly. Maintain suction at all time.

11. If at least a 2-cm core of tissue is obtained, transfer the specimen to the appropriate container. Perform a second or third biopsy if more tissue is necessary. Clean the biopsy site and apply a bandage.

12. Position the patient in the right lateral decubitus position to maintain constant body pressure on the biopsy site for about 2 hours. The patient then remains on bedrest for an additional 2 to 4 hours, while his or her vital signs are monitored every 15 minutes.

13. Discuss detailed and clearly written postprocedure instructions with the patient before discharge.

ADVERSE EVENTS

Pain is the most common adverse event of percutaneous liver biopsy, occurring in up to 84% of patients. This includes the development of mild discomfort. Pain can usually be managed with small doses of narcotics in the immediate postprocedural setting.[3] Moderate to severe pain should raise the concern for bleeding or gallbladder puncture, which occurs in 0.12% of liver biopsies.[5] Severe pain should warrant radiologic evaluation with liver ultrasound or abdominal computer tomography (CT) with contrast. Severe bleeding occurs in 1 in 2500 to 10,000 biopsies; this is defined as clinically significant bleeding requiring hospitalization, transfusion, or radiologic or surgical intervention.[3,6,7] Mortality related to liver biopsy is usually due to hemorrhage and the rate is less than 1 in 10,000 liver biopsies.[3,8] Less common adverse events include hemobilia, pneumothorax, colonic puncture, biliary peritonitis, and sepsis.[3,8]

References

1. Bravo AA, Sheth SG, Chopra S. Liver biopsy. *N Engl J Med*. 2001;344(7):495-500.
2. Tapper EB, Lok AS. Use of liver imaging and biopsy in clinical practice. *N Engl J Med*. 2017;377:756-768.
3. Rockey DC, Caldwell SH, Goodman ZD, Nelson RC, Smith AD. Liver biopsy. *Hepatology*. 2009;49(3):1017-1044.
4. Grant A, Neuberger J. Guidelines on the use of liver biopsy in clinical practice. *Gut*. 1999;45(suppl IV):IV1-IV11.
5. Piccinino F, Sagnelli E, Pasquale G, Giusti G. Complications following percutaneous liver biopsy. A multicentre retrospective study on 68,276 biopsies. *J Hepatol*. 1986;2(2):165-173.
6. Janes CH, Lindor KD. Outcome of patients hospitalized for complications after outpatient liver biopsy. *Ann Intern Med*. 1993;118(2):96-98.
7. Garcia-Tsao G, Boyer JL. Outpatient liver biopsy: how safe is it? *Ann Intern Med*. 1993;118:150-153.
8. Huang FJ, Hsieh MY, Dai CY, et al. The incidence and risks of liver biopsy in non-cirrhotic patients: an evaluation of 3806 biopsies. *Gut*. 2007;56:736-737.

PART ELEVEN

Tests of Gastrointestinal Function

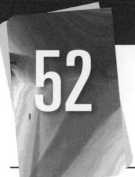

52

Esophageal Manometry

Joseph R. Triggs, MD, PhD
John E. Pandolfino, MD, MSCI

High-resolution esophageal manometry (HREM) and subsequent interpretation using the Chicago Classification (CC) is the gold standard for the diagnosis of esophageal motility disorders.[1] The procedure is performed by placing a catheter with a dense series of pressure sensors transnasally with the distal tip ending in the patient's stomach. Test swallows are then performed and recorded assessing contractile timing and intraluminal pressures. HREM studies are displayed as pressure topography plots or Clouse plots, named after the individual who developed them.[2,3] These plots place time on the x-axis, anatomic location on the y-axis, and pressure depicted as color, with warmer colors representing higher amplitudes. HREM replaced traditional line tracing manometry and has led to increased ease of use, uniformity, standardization of objective measures used in the diagnosis of motility disorders, improved interrater agreement, and improved diagnostic yield.[4-7] Despite these advances, HREM is a diagnostic tool that requires special expertise and training to reliably perform high quality studies.[8-10] Healthcare professionals reading these studies must be able to assess for technical adequacy, which includes ensuring proper placement, recognizing common artifacts and equipment failure, in addition to being able to accurately report the measurements used in the CC to allow for an accurate diagnosis.

INDICATIONS

Structural abnormalities should be ruled out prior to HREM with upper gastrointestinal endoscopy, esophagram, or other form of structural evaluation of the esophagus.

1. Nonobstructive dysphagia
2. Noncardiac chest pain, regurgitation, rumination, or belching
3. To aid in positioning for pH and pH-impedance testing
4. Prior to antireflux surgery for assessment of swallowing function

CONTRAINDICATIONS

1. Esophageal obstruction from an infiltrating process or high-grade constriction
2. Altered nasal passage anatomy preventing catheter insertion
3. High-grade oropharyngeal dysphagia
4. Significant coagulopathy

PREPARATION FOR STUDY

1. HREM catheters are made by several manufacturers and manufacturer instructions should be followed for catheter calibration and recording device setup prior to patient arrival.
2. Informed consent should be obtained and documented.[11]
3. Patients should have nothing to eat or drink for at least 6 hours before the HREM study to prevent aspiration.
   a. For patients with achalasia and esophageal retention, you may want to consider a clear liquid diet for 48 hours prior to the procedure.
4. Patients should be assessed for prior foregut surgery as this can alter interpretation during analysis.
5. The patient medication list should be reviewed specifically for opioids, calcium channel blockers, antispasmodics, nitroglycerin, and muscle relaxants as these can alter study results.

PRIMARY EQUIPMENT

1. HREM catheter (Fig. 52.1)
2. Computer workstation for data acquisition and storage

SECONDARY EQUIPMENT

1. Stretcher or exam table
2. Pillow
3. Towel or disposable underpads
4. Syringes with water (or saline for HREM with impedance)
5. Cup with a drinking straw
6. Emesis basin
7. Lubrication jelly
8. 2% viscous lidocaine jelly for topical anesthesia
9. Paper tape for securing the catheter in place
10. Gloves and protective eye wear
11. If provocative or postprandial testing will be performed, the appropriate viscous, solid, or meal items should also be on hand

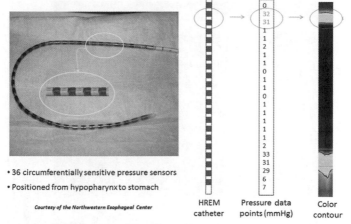

- 36 circumferentially sensitive pressure sensors
- Positioned from hypopharynx to stomach

Courtesy of the Northwestern Esophageal Center

HREM catheter | Pressure data points (mmHg) | Color contour

FIG. 52.1 HREM (high-resolution esophageal manometry) catheter with a depiction of the associated pressure data points and color contour.

PROCEDURE

Catheter Placement

1. Apply lidocaine 2% jelly to the inside of the nostril you will be using for catheter placement.
2. Tape a disposable underpad to the outside of the patient's clothing and have the emesis basin on hand.
3. Lubricate the catheter with jelly and place the catheter transnasally into the esophagus, through the esophagogastric junction (EGJ) and into the stomach.
   a. Instruct the patient to take small sips of water through a straw as the catheter is entering the nasopharynx.
4. Verify correct placement.
   a. Ideally there should be one sensor above the upper esophageal sphincter and 4 to 5 sensors in the stomach. If this is not possible due to the patient's esophageal length, prioritize having 4 to 5 sensors in the stomach (Fig. 52.2).
   b. To check whether the catheter has passed through the diaphragm, instruct the patient to take a series of slow deep breaths to identify the pressure inversion point. If the catheter has crossed the EGJ, there should be a drop in the intrathoracic pressure sensors during inhalation and an increase in the pressure for the gastric sensors. If there is difficulty visualizing the pressure inversion, instruct the patient to perform a leg raise during the deep breaths, or press on the patient's abdomen during inhalation to accentuate the increased abdominal pressure.

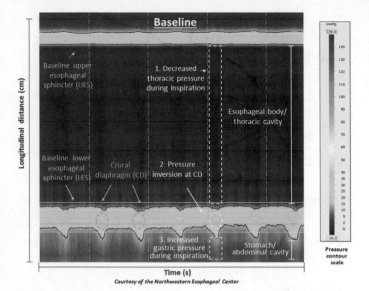

Courtesy of the Northwestern Esophageal Center

FIG. 52.2 Esophageal pressure topography plot of a baseline HREM (high-resolution esophageal manometry) assessment demonstrating the upper esophageal sphincter, lower esophageal sphincter, and changes in intrathoracic and intra-abdominal pressure signals during inspiration.

5. Tape the catheter in place.
6. In patients with difficult anatomy (e.g., large paraesophageal hernia or sigmoid esophagus), it can be difficult or even impossible to pass the manometry catheter. In these instances, the catheter will often fold back on itself generating a plane of symmetry, which is a hallmark of improper placement (Fig. 52.3). For these patients, it is possible to pass the manometry catheter under direct visualization during upper endoscopy. The catheter can then be left in place during recovery, and the study can commence when the patient is able to follow commands and swallow safely.

Baseline and Test Swallows

1. Recline the patient into the supine position (about 30° above horizontal). You can place a pillow behind their head to reduce discomfort caused by the catheter.
   a. Although the current classification system is based on 10 supine swallows, in the era of HREM, this is no longer a technical requirement for zeroing pressure and thus the procedure can be performed in the upright position. Of note, compared with supine, normative values are reduced in the sitting position.[12]

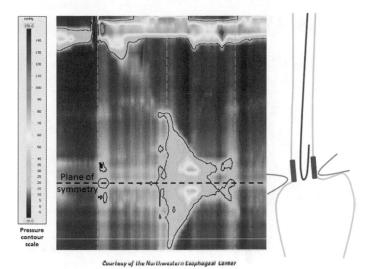

FIG. 52.3 Esophageal pressure topography plot demonstrating improper positioning of the HREM (high-resolution esophageal manometry) catheter with a plane of symmetry indicating catheter inversion; schematic of the same on the right.

2. Start recording the procedure.
3. Begin with a 2-minute baseline measurement during which time the patient does not swallow. If a 2-minute baseline cannot be obtained, a baseline of at least 30 seconds is sufficient (Fig. 52.2).
4. Instruct the patient to take three deep breaths following the baseline measurement to once again demonstrate correct catheter placement. Annotate the deep breaths.
5. Begin test swallows by administering 5 mL of water (or saline for HREM with impedance) and instruct the patient to swallow a single time. Each swallow should be annotated with the recording software (Fig. 52.4).
   a. Test swallows should be repeated if double swallows or other variations occur.
6. Perform this measurement 10 times with at least 30 seconds between swallows. This interval allows the lower esophageal sphincter pressure to return to baseline and avoids deglutitive inhibition of esophageal motor activity.
   a. In addition to the 10 supine test swallows, 5 upright swallows with 5 mL can be performed to eliminate artifact identified in the supine position. This is most relevant in ruling out esophageal outflow obstruction.
7. The patient can now be extubated.
8. Stop the recording and save the file after the catheter has been removed. This step is important for thermal compensation during the analysis process.

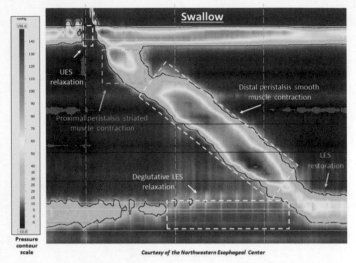

FIG. 52.4 Esophageal pressure topography plot with a normal test swallow. LES, lower esophageal sphincter; UES, upper esophageal sphincter.

Optional Provocative Testing

1. *Multiple rapid swallow*: administer 2 mL of water five times in succession with a 2- to 3-second interval. Instruct the patient to swallow each time with the goal of completing all five swallows within 10 seconds. Annotate this swallow. This test can be used to assess contractile reserve and identify defects in deglutitive inhibition.[13,14]
2. *Viscous/solid swallow*: 5 mL of apple sauce can be used for viscous swallows and graham crackers can be used for solid swallows. The patient should be instructed to chew the graham cracker thoroughly and to swallow one time for either. These test swallows can be repeated two to five times and should be annotated. There is some evidence that bolus consistency can alter esophageal function and increase the yield of detection for esophageal motor disorders.[15]
3. *Rapid drink challenge (200 mL drink)*: administer 200 mL of water (or saline for HREM with impedance). Instruct the patient to drink all of the fluid as quickly as possible while seated in the upright position. This test assesses EGJ function and therefore can aid in the identification of achalasia or outflow obstruction.[16] If an impedance catheter is used, this measurement can also be extended to 5 minutes to assess for esophageal retention similar to the timed barium swallow.[17]
4. *Postprandial*: after completion of the standard manometry, the patient should consume a meal consistent with their

typical diet. Annotate the study when the patient completes their meal as this commences the 30- to 90-minute observation period. During the waiting period, patient symptoms can be annotated on the study. Postprandial testing has been shown to aid in symptom evaluation, diagnosis of outflow obstruction, and esophageal spasm, as well as rumination and belching when HREM with impedance is used.[18-22]

POSTPROCEDURE

1. Provide the patient with discharge instructions and plan for follow-up.
2. There are no required postprocedure dietary or activity restrictions.

ADVERSE EVENTS

1. Common adverse events include nasal and oropharynx discomfort, sore throat, gagging, and retching. These can typically be managed with relaxation techniques but rarely can cause the procedure to be aborted.
2. Uncommon adverse events include epistaxis, chest pain, vasovagal syncope, or aspiration. If epistaxis occurs, this can typically be treated with conservative therapy and pressure.
3. Infection and perforation are theoretically possible; however, there are no case reports of these adverse events.

CPT CODES

91010—Esophageal motility (manometric study of the esophagus and/or gastroesophageal junction) study with interpretation and report

91037—Esophageal function test; gastroesophageal reflux test with nasal catheter intraluminal impedance electrode(s) placement, recording, analysis, and interpretation (can be added for HREM with impedance)

Suggested Reading

Gyawali CP, Bredenoord AJ, Conklin JL, et al. Evaluation of esophageal motor function in clinical practice. *Neurogastroenterol Motil.* 2013;25(2):99-133. Epub 2013/01/23.

Pandolfino JE, Kahrilas PJ. AGA technical review on the clinical use of esophageal manometry. *Gastroenterology.* 2005;128(1):209-224. Epub 2005/01/06. PubMed PMID: 15633138.

References

1. Kahrilas PJ, Bredenoord AJ, Fox M, et al, International High Resolution Manometry Working G. The Chicago classification of esophageal motility disorders, v3.0. *Neurogastroenterol Motil.* 2015;27(2):160-174. doi:10.1111/nmo.12477.

2. Clouse RE, Staiano A, Alrakawi A, Haroian L. Application of topographical methods to clinical esophageal manometry. *Am J Gastroenterol*. 2000;95(10): 2720-2730. Epub 2000/10/29. doi:10.1111/j.1572-0241.2000.03178.x. PubMed PMID: 11051340.

3. Clouse RE, Staiano A. Topography of the esophageal peristaltic pressure wave. *Am J Physiol*. 1991;261(4 Pt 1):G677-G684. Epub 1991/10/01. PubMed PMID: 1928353.

4. Grubel C, Hiscock R, Hebbard G. Value of spatiotemporal representation of manometric data. *Clin Gastroenterol Hepatol*. 2008;6(5):525-530. Epub 2008/04/15. doi:10.1016/j.cgh.2008.02.006. PubMed PMID: 18407799.

5. Soudagar AS, Sayuk GS, Gyawali CP. Learners favour high resolution oesophageal manometry with better diagnostic accuracy over conventional line tracings. *Gut*. 2012;61(6):798-803. Epub 2011/10/15. doi:10.1136/gutjnl-2011-301145. PubMed PMID: 21997554; PMCID: PMC4565504.

6. Roman S, Huot L, Zerbib F, et al. High-resolution manometry improves the diagnosis of esophageal motility disorders in patients with dysphagia: a randomized multicenter study. *Am J Gastroenterol*. 2016;111(3):372-380. Epub 2016/02/03. doi:10.1038/ajg.2016.1. PubMed PMID: 26832656.

7. Carlson DA, Ravi K, Kahrilas PJ, et al. Diagnosis of esophageal motility disorders: esophageal pressure topography vs. Conventional line tracing. *Am J Gastroenterol*. 2015;110(7):967-977; quiz 78. Epub 2015/06/03. doi:10.1038/ajg.2015.159. PubMed PMID: 26032151; PMCID: PMC4587659.

8. Carlson DA, Kahrilas PJ. How to effectively use high-resolution esophageal manometry. *Gastroenterology*. 2016;151(5):789-792. Epub 2016/10/04. doi:10.1053/j.gastro.2016.09.024. PubMed PMID: 27693348; PMCID: PMC5159243.

9. Yadlapati R, Keswani RN, Dunbar KB, et al. Benchmarks for the interpretation of esophageal high-resolution manometry. *Neurogastroenterol Motil*. 2017;29(4). Epub 2016/10/16. doi:10.1111/nmo.12971. PubMed PMID: 27739183; PMCID: PMC5367956.

10. Yadlapati R, Keswani RN, Ciolino JD, et al. A system to assess the competency for interpretation of esophageal manometry identifies variation in learning curves. *Clin Gastroenterol Hepatol*. 2017;15(11):1708-1714. Epub 2016/07/31. doi:10.1016/j.cgh.2016.07.024. PubMed PMID: 27473627; PMCID: PMC5272908.

11. Yadlapati R, Gawron AJ, Keswani RN, et al. Identification of quality measures for performance of and interpretation of data from esophageal manometry. *Clin Gastroenterol Hepatol*. 2016;14(4):526-534.e1. Epub 2015/10/27. doi:10.1016/j.cgh.2015.10.006. PubMed PMID: 26499925; PMCID: PMC4993017.

12. Xiao Y, Read A, Nicodeme F, Roman S, Kahrilas PJ, Pandolfino JE. The effect of a sitting vs supine posture on normative esophageal pressure topography metrics and Chicago Classification diagnosis of esophageal motility disorders. *Neurogastroenterol Motil*. 2012;24(10):e509-e516. Epub 2012/08/18. doi:10.1111/j.1365-2982.2012.02001.x. PubMed PMID: 22897486; PMCID: PMC3649008.

13. Fornari F, Bravi I, Penagini R, Tack J, Sifrim D. Multiple rapid swallowing: a complementary test during standard oesophageal manometry. *Neurogastroenterol Motil*. 2009;21(7):718.e41. Epub 2009/02/19. doi:10.1111/j.1365-2982.2009.01273.x. PubMed PMID: 19222762.

14. Shaker A, Stoikes N, Drapekin J, Kushnir V, Brunt LM, Gyawali CP. Multiple rapid swallow responses during esophageal high-resolution manometry reflect esophageal body peristaltic reserve. *Am J Gastroenterol*. 2013;108(11):1706-1712. Epub 2013/09/11. doi:10.1038/ajg.2013.289. PubMed PMID: 24019081; PMCID: PMC4091619.

15. Carlson DA, Roman S. Esophageal provocation tests: are they useful to improve diagnostic yield of high resolution manometry? *Neurogastroenterol Motil*. 2018;30(4):e13321. Epub 2018/04/01. doi:10.1111/nmo.13321. PubMed PMID: 29603510.

16. Ang D, Hollenstein M, Misselwitz B, et al. Rapid Drink Challenge in high-resolution manometry: an adjunctive test for detection of esophageal motility disorders. *Neurogastroenterol Motil*. 2017;29(1). Epub 2016/07/16. doi:10.1111/nmo.12902. PubMed PMID: 27420913.

17. Cho YK, Lipowska AM, Nicodeme F, et al. Assessing bolus retention in achalasia using high-resolution manometry with impedance: a comparator study with timed barium esophagram. *Am J Gastroenterol*. 2014;109(6):829-835. Epub 2014/04/09. doi:10.1038/ajg.2014.61. PubMed PMID: 24710506; PMCID: PMC4307753.

18. Ang D, Misselwitz B, Hollenstein M, et al. Diagnostic yield of high-resolution manometry with a solid test meal for clinically relevant, symptomatic oesophageal motility disorders: serial diagnostic study. *Lancet Gastroenterol Hepatol*. 2017;2(9):654-661. Epub 2017/07/08. doi:10.1016/s2468-1253(17)30148-6. PubMed PMID: 28684262.

19. Kessing BF, Bredenoord AJ, Smout AJ. Objective manometric criteria for the rumination syndrome. *Am J Gastroenterol*. 2014;109(1):52-59. Epub 2013/12/25. doi:10.1038/ajg.2013.428. PubMed PMID: 24366235.

20. Kessing BF, Bredenoord AJ, Velosa M, Smout AJ. Supragastric belches are the main determinants of troublesome belching symptoms in patients with gastro-oesophageal reflux disease. *Aliment Pharmacol Ther*. 2012;35(9):1073-1079. Epub 2012/03/21. doi:10.1111/j.1365-2036.2012.05070.x. PubMed PMID: 22428801.

21. Kessing BF, Bredenoord AJ, Smout AJ. Mechanisms of gastric and supragastric belching: a study using concurrent high-resolution manometry and impedance monitoring. *Neurogastroenterol Motil*. 2012;24(12):e573-e579. Epub 2012/10/18. doi:10.1111/nmo.12024. PubMed PMID: 23072402.

22. Yadlapati R, Tye M, Roman S, Kahrilas PJ, Ritter K, Pandolfino JE. Postprandial high-resolution impedance manometry identifies mechanisms of nonresponse to proton pump inhibitors. *Clin Gastroenterol Hepatol*. 2018;16(2):211-218.e1. Epub 2017/09/16. doi:10.1016/j.cgh.2017.09.011. PubMed PMID: 28911949; PMCID: PMC5794564.

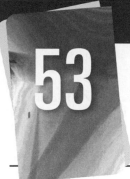

53

Ambulatory 24-Hour Esophageal pH Monitoring

Jason R. Baker, PhD

Ambulatory 24-hour esophageal pH monitoring is a study in which continuous esophageal intraluminal pH measurement allows the detection of changes in pH caused by gastroesophageal reflux disease (GERD) episodes. GERD has a prevalence of 8% to 33% impacting all age groups and both genders. Acid reflux episodes are defined as pH drops to below four in the distal esophagus, and reflux time is the elapsed time until the pH exceeds four. Normal subjects do experience reflux episodes primarily after meals, but they are not associated with GERD symptoms. A physiological range of esophageal acid exposure has been established in normal subjects. Prolonged ambulatory 24-hour esophageal pH monitoring enables identification of both symptomatic and asymptomatic reflux events in physiologic conditions.

The value of the test lies in its ability to diagnose GERD in patients with normal endoscopic findings, atypical and extraesophageal symptoms, and poor response to medical, surgical, or endoscopic therapy, as well as in identifying patients who have an increased risk for a complicated outcome (prolonged nocturnal reflux, significant asymptomatic reflux).

Development of thinner pH probes and a wireless pH-sensitive capsule has made the procedure more acceptable to patients, allowing for data collection while patients pursue their everyday activities.

Reflux evaluation may be performed on or off proton-pump inhibitors (PPIs) therapy. To assess acid-exposure time in the esophagus, pH ambulatory monitoring should be performed off PPI therapy in patients without previous markers for GERD. If patients have previous markers for GERD, pH ambulatory monitoring should be performed on PPI therapy to correlate symptomology and refractory symptoms.

Multiple pH sensor probes allow the assessment of high-reflux episodes, involving the proximal esophagus and pharynx, as well as the simultaneous measurement of gastric pH if needed.

Multiple technology is available to place an ambulatory pH catheter. However, a recent study depicted the difference between using high-resolution esophageal manometry data versus the Air Flow Sphincter Locator to determine accurate pH catheter location. The data illustrated that the Air Flow Sphincter Locator was inaccurate over 30% of the time. Thus, using high-resolution esophageal manometry data is recommended to accurately identify the proximal lower esophageal sphincter (LES) border for proper pH catheter placement.

INDICATIONS

1. Patients with nonerosive reflux disease who are being considered for surgical antireflux repair
2. Patients after antireflux surgery who continue to be symptomatic or are suspected to have ongoing abnormal acid reflux
3. Patients who continue to have GERD-related symptoms despite PPI therapy administered at least twice daily (the test is performed on treatment)
4. Patients with noncardiac chest pain who failed the PPI test or an empirical trial with a PPI administered at least twice daily (the test is performed on treatment)
5. Patients with suspected otolaryngologic manifestations of GERD who failed an empirical trial of PPI therapy administered at least twice daily (the test is performed on treatment)
6. Patients with adult-onset, nonallergic, refractory asthma who failed PPI therapy administered at least twice daily (the test is performed on treatment)

CONTRAINDICATIONS

1. Nasoesophageal obstruction or upper esophageal obstruction
2. Severe maxillofacial trauma and/or basilar skull fracture
3. Patients who are unable to cooperate or are high risk for pulling out the pH probe
4. For the wireless pH system, the test is also contraindicated in patients with coagulopathy, severe erosive esophagitis, esophageal ulceration, tight esophageal ring or a stricture, tumor (benign or malignant), varices, any obstruction in the gastrointestinal tract, pacemaker, or implanted cardiac defibrillator

PREPARATION

1. Inform the patient of the nature of the examination and that it entails two visits within 24 hours or 48 or 96 hours for the wireless pH system.
2. Discontinue food and liquids 6 hours prior to the study.
3. If the pH study is done off antireflux treatment, confirm that PPIs have been discontinued for at least a week. Prokinetics, H_2 blockers, and smooth-muscle relaxants should be stopped for 2 to 3 days prior to the test. Antacids are allowed until a day prior to the test. In contrast, if the test is used to monitor treatment response, the patient should continue all medications.
4. Obtain informed consent.

EQUIPMENT

1. Standard manometry equipment or LES locator (a pressure sensor added to the pH probe)
2. Flexible pH microelectrode with reference electrode or wireless pH capsule (mounted on a delivery device)
3. Dual-sensor catheter that permits assessment of proximal esophageal acid exposure in addition to distal esophageal acid exposure
4. Standard buffer solutions for calibration (pH 7.0 and pH 1.0)
5. Reference electrode (incorporated into the capsule in the wireless pH system)
6. Ambulatory data logger powered by a battery (9 V). For the wireless pH system, an external recorder device receives data signal via radiofrequency telemetry
7. Computer software for data transfer and analysis
8. For the wireless pH system, a custom-made vacuum unit capable of generating 600 mm Hg vacuum pressure to the well in the capsule, via the delivery system

PROCEDURE

Catheter pH System

1. Calibrate the pH electrode according to the supplier's instruction manual. If using a dual-sensor pH probe, immerse both sensors in the buffer solution during calibration. Zero the data logger using the software program. Connect the electrode to the data logger, and place it into the 7.0 pH buffer solution for 3 minutes (also place the external reference electrode if you are using a catheter with external reference). The device should read close to 7.0. Rinse the electrode(s) and repeat the procedure with the standard buffer solution at pH 1.0.
2. Locate the LES either by standard manometry (see Chapter 40) or by using LES locator.

3. If utilizing an LES locator, use the LES identification accessory kit. It consists of a pressurized water bag connected through a tubing system to the pH catheter and to a pressure transducer. Adjust the baseline pressure to gastric pressure and withdraw 1 cm at a time. Checking pressure changes with respiration is helpful (increasing below the diaphragm and decreasing above). A sudden rise in resting pressure identifies the LES. After a swallow, there will be a relaxation followed by a pressure wave.

4. Apply a local anesthetic to the patient's nostril (gel or liquid). After a few minutes, the catheter can be introduced via the nares into the stomach. After gently reaching the pharynx, flex the patient's head. Sipping water during insertion may help. To confirm that catheter is in the stomach and not curled in the esophagus, verify that the reading on the data logger is pH <4.

5. Withdraw the pH catheter to 5 cm above the proximal margin of the previously identified LES. Fix the catheter by taping it to the cheek and passing it behind the ear. Connect the reference electrode (if external) to the skin of the chest (the area over the manubrium sterni).

6. Connect the catheter to the portable data logger.

Wireless pH System

1. If the pH capsule is delivered after an upper endoscopy, then the proper location of placement is 6 cm above the gastro-esophageal junction. If the capsule is placed transnasally or per-orally, then identification of the LES is done by esophageal manometry.

2. Activate the capsule by the magnetic switch and calibrate in buffer solutions of pH 7.0 and 1.68.

3. Advance the delivery system with the capsule to 6 cm above the proximal margin of the LES. Connect the external vacuum pump to the delivery system. Apply suction by the vacuum pump for 30 seconds. Successful suction of the esophageal mucosa is achieved when the vacuum gauge on the pump stabilizes at a value >510 mm Hg for 10 seconds. Remove the plastic safety guard on the handle and then press the activation button. Subsequently, twist clockwise 90° the activation button and then reextend to release the delivery device from the attached capsule. Remove the delivery system.

PATIENT INSTRUCTIONS

1. Encourage patients to pursue their everyday activities.

2. Encourage patients to consume their regular diets. Most centers today do not apply diet restrictions on patients undergoing 24-hour esophageal pH monitoring.

3. Patients are allowed to smoke and drink alcohol.
4. Instruct the patient to keep a diary during the monitoring period. Data loggers display event buttons (markers) to record symptoms or other events. However, it is advisable that a written record be kept as well. A diary should include the following:
   a. Upright or recumbent time (awake or asleep)
   b. Meals and snacks (time of onset and ending)
   c. Exact time of symptoms of interest
5. Instruct patient to avoid getting the recorder device wet. Patients undergoing assessment with the wireless pH capsule can shower or sleep without the data receiver as long as it is kept at a range of 3 to 5 ft from the patient.

POSTPROCEDURE

1. Remove the catheter while the patient blows out through the nose. There is no need for the patient to fast for catheter removal.
2. Go over the symptom diary with the patient.
3. The patient can resume normal activities and restart discontinued medications.
4. Download the recorded data into the computer.
5. Wireless capsules usually self-detach within 7 to 10 days after placement. In rare cases, endoscopic removal is needed. Chest x-ray is a simple test that can help to determine the status of the capsule in patients with persistent chest discomfort suspected to be caused by the capsule. Avoid magnetic resonance imaging for 30 days after placement of the pH capsule.

INTERPRETATION

1. A completed test should last 24 hours. Short-duration examinations are sometimes performed but must include at least one postprandial and nighttime (supine) period.
2. Computer software analyzes the presence of pathologic esophageal acid exposure. Most commercially available software packages analyze data for the following variables:
   a. Percent total time pH <4
   b. Percent upright time pH <4
   c. Percent supine time pH <4
   d. Number of reflux episodes
   e. Number of reflux episodes ≥5 minutes
   f. Longest single episode of reflux
3. The Johnson and DeMeester composite score which is calculated based on the aforementioned variables.

TABLE 53.1	**Commonly Used Reference Values**		
		Catheter pH System	**Wireless pH Capsule (48-96 Recording Time)**
Percent total time pH <4		<4.2	<5.3
Percent upright time pH <4		<6.3	<6.9
Percent supine time pH <4		<1.2	<6.7
Number of reflux episodes		<50.0	<36.8 (±20.1)
Number of reflux episodes (≥5 min)		<3.0	<1.2 (±0.55)
Longest reflux episode (min)		<9.2	–
DeMeester and Johnson composite score		<14.7	–

4. Percent total time pH <4 is the most reliable and reproducible parameter and consequently widely accepted criteria to define an abnormal study.

5. Commonly used reference values (see Table 53.1).

6. Recently, an international group of GERD experts (Lyon Consensus) published the interpretation of esophageal results in the context of GERD (see Table 53.2). This new GERD consensus provides a contemporary criteria clinically diagnosing GERD.

7. Three main measurements have been created in an attempt to correlate episodes of acid reflux with symptoms. Those measurements are discussed below. Symptom correlation is particularly important in patients with atypical or extraesophageal manifestations of GERD.

8. Interpretation of symptom correlation: Symptoms are considered to be related to an acid reflux event when they occur in the 2- to 5-minute window following a reflux episode.

   a. Symptom index (SI): Percentage of symptoms reported during the study period that is associated with acid reflux event. If the value is >50%, then the symptom index is considered positive (the symptoms are due to acid reflux).

   $$\text{Symptom Index} = \frac{\text{Number of symptoms related to reflux} \times 100\%}{\text{Total number of symptoms}}$$

   b. Symptom sensitivity index (SSI): Percentage of reflux episodes that are associated with GERD-related symptoms.

TABLE 53.2 Esophageal Evaluation			
GERD Testing Results	**Endoscopy**	**pH or pH-Impedance**	**High-Resolution Manometry**
Conclusive evidence for pathologic evidence	LA grades C and D esophagitis Long-segment Barrett mucosa Peptic esophageal stricture	Acid exposure time >6%	
Borderline of inconclusive evidence	LA grades A and B esophagitis	Acid exposure time 4%-6% Reflux episodes 40-80	
Adjunctive or supportive evidence	Histopathology (score) Electron microscopy (DIS) Low mucosal impedance	Reflux-symptom association Reflux episodes >80 Low mean nocturnal baseline impedance Low post-reflux swallowed-induced peristaltic wave index	Hypotensive esophagogastric junction (EGJ) Hiatus hernia Esophageal hypomotility
Evidence against pathologic reflux		Acid exposure time <4% Reflux episodes <40	

This parameter quantifies a patient's sensitivity to acid reflux. A positive SSI results if the value is >10%.

$$\text{Symptom Sensitivity Index} = \frac{\text{Number of symptomatic acid reflux events} \times 100\%}{\text{Total number of acid reflux events}}$$

c. Symptom association probability (SAP): Calculates the probability that symptoms and acid reflux events are truly associated. Positive SAP (positive association) is determined if the calculated value is >95%. Calculating SAP requires a statistical program.

ADVERSE EVENTS

1. Catheter pH electrode: trauma to nasopharynx, epistaxis, throat pain/discomfort, nose pain, chest pain/discomfort, cough, and dysphagia. Catheter misplacement owing to bending or rolling has been reported in less than 5% of patients within the esophagus or pharynx. Generally, the pH test has been demonstrated to significantly affect patient's lifestyle (diet, activities, sleep, etc.).

2. Wireless pH capsule: nosebleed (transnasal placement), chest discomfort/pain, and premature or failure of capsule detachment.

CPT CODES

91034—Esophagus, gastroesophageal reflux test; with nasal catheter pH electrode(s) placement, recording, analysis, and interpretation, for gastroesophageal reflux testing

91035—Esophagus, gastroesophageal reflux test; with mucosal-attached telemetry pH electrode placement, recording, analysis, and interpretation, for scenarios in which the physician performs a gastroesophageal reflux test with a Bravo probe

91038—Esophageal function test, gastroesophageal reflux test with nasal catheter intraluminal impedance electrode(s) placement, recording, analysis, and interpretation; prolonged (greater than 1 hour, up to 24 hours)

Bibliography

1. American Gastroenterological Association Medical Position Statement. Guidelines on the use of esophageal pH recording. *Gastroenterology*. 1996;110(6):1981-1996.
2. Breumelhof R, Smout AJ. The symptom sensitivity index: a valuable additional parameter in 24-hour esophageal pH recording. *Am J Gastroenterol*. 1991;86(2):160-164.
3. Chen JW, Baker JR, Rubenstein JR, et al. Accuracy of the air flow sphincter locator system in identifying the lower esophageal sphincter for placement of pH catheters. *Dis Esophagus*. 2017;30:1-5.
4. Dhiman RK, Saraswat VA, Mishra A, Naik SR. Inclusion of supine period in short-duration pH monitoring is essential in diagnosis of gastroesophageal reflux disease. *Dig Dis Sci*. 1996;41(4):764-772.
5. El-Serag HB, Sweet S, Winchester CC, et al. Update on the epidemiology of gastroesophageal reflux disease: a systematic review. *Gut*. 2014;63:871-880.
6. Fass R, Hell R, Sampliner RE, et al. The effect of ambulatory 24-hour esophageal pH monitoring on reflux provoking activities. *Dig Dis Sci*. 1999;44:2263-2269.
7. Gyawali CP, Kahrilas PJ, Savarino E, et al. Modern diagnosis of GERD; the Lyon Consensus. *Gut*. 2018;67(7):1351-1362.
8. Johnson PE, Koufman JA, Nowak LJ, et al. Ambulatory 24-hour double-probe pH monitoring: the importance of manometry. *Laryngoscope*. 2001;111:1970-1975.

9. Pandolfino JE, Richter JE, Ours T, et al. Ambulatory esophageal pH monitoring using a wireless system. *Am J Gastroenterol*. 2003;98(4):740-749.
10. Streets CG, DeMeester TR. Ambulatory 24-hour esophageal pH monitoring: why, when, and what to do. *J Clin Gastroenterol*. 2003;37(1):14-22.
11. Weusten BL, Roelofs JM, Akkermans LM, et al. The symptom-association probability: an improved method for symptom analysis of 24-hour esophageal pH data. *Gastroenterology*. 1994;107(6):1741-1745.

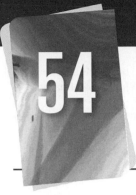

54 Small Bowel Motility Testing: Manometry and Scintigraphy

Kimberly N. Harer, MD
William L. Hasler, MD

If a patient's small bowel motility is in question after standard evaluation and imaging (plain films or barium studies), manometry and scintigraphy are the main tools to assess motor function in this gut region. Manometry does not provide information regarding transit time, but it does measure intraluminal pressure changes caused by occlusive contractions of the bowel wall, which are indirect measures of contractile activity. In contrast, scintigraphy allows for the noninvasive measurement of small bowel transit time, but contractile activity is not evaluated.

SMALL BOWEL MANOMETRY

This section will focus mainly on stationary techniques of small bowel manometry. Prolonging a stationary fasting manometry study to 6 hours provides the same accuracy as ambulatory 24-hour studies in more than 90% of patients and also provides manometric information about the antrum. If a lengthier recording or nocturnal study is needed, ambulatory systems are available.

Indications[1]

1. To assess for causes of gastric or small bowel dysmotility such as neuropathy, myopathy, or obstruction not identified by endoscopy or radiographic imaging
2. To assess unexplained nausea, vomiting, bloating, abdominal distention, or other symptoms suggestive of upper gastrointestinal (GI) dysmotility
3. To distinguish generalized from localized gastrointestinal dysmotility in patients with dysmotility elsewhere (i.e., chronic constipation, gastroparesis, gastroesophageal reflux)
4. To evaluate small bowel motility in patients with slow transit constipation undergoing consideration of total colectomy

5. To diagnose suspected chronic intestinal pseudo-obstruction (CIP) when the diagnosis is unclear
6. To provide information to help select the optimal approach to feeding CIP patients (oral, gastric, jejunal, total parenteral nutrition [TPN])
7. To assess potential therapeutic response to a medical intervention or medication
8. To help exclude small bowel motor dysfunction with an entirely normal study

Contraindications
1. Those associated with esophagogastroduodenoscopy (EGD)
2. Massively dilated small bowel is a relative contraindication due to risk of perforation
3. Known multiple duodenal or jejunal diverticula
4. Small bowel strictures or mechanical obstruction

Preparation
1. A 12-hour fast is required, with clear liquids for the evening meal on the day before testing. Some labs require up to 2 days of full liquid diet prior to testing.
2. Cessation of medications affecting motility for at least 48 to 72 hours prior to testing (including narcotics, macrolides, metoclopramide, anticholinergics, adrenergics). For diabetic patients, many centers will postpone study performance unless the blood glucose is <200 to 275 mg/dL at the start of testing due to effects of hyperglycemia to alter normal small bowel contractility.
3. If the patient is on TPN, discontinue the infusion 8 hours before the study.
4. If sedation for catheter placement is necessary, propofol or a short-acting benzodiazepine followed by a waiting period of at least an hour is recommended prior to proceeding with measurements in order to avoid possible drug-induced motility effects.

Equipment
1. Catheters
   a. Stationary systems: multilumen water-perfused catheter with side-holes, where water perfusion through the side-holes serves as sensors (Fig. 54.1). The catheter is continuously perfused with water by means of an infusion pump at a low rate and is connected to external pressure transducers and recorders. Some water-perfused catheters include transmucosal potential difference (TMPD) electrodes or a Dent sleeve which can improve fidelity of pyloric pressure measurements by (1) increasing the

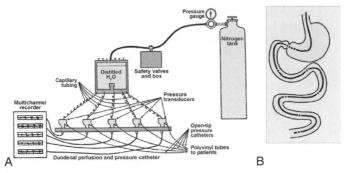

FIG. 54.1 Small bowel manometry. A, Pneumohydraulic perfusion system, linked to a multilumen manometric catheter via interposed strain gauges. B, The catheter placement involves at least 5 side-holes spaced a few mm to 1 cm apart within the gastric portion of the tube, and two to three side-holes placed 10 cm apart in the small bowel, with the midsensor placed at the level of the angle of Treitz to ensure that a segment of jejunum can be assessed with the distal sensor. (Reproduced by permission from Malagelada J-R, Camilleri M, Stanghellini V. *Manometric Diagnosis of Gastrointestinal Motility Disorders.* New York, NY: Thieme Publishers; 1986:41.)

    number of sensors across the pylorus and (2) helping to minimize catheter migration (see item number 6). Water-perfused catheters are widely available and relatively inexpensive; however, adequate dynamic performance of each catheter and transducer needs to be confirmed prior to each study.

b. Ambulatory systems: Teflon catheters with solid-state pressure transducers or impedance sensors combine solid-state miniaturized tube-mounted strain gauges with data loggers/recorders, similar to outpatient 24-hour pH monitoring.[2] These catheters are portable and typically are more comfortable for patients.

c. High-resolution manometry (HRM) systems: high-resolution manometry catheters with up to 36 circumferential pressure sensors located 1 to 2 cm apart with data output available as both standard pressure tracings and color contour plots. The HRM system provides superior pressure profile detail than the aforementioned systems, and it is the modality of choice to evaluate pyloric activity. HRM recordings also offer better definition of antegrade and retrograde propagation of individual duodenojejunal contractions and can quantify contractile coupling.[3]

2. Stationary pneumohydraulic system connected to the water-perfused catheter

    a. Degassed water in a reservoir is maintained at a high constant pressure (7.5 to 15 psi) by nitrogen oxide or carbon dioxide and is then reduced to atmospheric level by capillary tubing (providing high resistance) by the time the water enters the manometric assembly. Optimal perfusion rates of 0.05 to 0.3 mL/min per channel can be achieved either with a pneumohydraulic perfusion system and incorporation of steel capillary or other tubes that control rate of flow, or by use of commercially available external transducers that have a set flow rate.

3. Data acquisition
   a. A variety of computer-based systems are available with their own specifications. For example, for some computer software, the calibrations for peak pressure can be set to 50 to 100 mm Hg for small bowel contractions and 100 mm Hg for antral contractions.
4. Standard fluoroscopy equipment
5. Standard upper endoscope
6. Transmucosal potential difference (TMPD) electrodes or Dent sleeve
   a. Aids the evaluation of motor activity in sphincteric regions, in this case the pylorus. This consists of two saline-perfused intraluminal catheter channels, connected to an electrometer, placed on either side of the pylorus. An electrode is placed subcutaneously (ideally) or on the skin, and transmucosal potential differences are obtained. The device facilitates correct placement of pressure sensors in the terminal portion of the antrum by maintaining the potential difference between gastric and duodenal mucosa. To date, Dent sleeves have not been used extensively to evaluate the pylorus.

Procedure

1. Prepare the system for use. For the stationary system, connect each multilumen perfusion tube to strain gauges and flush with distilled water, set pressure in the tank drum of the pneumohydraulic system at 10 psi (nitrogen gas), connect tubing to the water tank, and label the tracing with patient information. The external strain gauges linked to the manometric assembly should be approximately at the same height above the floor as the sensors within the gut for accurate pressure determinations. This is easily achieved by having the patient lie on a bed that can be moved vertically up or down, with the head at a 45° angle.
2. Calibrate the equipment. For the stationary system, calibration of each strain gauge should precede every study. Before and during each study, the tracing needs to be monitored for uniformity of rate of rise of pressure peaks. A slow rate of rise

of waves mandates review of that sensor for potential blockage or air bubbles and flushing of the system with a bolus of degassed water. Ambulatory and HRM catheters should be calibrated based on the specified catheter protocol.

3. Place the catheter. The catheter can be placed either without or with endoscopy.

   a. Nonendoscopic catheter placement

      i. Pass the catheter with pressure sensors/transducers through the nose or mouth, guiding it with fluoroscopy beyond the pylorus into the duodenum and just past the ligament of Treitz. Steerable Teflon catheters are employed at some institutions. Radiation safety regulations at some centers recommend a maximum of 5 minutes of fluoroscopy time. If nonendoscopic placement does not achieve appropriate guidewire or catheter placement within 4 minutes of fluoroscopy time, upper GI endoscopy should be performed to secure proper guidewire placement. This leaves additional sufficient fluoroscopy time to ensure proper positioning of the catheter if needed.

   b. Endoscopic catheter placement

      i. A variety of methods are available for endoscopic placement of stationary or HRM catheters.

      ii. One method involves passing a guidewire through the biopsy channel of the endoscope into the third portion of the duodenum. The endoscope is removed and the manometry catheter is advanced over the guidewire with positioning of the tip beyond the ligament of Treitz.

      iii. Alternatively for catheters not designed to be passed over guidewires, sutures tied on the manometry catheter can be endoscopically carried into the duodenum using biopsy forceps. This method permits endoscopic visual confirmation of appropriate sensor positioning across the pylorus.

4. Position the sensors. The sensors should be spaced from the antrum across pylorus to the distal duodenum or proximal jejunum, starting 3 to 5 cm proximal to the pylorus (see Fig. 54.1). Prior to initiating recording, sensor positioning across the pylorus can be confirmed manometrically by identifying one of the three following patterns:

   a. A combination of distal antral peaks (duration >5 seconds and higher amplitude, typically >20 mm Hg, with a maximum frequency of 3 per minute) and duodenal peaks (duration <3 seconds and lower amplitude, typically <20 mm Hg, with a maximum frequency of 12 per minute)

   b. The presence of a high-pressure zone (tone)

   c. The lack of contractions in the tracing from the sensor adjacent to clear antral contractions, indicating quiescence recorded from a large diameter duodenal bulb

5. Complete the recording phase. There is variability among labs regarding the recording phase protocol. Some labs continue the study until an activity front (or clear-cut abnormality) is recorded; other labs focus on a 3- to 6-hour fasting period and a 2-hour postprandial period. Provocative testing trials with erythromycin or octreotide can be integrated at the end of a study. Compared with the stationary systems, solid-state ambulatory catheter systems allow for 24 hours of recording time. Both stationary and ambulatory systems are discussed below.

   a. Stationary system

      i. Step 1: Fasting phase (3 to 6 hours)

- The pyloric tracing should be kept in the center of the array of recordings from the antroduodenal junction sensors; this is more easily achieved by having at least three, but preferably five or more, closely spaced sensors across the antroduodenal junction.
- The location of the pyloric recording helps facilitate proper assessment of antral contractility. Careful monitoring of the waveforms is essential for optimal recordings. Catheter repositioning may be needed during a stationary study to ensure accurate distal antral recordings during the fasting and postprandial periods. If this cannot be achieved by monitoring the waveforms, brief repeat fluoroscopy may be needed to reposition the tube correctly. Alternatively, incorporating the aforementioned transmucosal potential difference (TMPD) apparatus into the tube assembly allows the operator to keep the tube at the pylorus by recording the difference in mucosal voltage between antral and duodenal bulb mucosa.

     ii. Step 2: Postprandial phase (2 hours)

- Make certain there is no migrating motor complex (MMC) activity (see below) starting just before you feed the patient.
- If needed, adjust the catheter depending upon position within the stomach, with the patient seated almost upright.
- The test meal should contain at least 400 kcal to ensure a postprandial small intestinal response lasting at least 2 hours. Ideally, the solid-liquid meal should be balanced and typical of the average US

diet with 20% to 25% fat, 20% to 25% protein, and 50% to 55% carbohydrate. The caloric content is important because a 2-hour duration of the intestinal fed response is critical in order to assess the possibility of extrinsic neuropathy. Insufficient caloric intake can result in return of MMCs before the end of the postprandial 2-hour period. The meal should be consumed in 30 minutes or less, with at least half of the solid meal consumed in 15 minutes. If the patient is unable to complete the solid meal, a commercially available supplemental caloric-rich liquid nutrient beverage can be used to ensure intake ≥400 kcal.

  iii. Step 3: Provocative testing phase (optional) (1 hour)
      • Erythromycin 50 to 125 mg intravenously over 20 minutes or octreotide 75 to 100 µg subcutaneously can be used to stimulate motor activity to aid in study interpretation.
      • Responses to medications administered during manometry are believed by some to potentially reflect if a patient may be responsive to prokinetic medication treatments.
  b. Ambulatory system
      i. Solid-state catheter is employed for ambulatory recordings, obviating the need for pneumohydraulic perfusion or pressure systems/tubing. The patient is instructed on meals and overnight fasting prior to leaving the lab. No adjustment to the catheter system is made once the patient has left the medical center. Thus, even when the tube incorporates antral recording sites, it is not guaranteed that these will remain in the right place during and after meals.

Postprocedure

1. Water-perfused stationary catheters including some HRM catheters
   a. Withdraw the stationary tube from the patient.
   b. Turn off the pressure tank, and disconnect the tubing from the tank.
   c. Clean the tube, flush all channels, soak in high-level disinfection solution, and force air-dry all channels (or as per catheter specified protocol).
2. Solid-state catheters for ambulatory (and some stationary) systems
   a. Withdraw the catheter from the patient.
   b. Clean catheter per the catheter's specified protocol.

Interpretation (See Fig. 54.2)

Assess the small intestine's functional integrity by analyzing the migrating motor complex (MMC), the presence/nature of the motor response to the meal, response to provocative medications, and any recognized abnormal patterns.[2]

Normal[1]

1. At least one complete MMC per 24 hours, demonstrating clearly identifiable Phase 1 (quiescence), Phase II (intermittent, irregular phasic pressure activity unassociated with significant baseline elevations), and Phase III (burst of propagated, rhythmic contractions) complexes. If the fasting recording is less than 6 hours, it may not be abnormal if a migrating motor complex is not appreciated.

2. Phase I (quiescent phase) will typically last 40 to 50 minutes. Phase II is variable in length and characterized by irregular contractions with an antral frequency typically below 3 cpm and duodenal frequency less than 11 cpm. Phase III typically lasts 5 to 9 minutes and demonstrates antral contractions at 3 cpm and duodenal contractions at 11 to 12 cpm, with amplitudes >20 mm Hg (average >10 mm Hg).

3. Conversion to the fed pattern after consumption of a 400 kcal meal, without return of MMC activity for at least 2 hours.

4. Postprandial pattern is induced 5 to 10 minutes after meal ingestion, with maximal contractile activity occurring 10 to 20 minutes after beginning the meal.

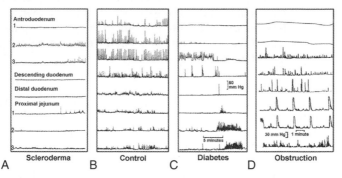

FIG. 54.2 Examples of classical gastroduodenal manometry tracings during the postprandial period. A, Low-amplitude contractions, a myopathic pattern. B, Control tracing-normal postprandial fed pattern. C, Normal amplitude but premature MMC (migrating motor complex) activity in the postprandial period, a neuropathic pattern. Note the absence of antral contractions. D, Simultaneous long-duration contractions above the level of the obstruction, and a normal fed pattern below the proximal jejunum.

Abnormal Patterns

1. Neuropathy[4]

   a. Definition: In intrinsic (enteric) neuropathic processes, the contraction pattern is disorganized and uncoordinated; however, the contraction amplitude remains normal. In extrinsic (autonomic) neuropathy, the fed response is impaired and postprandial antral hypocontractility is demonstrated. Distal postprandial antral contractile frequency <1 per minute during the first postprandial hour has been described with some neuropathic processes.[5]

   b. Variations: Antral hypomotility, abnormal propagation of phase III of the MMC, hypercontractility (bursts of non-propagated phasic activity or sustained uncoordinated pressure activity), and failure of the fasting to be converted to a fed response.

   c. Bursts are defined as groups of contractions occurring at the typical frequency and amplitude of phase III, lasting at least 2 minutes, and associated with tonic elevation of baseline pressure. They have been reported in extrinsic neuropathies and in chronic intestinal pseudo-obstruction.

   d. With regard to a finding of decreased frequency of MMCs, only the complete absence of MMCs over 24 hours is abnormal.

   e. Etiologies of neuropathy in small bowel dysmotility include diabetes mellitus, paraneoplastic, medications, Chagas disease, chronic idiopathic intestinal pseudo-obstruction, viral infections, Von Recklinghausen disease, spinal cord injury, and Parkinson disease.[6]

   f. Specific patterns

      i. The frequency of intestinal MMCs is increased (more than three per 3 hours) in extrinsic vagal neuropathy or after vagotomy.

      ii. Decreased or absent phase III activity has been associated with gastric bezoars.[7]

      iii. Bacterial overgrowth has been associated with hypomotility with rare phase III activity, weak and disorganized contractions.[4]

      iv. Rumination has a characteristic pattern with an artifactual increase in intra-abdominal pressure at all levels of the upper gut, typically postprandially. This appears as simultaneous contractions at all sensors during vomiting; whereas, vomiting caused by intestinal contractions may be associated with high-amplitude contractions (>30 mm Hg) and retrograde small intestinal peristaltic contractions preceding the vomiting episode.[8]

    g. Although most often displaying a myopathic pattern, amyloidosis, dermatomyositis, and systemic sclerosis may also exhibit neuropathic characteristics, which may reflect an earlier stage of disease affecting the gut.

2. Myopathy

    a. Definition: Small bowel demonstrates low-amplitude contractions (not exceeding 20 mm Hg, average < 10 mm Hg) with or without decreased frequency of contractions at the sites affected. There is often a poor response to enteric feeding, with distal postprandial antral contractile amplitude < 40 mm Hg suggestive of a myopathic process.[4,5]

    b. Because the sensitivity of the sensors depends on their contact with the intestinal wall, apparent reductions in contractile amplitude mimicking myopathy may be found in conditions with profound luminal dilation from extreme aerophagia, chronic intestinal pseudo-obstruction (CIP), or mechanical obstruction.

    c. Etiologies of myopathy in small bowel dysmotility include scleroderma/systemic sclerosis, chronic intestinal pseudo-obstruction, amyloidosis, muscular dystrophy, familial visceral myopathy, mitochondrial cytopathy, and dermatomyositis.[6]

3. Mechanical obstruction

    a. It is important to differentiate pseudo-obstruction from mechanical obstruction. Mechanical obstruction demonstrates in decreasing order of positive predictive value (PPV) (1) prolonged and nonpropagated intestinal contractions lasting >8 seconds (PPV 82%), (2) nonpropagated cluster contraction or bursts with a duration of >30 minutes (PPV 57%), or (3) a combination of the two patterns (PPV 56%).[9]

Adverse Events

1. Catheter placement and manometry recording adverse events include sore throat (common) and rare (<1%) risks of aspiration pneumonia, bleeding, and gut perforation.

2. Provocative medication administration (erythromycin, octreotide) adverse events include rare (<1%) allergic reactions, nausea, vomiting, abdominal discomfort, and diarrhea.

3. Adverse events of EGD for catheters placed endoscopically include rare (<1%) risks of anesthesia reactions, aspiration pneumonia, bleeding, and gut perforation.

SMALL BOWEL SCINTIGRAPHY

Indications[1]

1. Noninvasive method measuring small bowel transit and assessing the existence of a motility disorder. At institutions where it is available, scintigraphy may be performed to document delayed small bowel transit test prior to performing manometry
2. To assess unexplained nausea, vomiting, bloating, abdominal distention, or other symptoms suggestive of upper gastrointestinal (GI) dysmotility
3. To distinguish generalized from localized gastrointestinal dysmotility in patients with dysmotility elsewhere (i.e., chronic constipation, gastroparesis, gastroesophageal reflux)
4. To evaluate small bowel motility in patients with slow transit constipation undergoing consideration of total colectomy
5. To diagnose suspected chronic intestinal pseudo-obstruction (CIP) when the diagnosis is unclear
6. To provide information to help select the optimal approach to feeding CIP patients (oral, gastric, jejunal, TPN)
7. To help exclude small bowel motor dysfunction with an entirely normal study
8. Assess therapeutic response to a medical intervention or medication on serial scintigraphic testing

Contraindications

1. Pregnancy. Women of childbearing potential should undergo a pregnancy test[10]
2. Allergy to egg (if egg meal is being utilized)

Preparation

1. A 12-hour fast is required prior to testing.
2. Cessation of medications affecting motility for at least 48 to 72 hours prior to testing (including narcotics, macrolides, metoclopramide, anticholinergics, adrenergics). For diabetic patients, many centers will postpone study performance unless the blood glucose is <200 to 275 mg/dL at the start of testing due to effects of hyperglycemia to alter normal small bowel function.

Equipment

1. Radiolabeled solids or liquids. Examples are ^{99m}Tc-sulfur colloid labeled solid food particles and indium-111-diethylenetriamine penta-acetic acid (DTPA) in water.[11,12] Small bowel scintigraphy is often performed simultaneously with gastric and colonic transit scintigraphy, which typically guides the choice of radiopharmaceutical.
2. A large field-of-view gamma camera with a dedicated computer for analysis to detect the field of interest[1]

Procedure

1. The radiolabeled tracer is mixed with water or food and ingested by the patient.
2. The patient lies on a tilt table at 45° to the horizontal or stands.
3. Anterior and posterior planar static images with the large field-of-view gamma camera are obtained immediately after ingestion of the radiolabeled meal, and after 2, 4, and 6 hours for gastric and small bowel transit.
4. If colonic transit is subsequently being evaluated as part of a combined study, additional images are obtained at 24, 48, and 72 hours.

Postprocedure

1. For the small intestine, the proportion of radiolabeled meal reaching the colon at 6 hours is used as a surrogate marker for small bowel transit.[13]
2. Standard corrections for depth (geometric mean of anterior and posterior counts), isotope decay, tissue attenuation, and Compton scattering are necessary.[10,14]

Interpretation

1. Delayed small bowel transit is defined by colonic filling of <49% at 6 hours, and rapid small bowel transit is defined as significant transit to tracer into the mid to distal ascending colon prior to 5 hours, or no tracer visualized in the small bowel at 6 hours, though there may be marked intra-individual variance. However, normal values are method-dependant, and there is variability between institutional protocols.
2. Results may be altered by gastric emptying time, colonic dysfunction, or obstruction to defecation.

References

1. Camilleri M, Hasler WL, Parkman HP, et al. Measurement of gastrointestinal motility in the GI laboratory. *Gastroenterology*. 1998;115:747-762.
2. Kellow JE. Principles of motility and sensation testing. *Gastroenterol Clin N Am*. 2003;32:733-750, ix.
3. Baker JR, Dickens JR, Koenigsknecht M, et al. Propagation characteristics of fasting duodeno-jejunal contractions in healthy controls measured by clustered closely-spaced manometric sensors. *J Neurogastroenterol Motil*. 2019;25:100-112.
4. Hansen MB. Small intestinal manometry. *Physiol Res*. 2002;51:541-556.
5. Weston S, Thumshirn M, Wiste J, Camilleri M. Clinical and upper gastrointestinal motility features in systemic sclerosis and related disorders. *Am J Gastroenterol*. 1998;93:1085-1089.
6. Coulie B, Camilleri M. Intestinal pseudo-obstruction. *Ann Rev Med*. 1999;50:37-55.
7. Pimentel M, Soffer EE, Chow EJ, Kong Y, Lin HC. Lower frequency of MMC is found in IBS subjects with abnormal lactulose breath test, suggesting bacterial overgrowth. *Dig Dis Sci*. 2002;47:2639-2643.

8. Thompson DG, Malagelada JR. Vomiting and the small intestine. *Dig Dis Sci.* 1982;27:1121-1125.

9. Frank JW, Sarr MG, Camilleri M. Use of gastroduodenal manometry to differentiate mechanical and functional intestinal obstruction: an analysis of clinical outcome. *Am J Gastroenterol.* 1994;89:339-344.

10. Von der Ohe MR, Camilleri M. Measurement of small bowel and colonic transit: indications and methods. *Mayo Clin Proc.* 1992;67:1169-1179.

11. Charles F, Camilleri M, Phillips SF, et al. Scintigraphy of the whole gut: clinical evaluation of transit disorders. *Mayo Clin Proc.* 1995;70:113-118.

12. Bonapace ES, Maurer AH, Davidoff S, et al. Whole gut transit scintigraphy in the clinical evaluation of patients with upper and lower gastrointestinal symptoms. *Am J Gastroenterol.* 2000;95:2838-2847.

13. Camilleri M, Zinsmeister AR, Greydanus MP, et al. Towards a less costly but accurate test of gastric emptying and small bowel transit. *Dig Dis Sci.* 1991;36:609-615.

14. Camilleri M, Zinsmeister AR. Towards a relatively inexpensive, noninvasive, accurate test for colonic motility disorders. *Gastroenterology.* 1992;103:36-42.

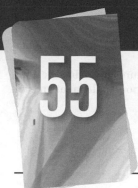

55 Anorectal Manometry and Biofeedback

Jason R. Baker, PhD

Anorectal manometry is a test of anorectal function that can provide useful information about disorders that affect defecation and continence. There are various methods of performing the studies,[1,2] and minimum standards of performance have been recommended.[3,4] The equipment used to perform anorectal manometry may also be used to provide biofeedback training for patients with constipation due to obstructed defecation and for those with fecal incontinence due to various causes. Before performing anorectal manometry or biofeedback, one should obtain hands-on instruction and supervision from someone experienced in manometry. Manometry training programs are available through some of the companies marketing manometric equipment (Medtronic, Minneapolis, Minnesota; Diversatek, Milwaukee, WI; Laborie, Williston, VT).

Prior to 2007, anorectal manometry was primarily performed using conventional methodology via water-perfused and solid-state catheters with three to six unidirectional sensors. Since 2007, high-resolution and high-definition catheters have become more prevalent to perform anorectal manometry. These catheters include tightly spaced circumferential sensors along a longitudinal axis illustrating a spatiotemporal depiction of the anorectum. Using these contemporary catheter designs, the anorectal manometry duration and resolution have become shorter and greater.[5,6] Conversely, the high-resolution and high-definition catheters are more fragile and expensive compared to conventional catheter designs.

INDICATIONS

1. Constipation
2. Fecal incontinence
3. Evaluation prior to biofeedback training for pelvic floor dyssynergia

4. Evaluation prior to biofeedback training for continence strategies
5. Preoperative evaluation before procedures involving the anus and/or rectum such as creation of a pouch, ileoanal anastomosis, and elective sphincteroplasty

CONTRAINDICATIONS

Use of latex balloons in individuals with latex allergy.

PREPARATION

In general, no preparation is required. If stool is present during a digital rectal examination, a rectal enema should be administered. A latency period of 30 minutes should be employed from the enema administration to the start of anorectal manometry. Patients may continue on their usual medications, and dietary modification is not required. Informed consent must be obtained.

The procedure should be explained to the patient. Afterward, the patient should be asked to change into a hospital gown.

EQUIPMENT

Required equipment includes the following:
1. A probe. Both water-perfused, solid-state probes, and closely spaced sensor catheters are commercially available for anorectal manometry. Pressure-sensitive transducers are arranged radially along the probe and spaced several centimeters apart. Reusable and disposable probes are available (Isle of Skye, Scotland; Medtronic, Minneapolis, Minnesota; Mui Scientific, Mississauga, Ontario, Canada; Sandhill Scientific, Highlands Ranch, Colorado)
2. A manometric recording device, a computerized recorder and storage device compatible with commercially available software, is recommended. Software programs are designed to perform study interpretation, but editing is required to ensure accuracy
3. A system to display the recording
4. A device to store the data
5. Cotton swab
6. Surgical tape
7. 4-in. × 4-in. gauze or washcloths
8. Gloves
9. Water-soluble lubricant
10. Hospital gown

PROCEDURE (HIGH-RESOLUTION AND 3D-HIGH-DEFINITION ANORECTAL MANOMETRY)

Before performing anorectal manometry, the equipment should be assembled and the probe and recorder calibrated according to the manufacturer's instructions. High-resolution and high-definition anorectal manometry catheters utilize closely spaced circumferentially pressure sensors for better spatio-temporal pressurization of the anorectum. Identify normative values pertaining to the specific anorectal manometry catheter and gender. The International Anorectal Physiology Working Group and the International Working Group for Disorders of Gastrointestinal Motility and Function protocol is listed below (47.1):

1. Lubricate the balloon with a water-soluble lubricant.
2. Position the patient on the left side with knees flexed. Inspect the buttocks, perineum, and the perianal area. Check the sensation of the anterior, posterior, and bilateral positions by rubbing the cotton swab in each location. The presence or absence of anal wink should be documented.
3. The high-resolution catheter is positioned with the posterior demarcation line on the catheter aligned with patient's dorsal anatomical region. The catheter should be positioned into the rectum approximately 10 cm post the attached balloon indicated by the reference line.
4. Following accurate placement, the patient should receive 3 minutes allowing anal sphincter acclimation.
5. Resting anal sphincter pressure should be assessed for at least 60 seconds.
6. Three short duration squeezes (5 seconds in duration) with 30 seconds recovery period in between each trial. These squeezes assess maximum anal sphincter pressure.
7. A maximum duration squeeze is performed for 30 seconds. This squeeze evaluates the sustainability of the maximum anorectal sphincter pressure.
8. Following a 60 seconds recovery period from the maximum duration squeeze, two cough responses are performed. A 30-second recovery period between each cough. The cough response assesses the spinal reflex pathways by illustrating the external anal sphincter contraction to increased abdominal pressure.
9. Following 30 seconds after the last cough response, instruct the patient to simulate defecation for 15 seconds. Three simulated defecation trials are performed with a 30-second recovery period.

10. The rectoanal inhibitory reflex (RAIR) is assessed by rapidly inflating the balloon with 50 mL of air to assess the relaxation of the internal anal sphincter. If reflex relaxation is not seen, the position of the probe should be confirmed and the rapid inflation repeated.

11. Rectal sensation measurements, first sensation, urgency to defecate, and maximum tolerated, are collected by inflating a nonlatex rectal balloon 10 mL/s. For threshold sensation, the balloon inflation is performed in increments of 10 mL. In relation to urgency to defecate and maximum tolerated, the balloon volume is increased in 30 mL increments. The maximum balloon inflation volume is 250 mL.

PROCEDURE (CONVENTIONAL ANORECTAL MANOMETRY)

Before performing anorectal manometry, the equipment should be assembled and the probe and recorder calibrated according to the manufacturer's instructions.

1. Inflate the rectal balloon with 50 mL of air for 30 seconds. All of the air should be withdrawn from the balloon. If less than 50 mL of air is recovered, the balloon should be tested for leaks by reinflating the balloon under water.

2. Lubricate the balloon with a water-soluble lubricant.

3. Position the patient on the left side with knees flexed. Inspect the buttocks, perineum, and the perianal area. Check the sensation of the anterior, posterior, and bilateral positions by rubbing the cotton swab in each location. The presence or absence of anal wink should be documented.

4. A careful digital rectal examination should be performed with notation made of the anal sphincter tone at rest, anal sphincter tone with squeezing, contraction of the puborectalis muscle, abdominal contraction, and perineal descent with Valsalva maneuver.

5. Gently insert the catheter 10 to 15 cm into the rectum (Fig. 55.1).

6. Allow the patient to rest for 3 to 5 minutes to give the patient time to adjust to the catheter and to allow the sphincter pressure to return to resting levels.

7. Identify the high-pressure zone with the continuous pull-through technique or the pressure will increase as the transducers enter the anal sphincter zone. Document the location, length, and pressure of the sphincter zone. The pressure will decrease as the transducers are pulled past the sphincter zone. Repeat the continuous pull-through twice, each time documenting the location, length, and pressure of the sphincter zone.

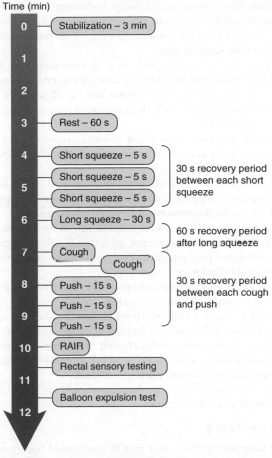

FIG. 55.1 The International Anorectal Physiology Working Group and the International Working Group for Disorders of Gastrointestinal Motility and Function: Standard Protocol for High-Resolution Anorectal Manometry. *RAIR*, rectoanal inhibitory reflex. (Reprinted from Carrington EV, Heinrich H, Knowles CH, et al. The international anorectal physiology working group (IAPWG) recommendations: standardized testing protocol and the London classification for disorders of anorectal function. *Neurogastroenterol Motil*. 2019:e13679. https://creativecommons.org/licenses/by/4.0/. Copyright © 2019 The Authors. Neurogastroenterology & Motility published by John Wiley & Sons Ltd.)

8. Allow the probe to remain undisturbed for 3 to 5 minutes to allow equilibration. Use the station pull-through technique to withdraw the probe into the high-pressure zone. The probe should be withdrawn 0.5 to 1.0 cm and the pressure recorded. Thirty seconds should be allowed before the pressure is recorded at each station.

9. Repeat the station pull-through technique to confirm the location and pressure of the high-pressure zone. Once the location of the high-pressure zone is confirmed, secure the probe with surgical tape.

10. Instruct the patient to perform a squeeze and hold maneuver by contracting the external anal sphincter as intensely as possible and holding the contraction for 30 seconds. Allow a 30-second rest period, then repeat the squeeze and hold maneuver twice.

11. Ask the patient to cough. A normal response is a reflex increase in the anal sphincter pressure as the intra-abdominal pressure increases.

12. Ask the patient to simulated defecation as if trying to defecate to test for pelvic floor dyssynergia. A normal response is a decrease in the pressure at the anal sphincter.

13. Rapidly inflate the balloon with 50 mL of air to assess the relaxation of the internal anal sphincter. If reflex relaxation is not seen, the position of the probe should be confirmed and the rapid inflation repeated.

14. Rectal sensation measurements, first sensation, urgency to defecate, and maximum tolerated, are collected by inflating a nonlatex rectal balloon 10 mL/s. For threshold sensation, the balloon inflation is performed in increments of 10 mL. In relation to urgency to defecate and maximum tolerated, the balloon volume is increased in 30 mL increments. The maximum balloon inflation volume is 250 mL.

15. After recording data, the balloon should be deflated and removed from the rectum.

AUXILIARY TESTS

1. The balloon expulsion test may be performed independently or at the time of anorectal manometry. This test evaluates whether the patient is able to evacuate a simulated stool. A lubricated balloon secured to a small-diameter catheter is placed into the rectum.
   a. The balloon is inflated with 50 mL of air or warm water.
   b. The patient is asked to sit on a commode and expel the balloon in privacy. The individual is given 3 minutes to expel the balloon.
   c. If expulsion is not successful, the balloon is deflated and removed.

2. Additional information may be obtained from the external anal sphincter electromyography (EMG). A surface EMG sensor may be placed directly into the anal canal or skin pads placed adjacent to the anus. Surface sensors do not provide information from the puborectalis muscle. Concentric

needle EMG provides data from the external anal sphincter or puborectalis but requires placement of a needle directly into the external anal sphincter or puborectalis muscle. Additional equipment including an oscilloscope is needed for concentric needle EMG.

POSTPROCEDURE

1. Wash the balloon and probe in warm, soapy water to remove fecal debris.
2. Disposable balloons and probes should be placed into appropriate waste receptacles.
3. Reusable equipment should be sterilized according to the manufacturer's guidelines.
4. Dry equipment thoroughly and store appropriately.

INTERPRETATION

Anorectal manometry measurements should be interpreted using the London classification.[7] This classification defines anorectal manometry impressions by major, minor, or inconclusive. The four-part classification depicts disorders of the following: (1) disorder of the RAIR, (2) disorders of anal tone and contractility, (3) disorders of rectal coordination, and (4) disorders of rectal sensation.

1. Resting sphincter pressure: The difference between the peak intrarectal pressure and maximum anal sphincter pressure in the basal state. The measurement should be stated as a range.
2. Maximum sphincter pressure: The mean maximum pressure among sensors at each centimeter depth. The measurement should be stated as a range.
3. Maximum duration squeeze: The measurement should be qualitatively assessed as the patient's ability to maintain 50% of their maximum squeeze pressure for 30 continuous seconds.
4. Cough reflex response: Evaluate the difference between baseline intrarectal pressure and increase in intrarectal pressure during a cough. Similarly, assess basal intra-anal pressure and increase in intrarectal pressure during a cough. These pressures should increase during the cough response. Also, dictate the presence of mucous, stool, and/or urine during the cough response.
5. Simulated defecation or response to straining should produce relaxation of the external anal sphincter and puborectalis muscle. Paradoxical contraction of the external anal sphincter and/or puborectalis muscle produces an increase in the pressure referred to as pelvic floor dyssynergia. Two

other indices should be calculated using simulated defecation metrics: Percentage of Anal Relaxation during Simulated Defecation and Defecation Index.

   a. Percentage of Anal Relaxation during Simulated Defecation: Anal relaxation pressure/anal relaxation pressure × 100.

   b. Defecation Index: Maximum rectal pressure during simulated defecation/minimum anal pressure during simulated defecation. A normal metric is greater than >1.5.

6. Rectoanal inhibitory reflex (RAIR): Following a rapid inflation into the balloon, a transient increase in sphincter pressure should be depicted followed by relaxation of the anal sphincter below the basal pressure. This relaxation pressure should return to the basal pressure state. Proper documenting of this metric is present or absent at a balloon inflation volume.

7. Rectal sensation: The measurements should be evaluated as hypersensitive or hyposensitive. Different normative ranges are published for specific catheter and balloon configuration.

ADVERSE EVENTS

Anorectal manometry is well tolerated. Serious adverse events have not been reported. Potential adverse events include rectal bleeding and perforation.

OTHER USES FOR THIS TECHNIQUE

Over the past 2 decades, visual and verbal biofeedback training for anorectal disorders have been commonly used: dyssynergic defecation, fecal incontinence, levator ani syndrome, rectal solitary ulcer syndrome, and abdominal metrics.[8,9] There is lack of standardization for biofeedback technique, but review of the literature supports effectiveness of biofeedback training for both constipation,[10] fecal incontinence,[11] and abdominal discomfort metrics.[8] Recently, the American Neurogastroenterology and Motility Society and the European Society of Neurogastroenterology and Motility task force determined that the evidence was strong for dyssynergic defecation and fecal incontinence but only fair for levator ani syndrome and rectal solitary ulcer syndrome.[9] Limitations to biofeedback for anorectal disorders relate to patient selection bias, lack of standardized protocols and evaluation metrics, and treatment compliance.

Biofeedback therapy may include pelvic floor exercises (strengthening and coordination), rectal sensory retraining, and pelvic floor alignment assessment. Commonly, biofeedback therapy is performed using manometric probes and/or EMG. The visual and/or auditory biofeedback in addition to pelvic floor exercises provides greater opportunities for improving anorectal function. Biofeedback has demonstrated positive impact on quality-of-life metrics for constipation and fecal incontinence patients.[12,13] Biofeedback therapy should be performed by a trained allied health professional to maximize effectiveness.

CPT CODES

51784—Electromyography (EMG) studies of anal or urethral sphincter, other than needle, any technique

91120—Rectal sensation, tone, and compliance (i.e., response to graded balloon distention)

91122—Anorectal manometry

90911—Biofeedback training, anorectal, including EMG and/or manometry

References

1. Diamant NE, Kamm MA, Wald A, et al. AGA technical review on anorectal testing techniques. *Gastroenterology.* 1999;116:732-760.
2. Wald A. Colonic and anorectal motility testing in clinical practice. *Am J Gastroenterol.* 1994;89:2109-2115.
3. Rao SSC, Azpiroz F, Diamant N, et al. Minimum standards of anorectal manometry. *Neurogastroenterol Motil.* 2002;14:553-559.
4. Lee TH, Bharucha AE. How to perform and interpret a high resolution anorectal manometry test. *J Neurogastroenterol Motil.* 2016;22:46-59.
5. Sauter M, Heinrich H, Fruehauf H, et al. Toward more accurate measurements of anorectal motor and sensory function in routine clinical practice: validation of high-resolution anorectal manometry and rapid baraostat measurements of rectal function. *Neurogastroenterol Motil.* 2014;26:685-695.
6. Jones MP, Post J, Crowell MD. High-resolution manometry in the evaluation of anorectal disorders: a simultaneous comparison with water-perfused manometry. *Am J Gastroenterol.* 2014;102:850-855.
7. Carrington EV, Heinrich H, Knowles CH, et al. The international anorectal physiology working group (IAPWG) recommendations: standardized testing protocol and the London classification for disorders of anorectal function. *Neurogastroenterol Motil.* 2019:e13679.
8. Baker JR, Eswaran S, Chey WD, et al. Abdominal symptoms are common and benefit from biofeedback therapy in patients with dyssynergic defecation. *Clin Transl Gastroenterol.* 2015;30(6):e105.
9. Rao SSC, Benninja MA, Bharucha AE, Chiarioni G, Lorenzo CD, Whitehead WE. ANMS-ESNM position paper consensus guidelines on biofeedback therapy for anorectal disorders. *Neurogastroenterol Motil.* 2015;27(5):594-609.
10. Heymen S, Jones KR, Scarlett Y, et al. Biofeedback treatment of constipation: a critical review. *Dis Colon Rectum.* 2003;46:1208-1217.
11. Heymen S, Jones KR, Ringel Y, et al. Biofeedback treatment of fecal incontinence: a critical review. *Dis Colon Rectum.* 2001;44:728-736.
12. Mazor Y, Kellow JE, Prott GM, Jones MP, Malcolm A. Anorectal biofeedback: an effective therapy, but can we shorten the course to improve access to treatment? *Ther Adv Gastroenterol.* 2019;12. doi:10.1177/1756284819836072.
13. Heyman S, Scarlett Y, Jones K, Ringel Y, Drossman D, Whitehead WE. Randomized controlled trial shows biofeedback to be superior to pelvic floor exercises for fecal incontinence. *Dis Colon Rectum.* 2009;52(10):1730-1737.

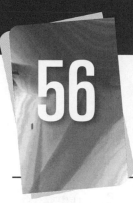

56

Hydrogen Breath Tests for Diagnosis of Carbohydrate Malabsorption and Small Intestinal Bacterial Overgrowth

Allen A. Lee, MD
Jason R. Baker, PhD

- Hydrogen breath tests (HBTs) are common, noninvasive, but indirect tests to aid in the diagnosis of common gastrointestinal conditions, such as carbohydrate malabsorption and small intestinal bacterial overgrowth (SIBO).
- The principal gases produced in the gastrointestinal tract include hydrogen (H_2), carbon dioxide (CO_2), and methane (CH_4) with lesser contributions from nitrogen (N_2) and oxygen (O_2).[1]
- HBTs are based on the principle that H_2 and CH_4 are produced exclusively by bacterial fermentation in the human gut.[2]
- An orally administered carbohydrate will be rapidly metabolized in the small intestine in the setting of SIBO or in the colon with carbohydrate malabsorption leading to production of H_2 and/or CH_4.
- These gases can then traverse the intestinal mucosa where it is absorbed into the systemic circulation, excreted into the lungs and can be measured in expired breath (Fig. 56.1).
- One of the main drawbacks of the HBT is the lack of a validated gold standard for diagnosing carbohydrate malabsorption and SIBO.
- In addition, there is lack of standardization regarding methodology of test across different studies and centers.
- This has produced considerable heterogeneity in terms of the indications, techniques, and interpretation of test results.
- Recently, European and North American consensus guidelines have been published in an attempt to standardize HBT.[3,4]
- This chapter will focus on the indications, methodology, interpretation, and limitations of HBT for the diagnoses of lactose malabsorption and SIBO.

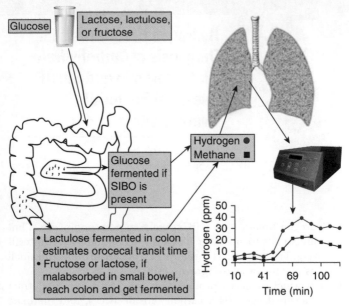

FIG. 56.1 A schematic diagram that shows principle of hydrogen breath test. ppm, parts per million; SIBO, small intestinal bacterial overgrowth. (Reproduced with permission from Ghoshal UC. How to interpret hydrogen breath tests. *J Neurogastroenterol Motil.* 2011;17(3):312-317.)

CARBOHYDRATE MALABSORPTION

- Lactose is a disaccharide found in milk and dairy products.
- In the absence of sufficient lactase, malabsorbed lactose passes into the colon where it leads to an increased osmotic load.
- Lactose is also readily fermented by colonic microbiota which results in production of H_2 and CH_4.
- Lactose malabsorption may manifest with gastrointestinal symptoms, such as abdominal pain, bloating, diarrhea, and flatulence.
- Lactase malabsorption may also occur secondary to other pathologic conditions in the small intestine, such as celiac disease, infectious gastroenteritis, or Crohn disease, which can lead to a decrease in lactase activity.
- Presence of SIBO may also cause false-positive results of lactose and fructose BT.[5] As such, tests to rule out SIBO are recommended prior to testing for carbohydrate malabsorption.
- Other carbohydrates, such as fructose, can also be tested for malabsorption. Fructose is a naturally occurring sugar and is widely used as high-fructose corn syrup in many foods and

beverages. Fructose is incompletely absorbed even in healthy volunteers while fructose malabsorption has been proposed as a potential cause of unexplained GI symptoms.[6,7]

- Sucrose, a disaccharide composed of fructose and glucose, is another important source of this carbohydrate.

SMALL INTESTINAL BACTERIAL OVERGROWTH

- SIBO is a condition of overgrowth of aerobic and/or anaerobic bacteria in the normally relatively sterile environment of the small intestine.[8]
- However, it remains a controversial topic as there is no universal agreement on the definition for SIBO.
- Symptoms are nonspecific and may include abdominal pain, bloating, diarrhea, malabsorption, and weight loss.
- Traditionally, SIBO was diagnosed by >10^5 cfu/mL on quantitative culture from small bowel aspirate.
- However, due to the invasiveness of the approach, high cost, difficulty avoiding oral contamination, and inability to sample further downstream in the small intestine, small intestinal culture has largely been replaced by noninvasive tests, such as HBT.

INDICATIONS
Lactose Malabsorption

- The lactose HBT is commonly performed in suspected cases of lactose malabsorption or intolerance.

Small Intestinal Bacterial Overgrowth

- Glucose or lactulose HBTs are commonly performed in suspected cases of SIBO, particularly related to its potential role in causing symptoms in irritable bowel syndrome (IBS) and other functional GI disorders.

TEST PREPARATION

- Based on North American Consensus guidelines,[4] patients should prepare for breath testing (BT) in the following ways:
  - Antibiotics should be avoided for at least 4 weeks prior to BT.
  - A firm position statement cannot be reached due to lack of conclusive data on stopping or continuing pro/prebiotics prior to BT.
  - Promotility drugs and laxatives should be stopped for at least 1 week prior to BT.
  - Fermentable foods, such as complex carbohydrates, should be avoided on the day prior to BT.

- Patients should fast for at least 8 to 12 hours prior to BT.
- Patients should avoid smoking on the day of BT.
- Physical activity should be limited during the BT.
- Proton-pump inhibitors may be continued during BT.

■ Our center also recommends that patients avoid bismuth-containing products (e.g., Pepto-Bismol) for at least 2 weeks prior to testing as bismuth has antibacterial properties.[9]

■ We further recommend that patients eat a diet low in fiber, poorly absorbed carbohydrates and dairy for 2 days prior to BT as these can affect baseline H_2 levels.[10,11]

■ Finally, poor oral hygiene can result in false-positive results. As a result, we administer an oral antibacterial mouthwash before ingestion of the carbohydrate substrate to minimize this risk.

METHODOLOGY

■ Approximately 36% of healthy adults contain enteric micro-flora which generate methane gas but little to no hydrogen production.[12]

■ Thus, it is important for breath analyzers to measure both hydrogen and methane production during BT.

■ Collection of CO_2 levels should also be obtained during BT. As samples should be collected at end-expiratory phase which most closely resembles alveolar air, CO_2 levels can be used to adjust for improperly collected breath samples.[13]

Carbohydrate Malabsorption

■ Earlier studies on lactose malabsorption were based on a 50 g dose of lactose.[14-16] However, this dose of lactose is equivalent to the amount of lactose in a liter of milk and is likely supraphysiologic.

■ More recently, studies have attempted to use a more physiologic dose of lactose with 25 g being the most widely utilized dosage (equivalent of 500 mL of milk).[17]

■ In children, the European guidelines recommend a dose of 1 g/kg up to a maximum of 25 g of lactose.

■ As sufficient time is required in order to ensure colonic fermentation of the lactose substrate, European guidelines recommend a test duration of 4 hours for adults and 3 hours in children, while the North American guidelines recommend at least 3 hours (Fig. 56.2).

■ While the optimal interval to collect samples is still unknown, the European guidelines recommend sample intervals of 30 minutes while the North American guidelines list this as one of the current gaps in knowledge.

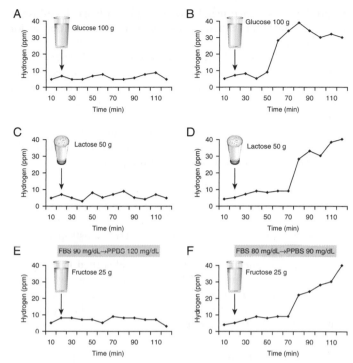

FIG. 56.2 Some typical hydrogen breath test graphs are shown. It shows glucose hydrogen breath test negative for small intestinal bacterial overgrowth (SIBO) (A), glucose hydrogen breath test positive for SIBO (B), lactose hydrogen breath test and tolerance test negative for lactose malabsorption (C), and lactose hydrogen breath test and tolerance test positive for lactose malabsorption (D). It shows a graph negative for fructose malabsorption (E) and a graph positive for fructose malabsorption (F). FBS, fasting blood sugar; PPBS, postprandial blood sugar; ppm, parts per million. (Reproduced with permission from Ghoshal UC. How to interpret hydrogen breath tests. *J Neurogastroenterol Motil.* 2011;17(3):312-317.)

Small Intestinal Bacterial Overgrowth Breath Tests
Lactulose Hydrogen Breath Test

- Glucose or lactulose are the most common substrates employed for diagnosis of SIBO.
- Lactulose is a nonabsorbable disaccharide which can be fermented by colonic bacteria.
- In the presence of SIBO, lactulose may be fermented by small intestinal bacteria to produce an early rise in H_2 and/or CH_4 before the substrate reaches the colon.
- Lack of standardization in the methodology and definition for positive studies has made it difficult to interpret lactulose BT.

- Most studies have utilized a loading dose of 10 g of lactulose.
- Breath samples are then measured every 15 to 30 minutes for 2 to 4 hours.
- Presence of a "double peak" was the original definition for a positive lactulose HBT whereby an initial early peak (rise in breath hydrogen ≥20 ppm) was seen indicating SIBO followed by a later peak at least 15 minutes later indicating colonic fermentation.[18]
- However, one study raised questions about the validity of this definition as these authors found that 50% of double peaks represented cecal fermentation in both peaks.[19]

Glucose Hydrogen Breath Test

- Meanwhile, glucose is readily absorbed in the proximal small intestine and rarely reaches the colon.[20]
- These properties make glucose an attractive substrate for diagnosing SIBO.
- However, as glucose is predominantly absorbed in the proximal small intestine, distal SIBO may be missed which may potentially lead to a higher false-negative rate.
- The dose of glucose used in HBT varies in the literature with most studies using 50 to 75 g of glucose.

PERFORMANCE OF BREATH TEST BASED ON NORTH AMERICAN GUIDELINES

1. We suggest that the correct dose of lactulose for BT is 10 g mixed with or followed by one cup of water.
2. We suggest that the correct dose of glucose for BT is 75 g mixed with or followed by one cup of water.
3. The correct dose of lactose for BT is 25 g mixed with or followed by one cup of water.
4. We suggest that the correct dose of fructose for BT is 25 g mixed with or followed by one cup of water.
5. We suggest that fructose and lactose BT should be performed for at least 3 hours.
6. We suggest that the presence of bacterial overgrowth should be ruled out before performing lactose of fructose BT.
7. We recommend that hydrogen, methane, and carbon dioxide should all be measured simultaneously during BT.

INTERPRETATION OF BREATH TEST RESULTS
Carbohydrate Malabsorption

- Both the European and North American guidelines recommend a cutoff value of breath hydrogen and/or methane excretion >20 ppm above baseline for test positivity.

- When compared to a single nucleotide polymorphism in the lactase gene (C/C_{-13910}) which is associated with lactase non-persistence and lactose malabsorption, lactose HBT showed 95% agreement (κ-statistic of 0.83).[21]

Small Intestinal Bacterial Overgrowth

- North American guidelines recommend a cutoff ≥20 ppm of H_2 by 90 minutes as suggestive of SIBO.
- Some patients have elevated baseline hydrogen levels >20 ppm. However, the clinical significance of this is still not clear and potentially may relate to lack of adherence to diet and fasting prior to the test. Alternatively, these subjects may have alterations in their gut microbiota or represent a variant of SIBO.

Lactulose Hydrogen breath test

- There is significant controversy regarding lactulose HBT and its ability to diagnose SIBO.
- Mean orocecal transit time using lactulose BT in healthy controls ranges from 94 to 97 minutes which suggests that 50% of healthy controls would be positive for lactulose BT.[22]
- Another study in IBS patients combined orocecal scintigraphy with lactulose HBT.[23] These authors demonstrated that in 88% of patients with a positive lactulose HBT, the rise in H_2 was explained by accelerated small intestinal transit rather than true SIBO.
- Compared with jejunal culture, the sensitivity and specificity of lactulose HBT have been found to be lower compared to other breath tests with one study reporting the specificity of lactulose HBT to be as low as 44%.[8,24]
- Moreover, several studies have demonstrated that lactulose HBT is not able to discriminate between IBS patients and healthy controls.[25-27]
- These observations suggest that lactulose HBT alone is not sufficient to make a definitive diagnosis of SIBO.

Glucose Hydrogen Breath Test

- The HBT is considered positive if there is an early rise in breath hydrogen ≥20 ppm after glucose ingestion.
- Comparing glucose HBT for diagnosis of SIBO with jejunal culture, glucose HBT showed a sensitivity and specificity of 62% and 83%, respectively.[24]
- However, similar to lactulose HBT, a recent retrospective review of 139 patients who underwent concurrent glucose HBT and scintigraphy demonstrated that almost half of all positive HBTs were falsely positive as a result of colonic fermentation.[28]
- These results suggest that both lactulose and glucose HBT have low specificity for diagnosing SIBO and raise questions about the role of breath tests in the diagnosis of SIBO.

INTERPRETATION OF BREATH TEST RESULTS BASED ON NORTH AMERICAN GUIDELINES

1. We suggest that a rise of ≥20 ppm from baseline in hydrogen during the test should be considered positive for fructose and lactose BT.
2. We suggest that until better data are available, for clinical and research purposes, a rise of ≥20 ppm from baseline in hydrogen by 90 minutes should be considered a positive test for SIBO.
3. We suggest that two peaks on breath test are not required for the diagnosis of SIBO.
4. Until further data are available, we suggest that a level of ≥10 ppm be considered positive for methane on a breath test.

CONCLUSION

- HBTs are simple, noninvasive tests that may provide important information on common gastrointestinal disorders, such as carbohydrate malabsorption and SIBO.
- However, despite efforts by the North American and European guidelines to standardize the methodology, questions remain regarding the significance of a positive test result.
- The use of HBT, particularly those using lactulose as a substrate, for the diagnosis of SIBO remains controversial.
- Furthermore, the utility of testing for carbohydrate malabsorption remains unclear.
- Ideally, future studies can combine HBT with different technologies, such as scintigraphy and next-generation DNA sequencing, to more clearly define the role of the enteric microflora in conditions, such as SIBO or functional gastrointestinal disorders.
- Moreover, new technologies, such as an ingestible electronic capsule, show promise in measuring intestinal gas production and deliver further insights into the complex host-microbiota relationship.[29]

ACKNOWLEDGMENTS

This work was supported by a grant from the National Center for Advancing Translational Sciences of the National Institutes of Health award KL2TR002241.

References

1. Levitt MD. Volume and composition of human intestinal gas determined by means of an intestinal washout technic. *N Engl J Med.* 1971;284(25):1394-1398.
2. Levitt MD. Production and excretion of hydrogen gas in man. *N Engl J Med.* 1969;281(3):122-127.

3. Gasbarrini A, Corazza GR, Gasbarrini G, et al. Methodology and indications of H2-breath testing in gastrointestinal diseases: the Rome Consensus Conference. *Aliment Pharmacol Ther*. 2009;29(suppl 1):1-49.

4. Rezaie A, Buresi M, Lembo A, et al. Hydrogen and methane-based breath testing in gastrointestinal disorders: the North American Consensus. *Am J Gastroenterol*. 2017;112(5):775-784.

5. Nucera G, Gabrielli M, Lupascu A, et al. Abnormal breath tests to lactose, fructose and sorbitol in irritable bowel syndrome may be explained by small intestinal bacterial overgrowth. *Aliment Pharmacol Ther*. 2005;21(11):1391-1395.

6. Rumessen JJ, Gudmand-Høyer E. Absorption capacity of fructose in healthy adults. Comparison with sucrose and its constituent monosaccharides. *Gut*. 1986;27(10):1161-1168.

7. Skoog SM, Bharucha AE. Dietary fructose and gastrointestinal symptoms: a review. *Am J Gastroenterol*. 2004;99(10):2046-2050.

8. King CE, Toskes PP. Small intestine bacterial overgrowth. *Gastroenterology*. 1979;76(5 Pt 1):1035-1055.

9. Thomas F, Bialek B, Hensel R. Medical use of bismuth: the two sides of the coin. *J Clin Toxicol [Internet]*. March 30, 2012;S3:004 [cited 2018 Jul 27]. Available at https://www.omicsonline.org/medical-use-of-bismuth-the-two-sides-of-the-coin-2161-0495.S3-004.php?aid=5343.

10. Brummer RJ, Armbrecht U, Bosaeus I, Dotevall G, Stockbruegger RW. The hydrogen (H2) breath test. Sampling methods and the influence of dietary fibre on fasting level. *Scand J Gastroenterol*. 1985;20(8):1007-1013.

11. Levitt MD, Hirsh P, Fetzer CA, Sheahan M, Levine AS. H2 excretion after ingestion of complex carbohydrates. *Gastroenterology*. 1987;92(2):383-389.

12. Levitt MD, Furne JK, Kuskowski M, Ruddy J. Stability of human methanogenic flora over 35 Years and a review of insights obtained from breath methane measurements. *Clin Gastroenterol Hepatol*. 2006;4(2):123-129.

13. Goldoni M, Corradi M, Mozzoni P, et al. Concentration of exhaled breath condensate biomarkers after fractionated collection based on exhaled CO_2 signal. *J Breath Res*. 2013;7(1):017101.

14. Newcomer AD, McGill DB, Thomas PJ, Hofmann AF. Prospective comparison of indirect methods for detecting lactase deficiency. *N Engl J Med*. 1975;293(24):1232-1236.

15. Metz G, Jenkins DJ, Peters TJ, Newman A, Blendis LM. Breath hydrogen as a diagnostic method for hypolactasia. *Lancet Lond Engl*. 1975;1(7917):1155-1157.

16. Szilagyi A, Malolepszy P, Hamard E, et al. Comparison of a real-time polymerase chain reaction assay for lactase genetic polymorphism with standard indirect tests for lactose maldigestion. *Clin Gastroenterol Hepatol*. 2007;5(2):192-196.

17. Saad RJ, Chey WD. Breath tests for gastrointestinal disease: the real deal or just a lot of hot air? *Gastroenterology*. 2007;133(6):1763-1766.

18. Rhodes JM, Middleton P, Jewell DP. The lactulose hydrogen breath test as a diagnostic test for small-bowel bacterial overgrowth. *Scand J Gastroenterol*. 1979;14(3):333-336.

19. Riordan SM, McIver CJ, Walker BM, Duncombe VM, Bolin TD, Thomas MC. The lactulose breath hydrogen test and small intestinal bacterial overgrowth. *Am J Gastroenterol*. 1996;91(9):1795-1803.

20. Sellin JH, Hart R. Glucose malabsorption associated with rapid intestinal transit. *Am J Gastroenterol*. 1992;87(5):584-589.

21. Almazar AE, Chang JY, Larson JJ, et al. Comparison of lactase variant MCM6-13910 C>T testing and self-report of dairy sensitivity in patients with irritable bowel syndrome. *J Clin Gastroenterol*. 2018;53(6):1.

22. Hasler WL. Lactulose breath testing, bacterial overgrowth, and IBS: just a lot of hot air? *Gastroenterology*. 2003;125(6):1898-1900.

23. Yu D, Cheeseman F, Vanner S. Combined oro-caecal scintigraphy and lactulose hydrogen breath testing demonstrate that breath testing detects oro-caecal transit, not small intestinal bacterial overgrowth in patients with IBS. *Gut*. 2011;60(3):334-340.

24. Corazza GR, Menozzi MG, Strocchi A, et al. The diagnosis of small bowel bacterial overgrowth. Reliability of jejunal culture and inadequacy of breath hydrogen testing. *Gastroenterology*. 1990;98(2):302-309.

25. Walters B, Vanner SJ. Detection of bacterial overgrowth in IBS using the lactulose H2 breath test: comparison with 14C-D-xylose and healthy controls. *Am J Gastroenterol*. 2005;100(7):1566-1570.

26. Posserud I, Stotzer P-O, Björnsson ES, Abrahamsson H, Simrén M. Small intestinal bacterial overgrowth in patients with irritable bowel syndrome. *Gut*. 2007;56(6):802-808.

27. Bratten JR, Spanier J, Jones MP. Lactulose breath testing does not discriminate patients with irritable bowel syndrome from healthy controls. *Am J Gastroenterol*. 2008;103(4):958-963.

28. Lin EC, Massey BT. Scintigraphy demonstrates high rate of false-positive results from glucose breath tests for small bowel bacterial overgrowth. *Clin Gastroenterol Hepatol*. 2016;14(2):203-208.

29. Kalantar-Zadeh K, Berean KJ, Ha N, et al. A human pilot trial of ingestible electronic capsules capable of sensing different gases in the gut. *Nat Electron*. 2018;1(1):79-87.

30. Ghoshal UC. How to interpret hydrogen breath tests. *J Neurogastroenterol Motil*. 2011;17(3):312-317.

Index

Note: Page numbers followed by "f" indicate figures and "t" indicates tables.

A

Abdominal paracentesis
adverse events, 516
analysis of aspirated fluid, 515, 515t–516t
diagnostic, 512–514, 513f
equipment, 512
indications and contraindications, 511
preparation of patient, 511–512
therapeutic, 514–515
Ablation therapy
adverse events, 98
contraindications, 87–88
CPT codes, 98
indications, 87
postprocedure, 97
preparation, 88
Acetaminophen, 495
Achalasia, pneumatic dilation for, 119–124
Acid-reducing agents, 387, 390
Acute variceal hemorrhage (AVH), 395
American Society for Gastrointestinal Endoscopy (ASGE), 15
American Society of Anesthesiologists (ASA) classification, 16
Ampullary adenomas, 172–174, 174f
Analgesia
endoscopy, 15–20
fasting guidelines, 17–20
sedation, 15–20
Anastomotic luminal stenosis, 447
Anastomotic stenosis/stricture
adverse events, 451
contraindications, 448
equipment, 449
indications, 447, 448f
postprocedure, 450–451
preparation, 449
procedure, 449–450, 450f
Anastomotic ulceration, 445
Anorectal manometry
adverse events, 568
auxiliary tests, 566–567
contraindications, 562
conventional anorectal manometry, 564–566, 565f
CPT codes, 569
high-resolution and 3D-high-definition anorectal manometry, 563–564
indications, 561–562
interpretation, 567–568
other uses for, 568–569
postprocedure, 567
preparation and equipment, 562
Anoscopy
contraindications, 204–205
CPT codes, 210
equipment, 205
examination, 207–208
indications, 203–204
position, 206–207
postprocedure, 209
procedure, 205–206
Antegrade stenting, 345
Antibiotics, 8–9
Anticoagulation management
bleeding risk, 29–30
bridging, 30, 32t
coronary stents, 32
direct-acting oral anticoagulants (DOACs), 32t, 33–34
dual antiplatelet therapy (DAPT), 32, 33t
polypectomy, 31
procedural risk, 27
reversal agents, 34–36, 36t
thrombosis risk, 28–29
Antiemetics, 416, 438, 495
Antispasmodics, 416
Antithrombotics management
bleeding risk, 29–30
bridging, 30, 32t
coronary stents, 32
direct-acting oral anticoagulants (DOACs), 32t, 33–34
dual antiplatelet therapy (DAPT), 32, 33t
polypectomy, 31
procedural risk, 27
reversal agents, 34–36, 36t
thrombosis risk, 28–29
APC. See Argon plasma coagulation (APC)

Apollo Endosurgery' Overstitch
    system, 428
Argon plasma coagulation (APC)
    adverse events, 376
    contraindications, 373
    CPT codes, 376
    definition, 372–373
    equipment, 374
    indications, 373
    postprocedure, 375–376
    preparation, 373
    procedure, 375
Ascites
    diagnostic abdominal paracentesis
        for, 511–516
    fluid
        profiles, 516t
        testing of, 515t
Atrial fibrillation (AF), 28–29
AVH. See Acute variceal hemorrhage
        (AVH)

B
Bacterial overgrowth, breath hydrogen
        test
    indications, 573
    methodology, 574–576
    test preparation, 573–574
Balloon sphincteroplasty, 281
Balloon tamponade
    adverse events, 407
    contraindications, 404
    efficacy, 408–409
    equipment, 405
    indication, 404
    postprocedure, 406–407, 408f
    preparation, 404–405
    procedure, 405–406
Barrett esophagus, 462
    ablation therapy, 87–98
Benzodiazepines, 18, 19, 396, 422
Betadine, 521
Biliary ductal obstruction
        management
    accessories, 288–289
    adverse events, 296–297
    contraindications, 288
    devices, 288–289
    endoprostheses, 289
    endoscopes, 288–289
    equipment, 288–289
    indications, 287–288
    nasobiliary catheter placement,
        295–296
    nasopancreatic drain placement, 296
    preparation, 288
    stent placement, 290–294
Biliary lithiasis
    adverse events, 285–286

    contraindications, 279–280
    equipment, 280
    indication, 279
    postprocedure, 285
    preprocedure, 280
    procedure, 281–285
Biliary/pancreatic pathology, endo-
        scopic retrograde cholan-
        giopancreatography (ERCP)
    adverse events, 455
    contraindications, 454
    equipment/procedure, 454–455
    indication, 454
    postprocedure, 455
    preparation, 454
Biliary sphincterotomy, 270t, 271–273,
        272f
Biofeedback therapy, 568
Biopsy
    esophagogastroduodenoscopy
        (EGD), 45–46
    FNA, EUS-guided, 311–323
    liver, percutaneous, 519–523
Bipolar/direct current electrocautery,
        220–221
Bipolar probe
    adverse events, 376
    contraindications, 373
    CPT codes, 376
    definition, 371–372
    equipment, 374
    indications, 373
    postprocedure, 375–376
    preparation, 373
    procedure, 374–375
Bleeding
    delayed bleeding, 238
    endoclips and endoloops for,
        379–383
    endoscopic submucosal dissection
        (ESD), 468
    esophageal EMR, 105
    esophageal peroral endoscopic my-
        otomy, 496
    gastric endoscopic submucosal dis-
        section (ESD), 479
    intraprocedural bleeding, 238
    patient-related factors, 29–30, 31t
    procedure-related factors, 29, 30t
    transoral outlet reduction (TORe),
        442
    variceal, 385
        balloon tamponade for, 403–409
Blunt objects, removal from upper GI,
        115–116
Bolus IV octreotide, 395
Boston Scientific Expect aspiration
        needle, 316

Botulinum toxin injection, 499
Bowel preparation
    capsule endoscopy, 22
    colonoscopy, 23–24
    deep enteroscopy, 22
    flexible sigmoidoscopy, 22–23
    general considerations, 21
    upper endoscopy, 21
Breath test, North American guidelines
    interpretation, 578
    performance, 576

C

Capsule endoscopy, 22
    adverse events, 185–186
    contraindications, 180
    CPT codes, 186
    equipment, 181–182
    indications, 179–180
    interpretation, 183–185
    postprocedure, 183
    preparation, 180
    procedure, 182
Carbohydrate malabsorption,
            breath hydrogen test for,
            572–573
    interpretation, 576–577
    methodology, 574, 575f
Cardiac disease, assessment prior to
            gastrointestinal procedures,
            5, 7t
Catheters, small bowel manometry,
            548–549
Ceftriaxone, 401
Central nervous system (CNS) embo-
            lism, 388
Chloraprep, 521
Chlorhexidine, 521
Cholangioscopy, 284
Cinching guide, 431f, 432
Ciprofloxacin, 489
Circumferential incision, 486, 487f
Clutch Cutter, 464
Coagrasper, 484
Colon endoscopic submucosal dis-
            section
    adverse events, 489
    contraindications, 481–482
    equipment, 482–485
    indications, 481, 482f
    procedural steps, 485–489, 485f,
            487f–488f
Colonic decompression
    adverse events, 245
    indications, 241
    patient approaches, 241–242
    procedure, 242–243
    surgical management, 246
    tube placement, 243–245

Colonic self-expandable metal stents
    adverse events, 251
    contraindications, 247
    equipment, 248
    indications, 247
    postprocedure, 251–252
    preparation, 247–248
    procedure, 248–251
Colonoscopy, 23–24
    adverse events, 199
    contraindications, 193
    CPT codes, 199–200
    diagnostics, 191–192
    equipment, 194–195
    indications, 191
    post procedure, 198–199
    preparation, 193–194
    procedure, 195–197
    therapeutic colonoscopy, 198
    therapeutics, 192–193
Cook Endoscopy, 428
Coronary stents, 32
CPT codes
    ablation therapy, 98
    anorectal manometry, 569
    anoscopy, 210
    argon plasma coagulation (APC),
            376
    bipolar probe, 376
    capsule endoscopy, 186
    colonoscopy, 199–200
    cyanoacrylate obturation, gastric
            varices, 391
    deep enteroscopy, 156–157
    endoscopic ultrasound (EUS),
            308–309
    endoscopic ultrasound (EUS)-
            guided FNA biopsy,
            322–323
    endoscopic variceal ligation, 401
    enteral self-expandable
            stents, 168
    esophageal manometry, 533
    esophageal pH monitoring, ambula-
            tory 24-hour, 544
    esophagogastroduodenoscopy
            (EGD), 48–49
    esophagus, dilation with wire-
            guided bougies, 57
    feeding tubes, 70
    Foreign bodies in upper GI
            tract, endoscopic
            management, 117
    heater probe, 376
    hemorrhoids, 222
    hemostasis, 369
    intraoperative enteroscopy,
            141–142

CPT codes *(Continued)*
  polypectomy, 239
  push enteroscopy, 141–142
  rigid sigmoidoscopy, 210
  spiral enteroscopy, 156–157
  through-the-scope (TTS) balloon
    dilators, 57
  transoral outlet reduction (TORe),
    443
Cryotherapy ablation
  equipment, 93
  liquid nitrogen spray cryotherapy,
    93–96
  liquid nitrous oxide balloon cryo-
    therapy, 96–97
  postprocedure, 97
  procedure, 93
Curved needle suturing system, 429
Cyanoacrylate injection, 386
Cyanoacrylate obturation, gastric
  varices
  CPT codes, 391
  equipment and additional prepara-
    tion, 388
  indications and contraindications,
    388
  other uses, 391
  postprocedure care, 390
  preparation, 388
  procedural-related complications
    and adverse events, 391
  procedure, 389–390, 389f–391f
Cytology, esophagogastroduodenoscopy (EGD), 46

D

Deep enteroscopy, 22
  adverse events, 155–156
  contraindications, 146
  CPT codes, 156–157
  double- balloon enteroscopy proce-
    dure, 149–151
  equipment, 146–147
  indications, 145–146
  preparation, 147–148
  single- balloon enteroscopy proce-
    dure, 148–149
Delayed bleeding, 497
Dermabond, 388
Dexamethasone, 418, 438
3D-High-definition anorectal manometry, 563–564
Diabetes, assessment preprocedure,
  9–10
Dilated gastrojejunal anastomosis,
  437, 438f
Dilation, pneumatic, for achalasia,
  119–124
Diphenhydramine, 19
Direct-acting oral anticoagulants
  (DOACs), 32t, 33–34

Direct percutaneous endoscopic jejunostomy
  equipment, 84
  placement, 83
  procedural steps, 84–85
Dual antiplatelet therapy (DAPT),
  32, 33t
DualKnife, 463, 483
Duodenal adenomas
  adverse events, 175
  endoscopic evaluation, 170
  equipment, 169–170
  follow-up, 172
  methods, 171
  outcomes, 172
  possible adverse events, 172
  postprocedure, 175
  preparation, 169
  special considerations, 171
Duodenum visualization
  EGD, 45
  EUS, 305–306

E

Eagle Claw, 429
Electrohydraulic lithotripsy (EHL),
  284–285
Electromagnetic placement device
  (EPMD), 64
Eleview, 474, 486
Endoclips
  contraindications, 379
  indications, 379, 380f
  postprocedure patient observation,
    383
  preparation and equipment,
    380–381
  procedure, 381
Endoloops
  contraindications, 379
  indications, 379, 380f
  postprocedure patient observation,
    383
  preparation and equipment,
    380–381
  procedure, 381–383, 382f–383f
Endoprostheses
  biliary endoprostheses, 290
  pancreatic endoprostheses, 290–291
Endoscopic knives, 463–464
Endoscopic mucosal resection (EMR),
  461, 481
  disease state, 99
  duodenal adenomas, 169–175
  risks, 105–106
  success rates, 106
  technique, 99–104, 100f, 101f
Endoscopic placement, 65–67
Endoscopic retrograde cholangiopancreatography (ERCP)
  contraindications, 255

equipment, 256–258
fluoroscopic imaging, 263–264
indications, 255, 256t
intraprocedural considerations, 259–264
patient positioning, 259
postprocedural considerations, 264–266
preprocedural considerations, 255–258
sedation, 258–259
technique, 259–262
Endoscopic sphincterotomy (ES)
adverse events, 275–276, 276f
contraindications, 269
equipment, 270–271
indications, 269
patient preparation, 269–270
techniques, 271–275
Endoscopic submucosal dissection (ESD)
contraindications, 462
equipment, 463–464
immediate adverse events, 468
indications, 461–462
postprocedural care, 468–469
pre-ESD lesion assessment, 462–463
procedural reimbursement, 469
procedure
anesthesia and airway protection, 464–465
gravity and traction, 467–468
inspection and marking, 465
submucosal dissection, 466–467
submucosal injection, 465
tips, for mucosal incision, 466
Endoscopic suturing
adverse events, 434
application, 427–428
current devices, 428
curved needle suturing system, 429
equipment, 429
figure of 8 suture, 433, 433f
flexible endoscopic stapling device suturing system, 428
hollow needle suturing system, 428
interrupted/simple, 432
patterns, 432, 433f
preparation, 429
procedure, 430–432
running, 433
suction-based device suturing system, 428
Endoscopic ultrasound (EUS), 386
coil embolization, 390, 390f
complications, 308
contraindications, 304
CPT codes, 308–309
definition, 301
equipment, 304–305
indications, 303

lower gastrointestinal tract, 306
preparation, 304
procedure, 305–307
types, 302
Endoscopic ultrasound (EUS)-guided biliary drainage
contraindications, 342
equipment, 342–343
indications, 342
preparation, 343
procedures, 343–345
Endoscopic ultrasound (EUS)-guided FNA biopsy
adverse events, 322
contraindications, 312
CPT codes, 322–323
equipment, 314–317
indications, 311–312
postprocedure, 321–322
preparation, 312–314
procedure, 317–321
Endoscopic ultrasound–guided gallbladder drainage, 350–351
Endoscopic ultrasound (EUS)-guided liver biopsy
adverse events, 329–333
focal liver lesions, 326–327
parenchymal disease, 327–328
sampling, 328–329
technique, 326–329
Endoscopic ultrasound (EUS)-guided pancreatic duct drainage
adverse events, 361
anatomy, 355
clinical manifestations, 354
contraindications, 355
devices, 356–357
diagnoses, 355
equipment, 356–357
follow- up, 361
indications, 353–354
postprocedure, 361
preparation, 355–356
procedure, 357–360
Endoscopic variceal ligation
adverse events, 401
CPT codes, 401
equipment and procedure, 396–400, 397f, 399f–400f
indications and contraindications, 395
postprocedure, 401
preparation, 395–396
Endoscopy
gastrointestinal procedures, 8t–9t
hemorrhoids, 213–222
management of foreign bodies in upper GI tract, 109–117
pregnancy, 11t
sedation and analgesia for, 15–20

Endoscopy band ligation, 403
Enteral self- expandable stents
    adverse events, 166–167
    concomitant biliary, 167
    contraindications, 160
    CPT codes, 168
    duodenal obstruction, 167
    indications, 159–160
    patient preparation, 161–162
    patient selection, 159–160
    postprocedure, 166
    techniques of insertion, 162–166
Erythromycin, 396, 552
ES. *See* Endoscopic sphincterotomy
    (ES)
Esophageal adenocarcinoma (EAC),
    462
Esophageal band ligation, 395
Esophageal manometry
    adverse events, 533
    baseline and test swallows, 530–
        531, 532f
    catheter placement, 529–530,
        530f–531f
    CPT code, 533
    equipment, 528, 529f
    indications and contraindications,
        527–528
    optional provocative testing,
        532–533
    postprocedure, 533
    preparation for study, 528
Esophageal perforation, 468
Esophageal peroral endoscopic my-
        otomy
    adverse events, 496–497
    contraindications, 491–492
    equipment, 492
    indications, 491
    postprocedure, 495–496
    preparation, 492
    procedure
        mucosal incision, 493, 493f
        myotomy, 494–495, 495f
        pre-POEM EGD, 492
        submucosal tunneling/dissec-
            tion, 493–494, 494f
        tunnel closure, 495, 496f
Esophageal pH monitoring, ambula-
        tory 24-hour
    adverse events, 544
    catheter pH system, 539–540
    contraindications, 538
    CPT codes, 544
    indications, 538
    patient instructions, 540–541
    postprocedure and interpretation,
        541–543, 542t–543t
    preparation and equipment, 539

    wireless pH system, 540
Esophageal self-expandable metal
        stent (SEMS)
    adverse events, 131–132
    contraindications, 127–132
    equipment, 128
    indications, 127
    postprocedure, 131
    preparation, 128
    procedure, 128–129
Esophageal trauma, 442
Esophageal varices, sclerotherapy, 387
Esophagogastroduodenoscopy (EGD)
    adverse events, 47–48
    biopsy, 45–46
    contraindications, 42
    CPT codes, 48–49
    cytology, 46
    equipment, 43
    indications, 41–42
    passing the endoscope, 44–45
    patient preparation, 42–43
    postprocedure, 47
    subacute bacterial endocarditis
        prophylaxis, 46–47
    visualization, 45
Esophagus
    dilation with wire-guided bougies
        adverse events, 57
        conditions, 52
        contraindications, 52
        CPT codes, 57
        equipment, 53
        indications, 52
        postprocedure, 57
        preparation, 53
        procedure, 53–55, 54f, 55f
    visualization
        EGD, 45
        EUS, 305–306
EsophyX, 428
Ethamolin, 385
Ethanolamine oleate, 385
Ethicon Endo-Surgery Inc, 428
Ethiodol, 386, 388
EUS. *See* Endoscopic Ultrasound (EUS)
EUS-guided coil embolization, 389
Expandable stent placement, 127–132

F
Fasting guidelines, 17–20
Feeding tubes
    adverse events, 68–69
    contraindications, 60
    CPT codes, 70
    indications, 60
    placement, 61–67
    post procedure, 68
    precautions, 60–61
    preparation, 60–61

Fentanyl, 43
Fine-needle aspiration (FNA) needle, 389–390
Flexible endoscopic stapling device suturing system, 428
Flexible sigmoidoscopy, 22–23, 203
Fluid aspirated analysis, 515
Fluoroscopic-guided placement, 65
Fluoroscopic imaging, 263–264
FlushKnife, 463, 484
Food impaction, esophageal, 114–115
Foreign bodies in upper GI tract, endoscopic management
    adverse events, 116–117
    contraindications, 110–111
    CPT codes, 117
    equipment, 112–113
    indications, 109–110
    postprocedure, 116
    preparation, 111–112
    procedure, 113–116
Fresh frozen plasma (FFP), 34
Functional lumen imaging probe (FLIP), 120

G

Gastric endoscopic submucosal dissection (ESD)
    additional treatment, 477
    adverse events, 477–479
    anesthesia and patient position, 473
    equipment, 473–476, 475f
    indications, 471–472
    preparation, 472–473, 474f
    procedure, 476–477, 478f–479f
Gastric per-oral endoscopic myotomy
    adverse events, 505
    contraindications, 500
    equipment, 501
    helpful tips, 506
    indications and patient selection, 500
    postprocedural care and follow-up, 504–505
    preparation, 501
    procedural outcomes, 505–506
    procedure team, 500
    techniques
        closure, of mucosal entry, 503–504, 504f
        mucosal incision and entry into the tunnel, 501, 502f
        pyloromyotomy, 502, 504f
        submucosal tunnel creation, 502, 503f
Gastroesophageal junction (GEJ), 119
Gastroesophageal reflux disease (GERD), 497
    and 24-hour esophageal pH monitoring, 537–544

Gastrointestinal procedures
    preprocedure assessment
        age-related alterations, 10
        cardiovascular and respiratory, 5
        coagulation status, 5–7
        diabetes, 9–10
        pregnancy, 10–11
Gastrointestinal surgery, 445
Gastrointestinal tract, upper, foreign bodies in, 109–117
Gastrointestinal (GI) variceal bleeding, 385
Gastrojejunal anastomosis (GJA), 437, 441f
Gastroparesis, 499
Gentamicin, 492, 495
Glucose hydrogen breath test, 576
G-Prox, 429

H

Heater probe
    adverse events, 376
    contraindications, 373
    CPT codes, 376
    definition, 371–372
    equipment, 374
    indications, 373
    postprocedure, 375–376
    preparation, 373
    procedure, 375
Hemorrhage, 523
Hemorrhoids
    adverse events, 215
    anatomy, 213
    contraindications, 214–215
    CPT codes, 222
    grade, 214
    incidence, 213
    indications, 214
    pathophysiology, 213
    post procedure, 221–222
    therapies, 215–221
Hemostasis
    adverse events, 369
    contraindications, 366
    CPT codes, 369
    equipment, 366
    indications, 365
    postprocedure, 368
    preparation, 366
    procedure, 367–368
Hespan, 486
Hiatal hernia, 45
High-resolution anorectal manometry, 563–564
High-resolution esophageal manometry (HREM), 527
High-resolution manometry (HRM) systems, 549
Hollow needle suturing system, 428

HookKnife, 463, 483
HybridKnife, 464, 484
Hydroxyethyl starch, 473
Hydroxypropyl methylcellulose
(HPMC), 473
Hyperosmotic agents, 24
Hypo-osmotic agents, 24

I
IGBs. *See* Intragastric balloons (IGBs)
Inadvertent mucosotomy, 496
Informed consent, 11–12
Infrared coagulation, 219–220
Injection therapy, 385–391
Integrative relaxation pressure (IRP),
119
Intragastric balloons (IGBs)
adverse events, 423, 424t
contraindications, 414–415
equipment, 416–417
follow-up, 423
indications, 413
postprocedure, 422–423
preparation, 415–416
procedure, 417–422
Intraoperative enteroscopy
CPT codes, 141–142
procedure, 141
Intraprocedural bleeding, 489
Intravenous ondansetron, 418
Isosmotic agents, 23–24
ITknife nano, 464, 483

J
Jejunal feeding, 80

L
Lactose malabsorption, breath hydro-
gen test, 573
Lactulose hydrogen breath test,
575–577
Laser lithotripsy, 285
Ligation, esophageal band, 395
Lipiodol, 386, 388
Liquid nitrogen spray cryotherapy,
93–96
Liquid nitrous oxide balloon cryother-
apy, 96–97
Liquid sucralfate, 447
Liver biopsy, percutaneous, 325–326
adverse events, 523
equipment and procedure, 521–522,
522f
indications and contraindications,
519–520
preparation, 520–521
Lower esophageal sphincter (LES),
119
Low-molecular-weight heparin
(LMWH), 30
Low-volume PEG preparations, 24

M
Magnetic resonance cholangiopan-
creatography (MRCP),
293–294
Malabsorption of carbohydrates,
breath hydrogen test for,
572–573
Mallampati classification, 16–17
Manometry
anorectal, 561–569
esophageal, 527–533
small bowel, 547–556
Marginal ulceration. *See* Anastomotic
ulceration
Mechanical lithotripsy, 282
Mediastinitis/peritonitis, 497
Methylene, 417
Metronidazole, 489
Midazolam, 18, 43
Minnesota tube
control of variceal hemorrhage,
403, 404f
efficacy, 408–409
flow chart for usage, 407, 408f
Minor papilla precut, 275
Minor papilla sphincterotomy,
274–275
Monitored anesthesia care (MAC), 18
Monitoring
esophageal pH, ambulatory 24-
hour, 537–544
oxygenation, during sedation, 17–18
MucoUp, 473

N
Nasoduodenal feeding tubes, 59–70
Nasoduodenal placement, 64–65
Nasogastric feeding tubes, 59–70
Nasogastric tube placement, 63–64
Nasojejunal feeding tubes, 59–70
Nasojejunal placement, 64–65
N-Butyl-2-cyanoacrylate, 386
NDO plicator, 428
Needles, liver biopsy, 521
Needle-type knife, 466

O
Obalon Balloon System, 413, 414f
equipment, 417
preparation, 415–416
procedure, 418–422, 419f, 421f
Obalon EZ fill dispenser, 418, 419f
Obalon Navigation System, 420–422,
421f
Obalon Touch Dispenser, 420, 421f
Obesity, 427
Octreotide, 552
2-Octyl cyanoacrylate, 386, 388
Olympus Optical LTD, 428
Opiate analgesics, 422

Opioids, 19
Oral quinolone, 401
Oral sodium sulfate, 24
Orbera Balloon, 413, 414f
   equipment, 416–417
   preparation, 415
   procedure, 417–418
OverStitch device, 428
Oxygenation monitoring, during
     sedation, 17–18

P

Pain, 523
Pancreatic ductal obstruction
   accessories, 288–289
   adverse events, 296–297
   contraindications, 288
   devices, 288–289
   endoprosthesis, 288
   endoscopes, 288–289
   equipment, 288–289
   indications, 287
   nasobiliary catheter placement,
     295–296
   nasobiliary drain, 288
   nasopancreatic drain placement,
     296
   preparation, 288
   procedure, 290–296
   stent placement, 294–295
Pancreatic fluid collections
   contraindications, 336
   endoscopic drainage, 336–339
   imaging, 335
   indications, 335–336
   postprocedure care, 339–340
   preprocedural considerations, 336
   treatment strategies, 340
Pancreatic sphincterotomy, 270t,
     271–273, 272f
Paracentesis, abdominal, 511–516
Patient assessment
   gastrointestinal procedures, 7,
     10–11
   sedation, 15–20, 16
PEG-3350 (Miralax), 24
Pepto-Bismol, 574
Percutaneous endoscopic gastrostomy
     (PEG), 9
   contraindications, 74
   ethical issues, 74
   indications, 73–74
   Ponsky pull technique, 75–78
   preparation, 74–75
   Russel introducer technique,
     78–80
   Sacks-Vine push technique, 75–78
Percutaneous endoscopic gastrostomy
     and jejunostomy (PEGJ)
   one-piece PEGJ, 82–83

two-piece PEGJ
   Johlin technique, 81–82
   Kirby technique, 80–81
Percutaneous liver biopsy, 325–326
Perforation
   in colon endoscopic submucosal
     dissection, 489
   endoscopic retrograde cholan-
     giopancreatography (ERCP),
     266
   polypectomy, 238
Periprocedural planning, 7–11
Per oral endoscopic myotomy (POEM),
     120, 465, 491
Placements
   biliary stent placement, 290–294
   colonic self-expandable metal
     stents, 247–252
   electromagnetic placement device
     (EPMD), 61–67
   enteral self- expandable stents,
     159–168
   esophageal self- expandable metal
     stents, 127–132
   feeding tubes, 61–67
   fluoroscopic-guided placement, 65
   nasoduodenal placement, 64–65
   nasogastric tube placement,
     63–64
   nasojejunal placement, 64–65
   radiographic placement, 65
Pneumatic dilation for achalasia
   contraindications, 120
   definition, 119
   equipment, 122
   esoFLIP, 124
   pneumatic dilation, 124
   preprocedural planning, 120–122,
     121t
   procedure, 122–124
Polyethylene glycol (PEG-ELS),
     23–24
Polypectomy
   adverse events, 238–239
   antithrombotics, 31
   cold snare polypectomy, 231–232
   contraindications, 229
   CPT codes, 239
   endoscopic mucosal resection,
     233–235
   equipment, 230
   evaluation, 227
   hot snare polypectomy (HSP),
     232–233
   indications, 228–229
   interpretation, 237–238
   postprocedure, 236
   preparation, 229
   procedure, 230–231

Post- ERCP pancreatitis (PEP), 264
Postsurgical adverse events, endo-
     scopic management
  anastomotic stenosis/stricture,
     447–451
  anastomotic ulceration, 445
  biliary/pancreatic pathology, en-
     doscopic retrograde cholan-
     giopancreatography (ERCP),
     454–455
  diagnosis
     adverse events, 447
     contraindications, 446
     equipment, 446
     indications, 445
     postprocedure care, 447
     preparation, 446
     procedure, 446
  postsurgical leaks, 451
  self-expandable metal stent place-
     ment, 452–453
Postsurgical leaks, 451
Power Medical, 428
Precut sphincterotomy, 273–274
Pregnancy, endoscopy, 11t
Prophylactic antibiotics, 8–9
Prophylaxis, subacute bacterial endo-
     carditis, 46–47
Propofol, 19
Proton pump inhibitor (PPI), 106
Pulmonary disease, assessment prior
     to gastrointestinal proce-
     dures, 5, 7t
Push enteroscopy
  adverse events, 140
  contraindications, 137
  CPT codes, 141–142
  equipment, 137
  indications, 136
  preparation, 137–138
  procedure, 138–140
P2Y12 inhibitor, 31–32
Pyloromyotomy, 502, 504f
Pylorus-directed therapies, 500

R

Radiofrequency ablation
  Barrx 90/60 catheters, 91–92
  Barrx Channel RFA Endoscopic
     Catheter, 92–93
  Barrx 360 Express RFA Balloon
     Catheter, 91
  equipment, 88–89
  procedure, 89–90
Radiographic placement, 65
Rapid on- site evaluation (ROSE),
     320–321
Rectoanal inhibitory reflex (RAIR), 564
Rendezvous technique, 343–345
ReShape Integrated Dual Balloon
     System, 413

Reversal agents, 34–36, 36t
Rigid sigmoidoscopy
  contraindications, 204
  CPT codes, 210
  equipment, 205
  indications, 203–204
  postprocedure, 209
  preparation, 204–205
  procedure, 205–209
RigiFlex balloons, 121
Roux-en-Y gastric bypass (RYGB),
     437, 445
Roux limb, 437
Rubber band ligation (RBL), 215–218

S

SB Knife, 464
Scintigraphy, role in small bowel,
     557–558
Scleromate, 385
Sclerosants, 385
Sclerosis, 385–386
Sclerotherapy, 218–219
  indications and contraindications,
     387
  postprocedure care, 387
  preparation and equipment, 387
  procedure, 387
Sedation
  analgesia, 15–20
  fasting guidelines, 17–20
  safety, 15
Selective cannulation, 260–262
Self-expandable metal stent (SEMS)
     placement, 452
  adverse events, 453
  contraindication, 452
  equipment, 452
  indication, 452
  postprocedure, 453
  preparation, 452
  procedure, 452–453
Sharp objects, removal from upper GI,
     115–116
SIC-8000, 474
Simethicone, 439
Single fluid-filled balloon, 413, 414f
Small bowel enteroscopy
  deep enteroscopy, 145–157
  push enteroscopy, 135–142
Small bowel manometry
  adverse events, 556
  contraindications, 548
  equipment, 548–550, 549f
  indications, 547–548
  interpretation, 554–556, 554f
  postprocedure, 553
  preparation, 548
  procedure, 550–553
Small bowel scintigraphy
  contraindications, 557

equipment, 557
indications, 557
interpretation, 558
postprocedure, 558
preparation, 557
procedure, 558
Small intestinal bacterial overgrowth (SIBO)
breath tests, 575–576
indications, 573
interpretation, 577
Sodium hyaluronate, 473
Sodium morrhuate, 396
Sodium phosphate, 24
Sodium tetradecyl, 396
Sodium tetradecyl sulfate, 385
Sotradecol, 385
Sphincterotomy, 262
Spiral enteroscopy
adverse events, 155–156
CPT codes, 156–157
insertion, 152–153
novel motorized spiral endoscope, 155
procedure, 152–153
retrograde (perrectal) spiral enteroscopy, 155
special preparation, 152
technique, 153–154
withdrawal, 154
Squamous cell carcinomas (SCCs), 461–462
Steerable Teflon catheters, 551
Stenting, esophageal cancers, 127–132
Stents
biliary placement, 290–294
colonic self-expandable metal stents, 247–252
enteral self- expandable stents, 159–168
self-expanding metals, 127–132
Stomach visualization
EGD, 45
EUS, 305–306
Sucralfate, 387, 390
Suction-based device suturing system, 428
Sulfate-free PEG-ELS, 24
Swallowable gas-filled intragastric balloon system, 413, 414f
Symptom association probability (SAP), 543
Symptom index (SI), 542
Symptom sensitivity index (SSI), 542–543

T

Tamponade, balloon, 403–409
Tattooing, endoscopic, 235–236

Teflon catheters, 549
Tension pneumoperitoneum/pneumothorax, 496
Therapeutic privilege, 12
Thrombosis risk, 28–29
Through-the-scope (TTS) balloon dilators
adverse events, 57
conditions, 52
contraindications, 52
CPT codes, 57
equipment, 55
indications, 52
postprocedure, 57
preparation, 53
procedure, 55–56
Tissue suturing guide, 430f, 431–432
Transjugular intrahepatic portosystemic shunt (TIPS), 403
Transmucosal potential difference (TMPD), 548
Transmural drainage, 345
Transoral outlet reduction (TORe)
adverse events, 442–443
contraindications, 437
CPT codes, 443
equipment, 438–439
follow-up, 442
indications, 437, 438f
postprocedure, 441–442
preparation, 437–438
procedure, 439–441, 440f–441f
Triangle Tip knife, 463

U

Ultrasound, endoscopic (EUS)
biliary drainage, 342–345
FNA biopsy guided by, 311–323
gallbladder drainage, 350–351
liver biopsy, 326–333
pancreatic duct drainage, 353–361
Upper endoscopy
bowel preparation, 21
cryotherapy ablation, 93

V

Variceal hemorrhage (VH), 385
Varices
bleeding, balloon tamponade for, 403–409
cyanoacrylate obturation of gastric, 388–391, 389f–391f
esophageal, sclerotherapy, 387
Vitamin K-dependent coagulation factors, 34
Voluven, 473, 486

Z

Zinc oxide-based tape (HyTape), 501
Z- tract, 513